Surviving Health Care

A Manual for Patients and Their Families

This book serves as a tool to help patients and their families deal rationally with the perplexing and often irrational world of health care. It covers the topics and addresses the challenges that experts in a variety of health care fields believe are the most vital to meeting the challenges of decision making when people feel most vulnerable. With contributions from leading health care specialists, *Surviving Health Care: A Manual for Patients and Their Families* examines a wide array of topics, including advance planning for health care, medical emergencies, genetic testing, pain management, and care of elders. It is a unique resource that aims above all to help patients reach their best health care decisions.

Thomasine Kushner is co-editor of the *Cambridge Quarterly of Healthcare Ethics* and a bioethicist with the California Pacific Medical Center Program in Medicine and Human Values in San Francisco. She taught bioethics at the University of California, Berkeley, for fifteen years and is the author (with David Thomasma) of *Birth to Death: Science and Bioethics*, *Asking to Die: Inside the Dutch Debate about Euthanasia*, and *Ward Ethics: A Case Book for Doctors-in-Training*, along with several books on aesthetics and design.

Surviving Health Care

A Manual for Patients and Their Families

Edited by

Thomasine Kushner

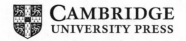

CAMBRIDGE
UNIVERSITY PRESS

CAMBRIDGE UNIVERSITY PRESS
Cambridge, New York, Melbourne, Madrid, Cape Town, Singapore,
São Paulo, Delhi, Dubai, Tokyo

Cambridge University Press
32 Avenue of the Americas, New York, NY 10013-2473, USA

www.cambridge.org
Information on this title: www.cambridge.org/9780521744416

© Cambridge University Press 2010

First published 2010

Printed in the United States of America

A catalog record for this publication is available from the British Library.

Library of Congress Cataloging in Publication data
Surviving health care: a manual for patients and their families / edited by
Thomasine Kushner.
   p.   cm.
Includes bibliographical references and index.
ISBN 978-0-521-76796-5 (hardback) – ISBN 978-0-521-74441-6 (pbk.)
1. Patient participation – Handbooks, manuals, etc.   2. Patients – Decision
making – Handbooks, manuals, etc.   3. Patient education – Handbooks,
manuals, etc.   I. Kushner, Thomasine Kimbrough.   II. Title.
R727.42.S87   2010
610.69′6 – dc22   2009042399

ISBN 978-0-521-76796-5 Hardback
ISBN 978-0-521-74441-6 Paperback

To William S. Andereck and Dena M. Bravata, physicians for all seasons

Contents

Contributors

Bette Anton, MLS, is Head Librarian for the Pamela & Kenneth Fong Optometry and Health Sciences Library of the University of California, Berkeley. This library serves the University of California, Berkeley School of Optometry, and the University of California, Berkeley–University of California, San Francisco, Joint Medical Program.

Paul Ford, PhD, is Associate Staff in Bioethics and Neurology at the Cleveland Clinic Foundation and Assistant Professor, Cleveland Clinic Lerner College of Medicine of Case Western Reserve University, Cleveland, Ohio. He is co-editor, with Denise M. Dudzinski, of *Complex Ethics Consultations: Cases That Haunt Us* (Cambridge University Press, 2009).

Erica S. Friedman, MD, is an internist and rheumatologist with Mount Sinai School of Medicine in New York City, where she is also Associate Dean for Undergraduate Medical Education.

Leonard C. Groopman, MD, PhD, is Assistant Professor of Clinical Psychiatry and Medical Ethics at Weill Cornell Medical College, where he also is active in the Institute for the History of Psychiatry.

Judy Illes, PhD, is Professor of Neurology and Canada Research Chair in Neuroethics, National Core for Neuroethics, at the University of British Columbia. Her book, *Neuroethics: Defining the Issues in Theory, Practice and Policy*, was published by Oxford University Press in January 2006.

Kenneth V. Iserson, MD, MBA, FACEP, FAAEM, is Professor Emeritus of Emergency Medicine, University of Arizona College of Medicine, Tucson.

Claudia Jacova, PhD, is a Postdoctoral Fellow in Neurobiology and Behavior, University of British Columbia, Canada.

Claudia Landau, MD, PhD, is Associate Clinical Professor of Medicine and Coordinator of the Geriatric Curriculum in the University of California, Berkeley–University of California, San Francisco, Joint Medical Program, Berkeley, and Chief of Geriatrics and Palliative Care in the Department of Medicine at the Alameda County Health Center, Oakland, California.

Alexis Lopez, BA, is a Research Technician with the Program in Medicine and Human Values, California Pacific Medical Center, San Francisco, California.

J. Westley McGaughey, BA, is Research Analyst, Grants and Study, in the Program in Medicine and Human Values, California Pacific Medical Center, San Francisco, California.

Eric M. Meslin, PhD, is Director of the Indiana University Center for Bioethics, Associate Dean for Bioethics, and Professor of Medicine and of Medical and Molecular Genetics at Indiana University School of Medicine. He also is Professor of Philosophy at the School of Liberal Arts and Co-Director of the Indiana University–Purdue University, Indianapolis, Signature Center Consortium on Health Policy, Law, and Bioethics. He has more than eighty publications on topics ranging from international health research to science policy, including *Belmont Revisited: Ethical Principles for Research with Human Subjects*, co-edited with James F. Childress and Harold T. Shapiro.

Guy Micco, MD, is a Clinical Professor in the University of California, Berkeley–University of California, San Francisco, Joint Medical Program; Director of the University of California, Berkeley, Academic Geriatric Resource Center (Center on Aging); and Co-Director of the University of California, Berkeley, Center for Medicine, the Humanities, and Law, Berkeley, California.

Ruchika Mishra, PhD, is editor of the Ethics Committees at Work section of the *Cambridge Quarterly of Healthcare Ethics* and a 2008–2009 Postdoctoral Fellow in the Program in Medicine and Human Values, California Pacific Medical Center, San Francisco, California.

William A. Norcross, MD, specializes in family practice and geriatric medicine in the Department of Family and Preventive Medicine at the University of California, San Diego. He is the founder of the Physician Assessment and Clinical Education (PACE) program.

Timothy E. Quill, MD, is Professor of Medicine, Psychiatry, and Medical Humanities and Director of the Center for Ethics, Humanities, and Palliative Care at the University of Rochester School of Medicine. He is the author of numerous books and articles on issues related to palliative care and end-of-life concerns.

Rosamond Rhodes, PhD, is Professor of Medical Education and Director of Bioethics Education at Mount Sinai School of Medicine and Associate Professor of Philosophy at the Graduate School, City University of New York. She is co-editor of the *American Philosophical Association Newsletter on Philosophy and Medicine* and co-editor of *Medicine and Social Justice: Essays on the Distribution of Health Care* (Oxford University Press, 2002).

Ben A. Rich, JD, PhD, is Professor and Chair of the Bioethics Program, University of California, Davis, Sacramento, California. He is the author of *Strange Bedfellows: How Medical Jurisprudence Has Influenced Medical Ethics and Medical Practice* (Kluwer Academic/Plenum Publishers, 2001).

Peter H. Schwartz, MD, PhD, is a core faculty member of the Indiana University Center for Bioethics, Assistant Professor of Medicine at the Indiana University Medical Center, and Assistant Professor of Philosophy at the Indiana University School of Liberal Arts at Indianapolis. He also practices adult outpatient medicine at the Primary Care Clinic at Wishard Hospital.

Mindy Shah, MD, is an attending physician on the inpatient palliative care consult service at the University of Rochester Medical Center, Strong Memorial Hospital.

Robyn S. Shapiro, JD, is editor of the Bioethics Education section in *Cambridge Quarterly of Healthcare Ethics* and a health law partner with Drinker Biddle & Reath LLP. She recently completed her twenty-six-year-tenure as Professor of Bioethics and Director of the Center for the Study of Bioethics at the Medical College of Wisconsin.

Ilina Singh, PhD, is Wellcome Trust Lecturer in Bioethics and Society at the London School of Economics, London, England.

Steven Smith, MD, is a transplant nephrologist and Associate Professor in the Division of Endocrinology, St. Luke's Roosevelt Hospital, New York.

Aaron Spital, MD, is an academic nephrologist at Elmhurst Hospital Center in Elmhurst, New York, and Clinical Professor of Medicine at Mount Sinai School of Medicine. He has had a longtime interest in ethical issues in organ transplantation and edits the Ethics section of *Seminars in Dialysis*.

James J. Strain, MD, is Professor in the Department of Psychiatry, Mount Sinai Medical Center in New York City.

Griffin Trotter, MD, PhD, is Associate Professor in the Center for Health Care Ethics at Saint Louis University, where he also holds an appointment in the Department of Surgery, Emergency Medical Division. He is the author of *The Loyal Physician* (Vanderbilt University Press, 1997) and *The Ethics of Coercion in Mass Causality Medicine* (Johns Hopkins University Press, 2007).

Mark R. Wicclair, PhD, is Professor of Philosophy and Adjunct Professor of Community Medicine, West Virginia University, and Adjunct Professor of Medicine and a part-time instructor of bioethics at the Center for Bioethics and Health Law Faculty, University of Pittsburgh. He is author of *Ethics and the Elderly* (Oxford University Press, 1993).

Timothy S. Yeh, MD, is Director of the Division of Critical Care Medicine and Vice Chairman of the Department of Pediatrics, Children's Hospital of New Jersey at Newark Beth Israel Medical Center. As Administrative Director of Critical Care, he supervises the operation of the Pediatric Intensive Care Unit, and as Vice Chairman, he assists in program development and planning for the Department of Pediatrics. He lectures extensively and is the author of numerous abstracts, articles, and book chapters.

Preface

Alice's lament after falling down the rabbit hole captures what most of us feel when we are catapulted into the world of illness: "How queer everything is today! And yesterday things went on just as usual. I wonder if I've been changed in the night?" Suddenly, like Alice, you find yourself struggling in an alien environment, with an unfamiliar culture, where even the language is strange. How do you cope? How do you manage? How do you find your way? Like Alice, it's natural to think, "It would be so nice if something made sense for a change."

Making sense of and surviving the powerlessness produced by illness are what this book is about, and it had its beginning where all medical encounters start – with the patient. In this case, HK, a vibrant man in his fifties who had achieved every worldly success, in large part because of the power of his personality and his ability to tackle difficult problems and solve them in creative ways. When he began to notice a persistent pain in his shoulder and arm, he attributed it to strain from physical activity. However, it did not decrease, and when he met a colleague for lunch, he complained of having trouble climbing the steep steps outside the restaurant. Alarmed, his friend urged him to go directly to an emergency department, where it was immediately clear he was having a heart attack. That began what HK later described as a descent into chaos in which he felt powerless, frightened, and totally at the mercy of a system he did not understand. Several years after open heart surgery, bouts in intensive care, and rehabilitation, HK urged the writing of a guide for patients – present and future – to help them navigate the unfamiliar world of health care and survive on their own terms and with their dignity intact.

There is a surfeit of self-help information on health: how to reach and maintain maximum health through diet, exercise, lifestyle regimens, and so forth. Such measures are all for the good, but what has been missing – and critically needed – is what HK wanted, a survival kit with tools to help patients and their families deal rationally with the perplexing and often irrational world of health care. Physicians tell us they find the health care system frustrating and even befuddling; it takes no imagination to discern how those of us outside the health care system feel! This manual is intended as a survival guide to help you find your way and regain control in a seemingly uncontrollable situation at a time when patients and families are at their most vulnerable.

All of us are united by our common desire to find useful information to meet inevitable health care challenges. However, it should be noted that when it comes to individual health care, one size does not fit all. Determining your own health care decisions must remain, as it should, an essential part of your relationship with your physician. Instead, what you will find here are practical suggestions to guide you through the *Terra Incognita* created by illness. Rather than solutions, the goal here is to afford you the kind of information and perspectives a variety of health care experts believe are your best navigational tools for reaching the best possible decisions for yourself and your family.

Because of the wide range of issues that need to be covered, as well as the breadth of information required to address them, my task as editor was to get contributors who are experts in the most challenging issues patients have to face. This volume includes chapters written by individuals not only from my own discipline (philosophy), but also from medicine, bioethics, public policy, psychology, and the law. These writers give you their personal perspectives and engage you directly and informally, as they might a friend or family member. They discuss aspects of health care planning and management both in and out of institutional settings. Their goal is to provide the resources and fill in the gaps. By knowing what to expect, how to access the environment, and what options are available, you will be better able to combat the fears and feelings of impotence and inadequacy that threaten clear decision making at the very time you need to be most effective.

You will find that just as medicine is said to be an art, there also is an art to being a patient. That means there is a time to push forward to ensure you get the answers and information you need, but there also is a time to put yourself in the hands of others. The art of being a patient comes in knowing when the moment is right for each. The following chapters serve as a compass to guide you in determining that balance for yourself and your family.

ONE

Letter to Patients

On Becoming the "Good" Patient and Finding the "Right" Doctor

– Leonard C. Groopman

I'm sorry to learn that you're sick. Your doctor has diagnosed you with an illness, has said it may be serious, and told you that you need treatment. You have become a patient. Being sick is difficult enough; being a patient comes with its own set of challenges.

You ask me (a physician and psychiatrist) what to do, how you can be a good patient, and how to choose the right doctor. You're hoping for a prescription, a set of clear instructions, maybe a checklist. I wish I could provide them, but in all honesty, I can't.

Fifty years ago, I could have told you simply to let your doctor make the decisions, both big and small, and to follow his or her orders. However, our culture and our technology have both changed since then, and with them, our ideas, choices, and practices regarding illness and medicine and doctors and patients have changed as well. No longer do we accept or believe that passive compliance is necessarily the best response (although for any given person and medical situation, it might be). Doctors, too, have come to see their role differently, no longer as parents who know best what's good for their patients and what the right decisions are for their lives.

Twenty years ago, I might also have been able to respond quite easily, although quite differently, as to how you can be a good patient:

inform yourself as best you can about your illness and its treatment, and make your own decisions. Such an approach, which placed patient choice at the heart of the medical process, brought many benefits, most notably the patient's right to informed consent. However, it also generated problems of its own. Many patients felt emotionally abandoned by their doctors. While caught in the psychological storm of their sickness, they were adrift in an ocean of confusing medical and moral choices, without the compass or the comfort of an experienced physician's hand at the helm. In turn, doctors often felt their role had been reduced to that of a technician, and they worried about encroaching too much upon the sacred sea of patient autonomy.

We currently are living in the historical wake of the patient autonomy movement. We're seeking better ways to be good doctors and good patients, ways that avoid the excesses of both medical paternalism and patient autonomy. The absence of a clear cultural answer to the question of how to be a good patient is partly what brings you to me today.

We seem to be moving toward a collaborative picture of the doctor–patient relationship, in which patient and doctor work together and each has a role in defining and negotiating the treatment, not only in its biological aspect, but especially in its psychological and social aspects.

We're also moving toward a pluralistic conception of the doctor–patient relationship, in which there is no one "good" way to be a patient and in which there is no one "right" relationship between doctor and patient. **When it comes to the doctor–patient relationship, one size does not fit all.** Each patient must find the proper fit for himself or herself.

For some, the more traditional, paternalistic doctor who explains little, chooses the course of treatment, and tells you what to do to get better fits best with their needs as patients. For others, a doctor who gives details about the illness, sets out treatment options, answers lots of questions, and then leaves it up to the patient suits their personality. Still other people want a sense of collaboration, of working together with their doctor each step of the way. Although the last of these three types may be the most fashionable these days, that doesn't mean it's the right approach for you. Look at yourself in the mirror and ask yourself what you want in your physician – do you prefer to be told which treatment to take, to choose which treatment you want, or to share both the power and the responsibility for your treatment and your health with your doctor?

So, I do not have easy answers, either to how to be a "good" patient or how to choose the "right" doctor. However, I think I have something valuable to offer you nonetheless: I want to give you an emotional and psychological map to help you navigate the foreign waters of illness and patienthood.

Let me be direct: **Your life has changed now that you are ill.**

I see you don't like the word *change*. You don't want your life to change, at least not because of illness. I can't blame you. Illness is mysterious, frightening, and uncertain, outside your control. Illness is a crisis. Like all crises, it's dangerous. It's a biological crisis, threatening your physical capacity to control your body and to function fully. It's a psychological crisis, stirring up strong and unwanted reactions, perhaps challenging your internal equilibrium and your sense of who you are emotionally. It's a social crisis, because your identity in the outside world, in the social world, is likely to be affected by the fact of your illness. A sick person often is treated differently by family and friends and co-workers and strangers – and by himself or herself – from how a healthy person is treated. It helps to be aware of this ahead of time rather than to be taken by surprise. That way, you can be prepared for some of what may lie ahead.

Sometimes you will feel frightened, even overwhelmed at times, about being sick. At other times, you may hardly be aware of it. You go about your daily life and seem not to know – or seem to forget – that you're ill. You wonder whether you're in denial about your illness, and the one thing our culture tells us not to be is in denial. Don't worry; you're not in denial. I know that because you're here, consulting me. Just because you're going about your life doesn't mean you're in denial. More likely, it means you're coping with your illness.

Embedded in the word *patient* are the notions of patience and passivity. These are the traditional virtues of the patient. Yet, when we're sick, we feel an urgent desire to be well, so patience is hard to come by as a patient. Also, as patients, we're expected to put ourselves in the hands of others – doctors and nurses, family and friends. It's difficult for many of us to depend on others so heavily, to be passive as well as patient. It certainly has been difficult for me when I've been sick. For many people, it's this passivity, this dependency, that's the most difficult aspect of their illness.

There's no denying that your life has changed and will change further as a result of your illness, especially if it's serious. It's worth recognizing this so you won't be surprised or feel bad about how you react along the way, especially if it's a long way, an odyssey you didn't ask for. Also, if you get used to the idea that your life has changed, you may be able to participate in that change rather than expend your energy to resist it. You might be able to influence the course and process of change and regain some of the lost control that comes with being a patient. Moreover, if you recognize the ways in which your life has changed, you'll be able to see the ways in which your life – and you – remain the same, the ways in which you remain yourself. Remember, **you're ill, but you're not your illness.**

Don't get me wrong: accepting that you're ill often is a long and difficult process. It's usually not smooth: at times you believe it; at other times you can't or won't. At times during the day – or in the quiet of the night, when our fears bubble up to the surface – it may suddenly hit you that you're sick. It may be hard to believe. Sickness is what happens to other people, not to me! At other times, the fact that you're ill may seem like the most important fact about you. It may even seem to define you. Many people struggle with these conflicting feelings for some time before they arrive at an equilibrium, before they can accept their illness as a part of themselves, without losing the sense of still being themselves. For many of us, it's an ongoing balancing act.

Being sick may be filled with strong and sometimes conflicting emotions, with contradictory and confusing impulses. At times, you may experience two opposing ideas, wishes, or reactions, simultaneously or in succession. You may feel reassured and safe one minute and anxious and vulnerable the next, angry at times and guilty at others, determined yet exhausted, supported but alone, protected although isolated, progressing and losing ground, hopeful and despairing, encouraged and powerless. Although it's challenging and difficult to cope with such contradictory emotions, they're normal and even to be expected.

Many people, upon receiving a medical diagnosis, feel nothing at all at first. It's shocking to be told you're sick, and it's not unusual to shut down emotionally, to go numb. This, too, may be confusing and distressing, because it's strange to not know how you're feeling, or to feel nothing at all. However, this is our way of protecting ourselves, of letting the reality of being sick sink in slowly, so we can get used to it gradually and to begin accepting and adjusting to it.

I'm reminded of a patient of mine, a lawyer in her fifties, who after many years of hard work, had finally pulled back from her busy legal practice to pursue the artistic interests she left behind many years previously. The eldest of four children, she had grown up as the surrogate mother of the family, taking care of her brothers and sisters.

She proudly told me she was known among her siblings as the family driver, because it was she who drove them all to their various activities when she was a teenager. She was the family driver both literally and metaphorically. She was equally proud of having raised her son on her own after her divorce, at the same time as she was building her legal practice and earning her professional reputation. Finally she had arrived at the point in her life when her work as a lawyer and a mother was largely behind her. Now it was time for her.

Then she was diagnosed with breast cancer. She took it in stride, of course. She was most concerned about protecting her son, her brothers and sisters, and her friends. She didn't want to upset them. She would tell them the news of her diagnosis and then reassure them that she was fine and they needn't worry. She couldn't allow herself to be taken care of. Friends offered to help her – she lived far away from the hospital where she was being treated, so they invited her to stay with them the nights before and after her chemotherapy treatments. She preferred a hotel. Underneath her composed exterior, however, she was frightened, angry, and lonely. She struggled with accepting that her own needs had changed, and that her need – and desire – for the help of others had increased. It was difficult for her, because she had spent her life priding herself on her independence and on her ability to take care of others. She was the big sister, after all. She felt weak because she wanted to be taken care of. Over time, she was able to open up to one sister, to cry to her, and to tell her how frightened and lonely she felt. Her anger subsided, along with her isolation, but she continued to feel uncomfortable about turning to her younger sibling for comfort.

You ask me how you can be a good patient. Why do you want to be a good patient? Is it because you're afraid? It's natural to be afraid in the face of illness, and one response to being afraid is to try to be good, because we believe if we're good, we'll be taken care of, be protected and safe. Neither the gods nor our well-meaning fellow humans, such as doctors, will willfully harm us if we're good. They'll take care of us. Therefore, you've made being good a top priority.

Sometimes we want to be good because we feel we've been bad, and we feel guilty and remorseful for having been bad. Not uncommonly, people who become sick feel responsible and blame themselves for their illness. They believe they did things they shouldn't have, or didn't do things they should have, and that's why they've become sick. Although doctors, family, and friends may try to convince them otherwise, the feeling of having in some way caused their illness may be tenacious, even when it's irrational. Sometimes people experience their illness as punishment for some earlier "crimes" or "sins" they feel they committed, either in their behavior or in their thoughts. You don't have to be religious to feel this way; you may not even be conscious that you're feeling this way, and that that's why you feel guilty or blame yourself or otherwise feel bad about yourself for being ill.

Sometimes people feel responsible and guilty for being sick because they (unconsciously) find it psychologically preferable – easier – than feeling helpless and powerless. If I brought this on myself somehow – so the logic goes – well, then I'm not simply helpless (an intolerable feeling for many people) and I do have some power, some control, over my illness.

These psychological maneuvers are attempts to make sense of being ill, which in one way or another just about everybody tries to do. As human beings, we seek to make sense of our experiences, to find meaning in the world and in our lives. We do this with illness just as we do with other aspects of life. At this point, the sick person often parts company with his or her doctor. Doctors, trained to think about disease scientifically, generally don't consider an illness as "meaning" anything at all. For physicians, illnesses first and foremost are biological facts and pathological processes. However, for a sick person, the illness also is a subjective – a physical, mental, and social – experience that must be understood in the context of his or her life. Therefore, for many patients, their illness must take on meaning, to be made sense of. As I mentioned earlier, sometimes people interpret their illness as a punishment. Others might take it as a "sign" or a message. Again, you don't have to be religious to interpret it this way. Illness may be interpreted as a message from your body that, for example, you need to change your lifestyle, take better care of yourself, stop drinking or smoking, or live differently or more fully because your illness reminds you you're actually mortal. It may be experienced as a "wake-up call" about life and how you're living it or want to live it. In this way, illness serves for some as an opportunity and an occasion for change.

I said earlier that illness is a crisis, and it is often said that in every crisis, both danger and opportunity exist. I'm no Pollyanna about illness. It's not something you wish for, or that's a good thing to have happen. Yet, our popular culture has become saturated with stories about how people change their lives as a result of their illness, discovering their true calling or their true meaning. Although some people experience epiphanies or make significant changes in their lives as a result of illness, I've found that these stories, so prevalent in our culture, create an expectation among many sick people that they, too, should experience self-transformation through their illness. Not only must they deal with the realities of their sickness, in all its physical, emotional, and social dimensions, they also feel they're failing if they don't experience spiritual enlightenment. This is an added burden that no sick person should have to bear.

Illness often does force people to stop and consider, to evaluate their lives and their priorities, and sometimes to make new resolutions – which, like most resolutions, rarely are kept after the crisis has passed. However, illness can inform you about yourself – how you react, what you feel, what matters to you – and that self-knowledge may be valuable and useful to you both during and after your illness.

As I said, feelings of guilt and responsibility sometimes accompany illness. Conversely, many sick people feel like victims. Why me?, we ask. What have I done to deserve this? If we can't come up with a satisfactory answer (and if we do, then we usually feel guilty), we're left with a sense of injustice and associated feelings of anger. For many patients, anger is the emotion they find most difficult to deal with while they're sick. It frightens them – they fear it will alienate others – and they feel "bad" for feeling it, especially when they feel angry toward family members, friends, or their doctors and other caretakers. Hence, they end up feeling guilty about feeling angry.

Many patients feel angry because they feel they're misunderstood by, or isolated from, family and friends and they're being treated differently because of their illness. Such feelings of isolation, whether emotional or social, add to patients' suffering. Sick people describe feeling as if they're on the other side of a thick glass wall, watching as healthy people go about the business of leading their lives, while they, the sick, live from doctor visit to doctor visit, from scan to scan, from blood test to blood test, from treatment to treatment. Illness invades and sometimes takes over their lives. The lives of the well and those of the sick may diverge. The daily worries of the sick are different from those of the healthy (or the temporarily well) person. Sick people may feel as if they have been robbed of their normal lives, and they resent it. They also may resent the people who have not been robbed of their lives.

Such feelings are common and natural. Again, it is worth accepting them and not feeling bad about feeling them. Also, after cataloguing the ways in which illness has changed your life, think about the ways in which it hasn't. Think again about how you and your life haven't changed.

I offer you a paradox: **the good patient is the patient who's not too concerned about being good.**

Don't worry too much about being good. It's more important that you get the help you need, in terms of both the medical treatment and the emotional, moral, and social support you require. Although you're a patient, you remain first and foremost a person. Moreover, if you're with the "right" doctor for you, he or she won't need or even want you to be "good" in the sense of aiming simply to be compliant or to please him or her. He or she will want you – need you – to let him or her know how you're feeling and what you're doing.

Sure, you want your doctor to like you, and doctors, being people themselves, would rather deal with people they like than with people they don't like. It would be naïve to suggest that whether your doctor likes you doesn't matter in the treatment you receive. Put differently, being actively disliked by your doctor might well have an adverse effect on your treatment. Most doctors, like most people, would rather avoid interactions that are frankly adversarial or hostile. However, doctors – at least those worth their salt – also understand that anger, fear, and distrust come with the territory of illness, and that it's part of their job to accept and respond to their patients' emotional state in the course of treatment. So, without ignoring the fact that doctors are people too, don't become too worried about hurting the doctor's feelings.

This is often easier said than done, as I know from personal experience. Not long ago, I had abdominal surgery for a condition known as diverticulitis and ran into some serious complications, including the need for a second operation five days after the first. Despite this and a few other serious untoward complications, I was reluctant to seek a second opinion from another surgeon when I was facing a therapeutic decision about the possible need for yet a third surgical procedure. Despite the urging of all my family and friends, I felt disloyal and ungrateful in going to another surgeon. After all, I felt my surgeon had done his best, that the complications were bad luck but not his fault, and I was afraid to insult, anger, and alienate him. I think I was even afraid to feel angry with him, although many of those around me had no problem doing so on my behalf. Although, as a physician, I know the best doctors welcome second opinions from colleagues, and often are happy to have another doctor consult on a difficult or complicated case, I still felt apprehensive and guilty about going to see another surgeon. I was anxious about calling my surgeon's office to ask for my records and scans, and I interpreted any delay in hearing back from his secretary as a sign of his displeasure. Like so many patients, I feared abandonment by my doctor because I felt both grateful to and dependent on him. Ultimately, I did seek a second opinion, and it proved reassuring and helpful. I didn't seem to hurt my surgeon's feelings (although to this day, I'm not quite sure), and he continues to follow up on my original condition.

I can attest to the fact that our thoughts, as well as our emotions, may be affected when we're sick. After my second operation for diverticulitis, while still in the hospital, I felt both physically and emotionally exhausted. Never in my life had I felt so depleted of energy. Thought itself was a physical effort. In that state of exhaustion, I began to distrust my caretakers, both the professionals and my family members. As one postoperative side effect was followed by another, I became focused on controlling my body and my environment and increasingly resistant to intrusions of any kind by others. I began to expect that another complication was just around the corner, and that the next one could be my last. I summoned whatever internal energies I could muster to anticipate and prevent the next complication from happening. I had lost confidence in my caretakers and felt that I could trust my care only to myself. This feeling gradually dissipated as I recovered my energy and my health, but I haven't forgotten the vivid sense that I was fighting for my life (whether I was or not, I'm still uncertain) and that I had to summon all my diminished powers to protect myself. Such feelings existed side by side with a sense of total dependence on those in whose hands I had placed myself, and with the fear of abandonment by them. Such an emotional cocktail isn't rare in the course of an illness, just as complications and side effects of any treatment aren't rare. Yet despite the fact that complications and side effects are frequent and even likely occurrences, when you experience one or more problems as a result of your treatment, it can shake your confidence and generate distrust.

Recovery may be almost as challenging as the illness itself. I probably have had more patients referred to me at the conclusion of successful medical treatment than I have during their treatment. Ending treatment may be a crisis on its own because it involves losing or, at the very least, reducing the care and attention the patient has been receiving from doctors and others. Moreover, so long as patients are actively being treated, they have the feeling that doctors and others are doing something to help. When treatment ends, anxieties may increase, because now nothing is being done to fight the disease. Patients may again feel frightened, abandoned, and alone, and it can take time to adjust back to a state of non-sickness and non-patienthood.

Because of medical progress, many diseases these days are chronic, and many people with chronic illnesses – from arthritis to heart disease to cancer – live in a limbo state between feeling recovered and awaiting recurrence. Appointments with doctors, blood tests, and periodic body scans conjure up memories of the past and fears of the future. Some side effects from prior treatments or ongoing medications may never fully disappear, so patients often are reminded by their body that they have been sick and could become so again. A patient of mine, whose metastatic cancer responded fully to the chemotherapy she received, still lives with painful feet and tearing eyes as reminders of her illness. Her oncologist quite understandably considers her treatment a success, as does she, but for him, her side effects are minor nuisances in the larger scheme of his work, whereas for her, they are impediments to living her daily life. Although she's grateful for the outcome of her cancer treatment, she also is angry that neither her body nor her life has returned to its premorbid state.

She also seems afraid of feeling well. She was shocked by the initial diagnosis of her cancer, which took her totally by surprise because it was made during a routine office visit. She entered her doctor's office a healthy woman – or so she thought – and came out a cancer patient. She won't allow herself to be taken by surprise again, so it's difficult for her to feel well. She distrusts her own body and her ability to interpret it. Is an ache a sign of recurrence? Although she gradually learned to tolerate these anxieties, she remains frightened before her periodic scans, imagining the worst for weeks beforehand. Her husband, who hears her doctor say she's cancer-free, tries to convince her all is well but ends up frustrated and angry at what appears to him to be utter irrationality. These episodes distance them from each other. She ends up feeling more emotionally alone. As she has recognized her fears, and as we have explored her wishes regarding her marriage and her life, it has become easier for her to accept her own emotional responses, as well as her husband's, and the isolation between them has decreased considerably.

We see, then, that being sick may be emotionally challenging, which makes finding the right doctor all the more important. I highlighted earlier that when it comes to doctors, one size doesn't fit all. No one doctor is right for all patients. However, the most important factor for choosing the right doctor is finding one who is knowledgeable about and competent with your illness. No matter how wonderful a bedside manner a doctor may have – and I would be the last person to underestimate the importance of bedside manner – competence is essential in a physician. It isn't always easy to assess a doctor's level of competence, however, so we generally choose on the basis of referrals, either from other physicians such as our internist or general practitioner or from friends, or on the basis of reputation, either of the doctor or of the medical institution with which he or she is affiliated. None of these criteria is foolproof, of course. A highly esteemed hospital may have doctors on its staff whose technical competence doesn't match the hospital's reputation. Nonetheless, as an initial means of choosing the "right" doctor, referrals and reputation are good approaches.

When choosing a specialist who likely will become your treating physician – whether a surgeon, cardiologist, oncologist, or psychiatrist – I recommend, if at all feasible, that you meet with more than one doctor before deciding. This will give you an opportunity to experience more than one physician's style, to hear more than one physician's clinical assessment and treatment recommendations, and to ask questions and receive responses from more than one doctor. Not only will you gather more information about your illness, you also will experience more than one doctor's treatment style. You will get your first taste of what it would be like to be treated by that doctor. Your experience during the consultation – from the initial phone call and interaction with the office staff to the doctor's manner of taking a history, performing a physical exam, and communicating with you afterward – may serve as a sample of what treatment by that doctor would be like. Do you feel respected and listened to? Does the doctor speak plainly and clearly so that you can understand him or her? Does he or she provide you with a framework that gives you a sense of what comes next, of what to expect? Did you feel comfortable asking questions? Did you feel you were taken seriously, or did you feel dismissed?

After leaving the office, think about the consultation appointment and your reactions. Ask yourself whether you got a sense that this doctor understood the importance to you of the appointment. I think a hallmark of good physicians is understanding that although they may see many patients in the course of a week, each patient will see the doctor only occasionally and that every appointment is a significant event in that patient's life even if it's a routine event in the life of the doctor.

Also ask yourself how you think this doctor would deal with complications or side effects, because problems of some kind likely will arise in the course of most treatments. It's important to remember that to be a good patient, you shouldn't strive to be too "good" a patient. So, again paradoxically, one criterion for finding the "right" doctor is finding a doctor who doesn't require that you be too "good" a patient if "good" means pleasing, passive, unemotional, or inexpressive. How do you think this doctor would deal with a challenge coming from you, be it in the form of a question, a complaint, or an expression of anger?

These questions are difficult, if not impossible, to answer after just one appointment and probably will be answered only during the course of treatment. You might seek a second opinion along the way if you run into difficulties, as I did. However, keep in mind that just as no one doctor is right for all patients, no doctor is perfect for any patient. Even with the "right" doctor for you, there may be bumps in the road. Tensions and conflicts may well arise, and at times you may feel dissatisfied. If you're feeling dissatisfied frequently, you probably should get a second opinion. (If you're feeling more than dissatisfied – highly anxious or depressed or in other ways inconsolably distressed – consult your physician and consider getting help from a psychiatrist or psychotherapist.) However, don't expect your doctor to understand or respond to you perfectly. As we saw in some of our earlier examples, sometimes doctors and patients diverge in their perspectives and concerns, and it's a mistake to expect your doctor to always understand you. Doctors, too, have their strengths and weaknesses, and your relationship with your doctor, like relationships in general, may function well in some ways and not so well in others.

In today's world, patients could use a survival manual to help them navigate the frightening and confusing terrain of both illness and medical care. Despite the many medical advances of the past half-century – or perhaps because of them – being sick seems to have become more, rather than less, complex. No longer can we rely on a single good or right way of being either a patient or a doctor. The old certainties of medical paternalism have run their course, just as the new certainties of patient autonomy to which they gave way also have exhausted themselves. I've tried to sketch the emotional and social landscape of being a patient, emphasizing the value of self-awareness, so that when you encounter a pitfall, you're not completely unprepared. Even so, unwelcome surprises likely will occur along the way. For those, you'll have to rely on yourself and those around you for guidance.

TWO

Becoming an Active Member
of Your Health Care Team

– William A. Norcross

You wouldn't be reading this book if you were perfectly happy with the health care you are receiving and the system that delivers it to you. The U.S. health care system is vexing and frustrating to physicians, nurses, and patients alike. Worse yet, many of our most important health outcomes are dramatically inferior to those of other Western nations that spend much less on health care.

Social, cultural, and legal factors indigenous to the United States have produced a unique health care system comprising many competing insurers and plans, each with its own bureaucracy. At its best, our health care is unsurpassed, but when examined across the entire American population, it's severely flawed. About 15% of the U.S. population has no health insurance whatsoever, yet when members of this group become ill (sometimes when a disease has progressed further than it might have if medical attention had been readily available), they receive care too, and someone must pay for that care. Moreover, most (but not all) health insurance plans reimburse at proportionately higher levels of health care for the highest "acuity" (e.g., surgical procedures, intensive care) of disease. This creates a system that rewards surgery and care for the sickest patients, rewards the outpatient management of disease less, and sometimes even provides disincentives for

13

providing preventive health care. Consequently, fewer and fewer U.S. medical school graduates are choosing careers in primary care, and those primary care physicians in practice are pushed to the limit. Little is done in the United States to incentivize medical students to pursue careers in specialties or generalist medicine in keeping with projected national health staffing needs; therefore, every year we produce a surplus of highly paid specialists who practice in urban or suburban areas. The conventional market economic principles of capitalism normally predict that oversupply will result in falling prices (this presumes that the "demand" for subspecialized medical services should remain steady over any population). However, studies have consistently shown that this is not the case: there are great geographic variations in expenditure for health care, and spending more money doesn't buy better health outcomes (in fact, the opposite may be true). What happens in American health care is called the "field of dreams" paradigm because it's true: If you build it, they will come. Communities with more hospital beds will have a populace that spends a higher number of days in the hospital per capita. Communities with more specialists receive, on average, more specialty procedures. The reason for this is that, unlike other sectors of the American economy, at some level, doctors themselves control the rate of utilization of health care services. Doctors choose whether or not to admit a patient to the hospital. Cardiologists choose whether or not to perform coronary angiography, angioplasty, and coronary artery stent placement, as well as which stent to use. Of course, doctors must provide informed consent, but how many patients in the emergency room with chest pain are going to ask for a deeper discussion with more hard data if their doctor recommends an immediate angioplasty? The geographic differences in health care expenditure are by no means trivial: If all geographic areas performed at expenditure levels of the lowest quintile of communities, about 30% would be lopped off the annual U.S. health budget (2.6 trillion dollars in 2006) with no change in health outcomes. The geographic areas with the highest health expenditure tend to have the most specialists, the most hospital beds, and the fewest primary care physicians. This situation is reversed for geographic areas with the lowest expenditures. (Again, the studies suggest a slight improvement in health care outcomes in the areas with the lowest expenditures.) Because of all the aforementioned reasons, the current U.S. physician workforce comprises 75% specialist physicians and 25% primary care physicians. Most economic models suggest that a health care system would work optimally with a 50–50 balance. (I speak in terms of "doctors" and "physicians," but nurse practitioners and physician assistants are part of the health staffing equation and probably should play an increasing role in helping America respond to the primary care shortage.)

Carefully performed studies have shown that primary care physicians should devote the following amounts of time to their practices on a daily basis to ensure their patients get all the care they require: chronic care illnesses: 10.6 hours; preventive health care: 7.4 hours; and acute care delivery: 4.6 hours. This totals 22.6 hours per day, a clear impossibility. About half of a primary care physician's workday is spent "outside the exam room," and much of this time is consumed by the paperwork and procedures necessary to get patients the things they need. The insurance companies that ultimately pay for patient services have an incentive to make this paperwork and bureaucracy as byzantine as possible because this makes it less likely they will have to provide these goods and services, and the blame for the failure to make this happen will rest squarely on the shoulders of the primary care physician.

In an effort to learn more about the factors that explain the disparity among Western nations, the Commonwealth Fund undertook one of the most detailed studies of its kind, comparing care in the United States, Australia, Canada, Germany, Great Britain, and New Zealand. Compared with people in other countries, Americans were 1) less likely to have "a regular doctor," 2) less likely to have seen the same primary physician for five years or more, 3) more likely to find difficulty obtaining health care in the evening or on weekends (excluding emergency room care), and 4) more likely to wait six days or more for an appointment for an acute medical problem. Perhaps saddest of all, half the American patients surveyed reported they had forgone health care at some time over the past two years because of concerns about cost. This was more than twice the percentage reported by patients in any of the other countries.

So, here are the facts plain and simple:

1. Things are not going to get better on a national basis anytime soon. Our 2.6 *trillion* dollar annual health care budget (2006 federal estimate) will not turn on a dime. Moreover, the U.S. Constitution, which guarantees competition among businesses, is not likely to be amended in that regard. Lastly, based on our recent political history, the political mood of America at present is "right of moderate." Although health care will be the subject of much political debate for years to come, it is unlikely that a major reshaping of our health care system will take place soon.

2. We need to spend *less*, not more, on health care, and we must obtain better outcomes. The way to better health outcomes will not be through throwing money at the problem. Counterintuitive as it may sound, that's what got us in this pickle.

The good news is that some of the best minds in the helping professions have been working on solutions for years. (The American Academy of Pediatrics [AAP] first put forward the concept of a *medical home* in 1967!) One of the best concepts to emerge is that of the patient-centered medical home. The following summary statements are from a March 2007 document titled "Joint Principles of the Patient-Centered Medical Home," written and published jointly by the American Academy of Family Physicians (AAFP), the AAP, the American College of Physicians (ACP), and the American Osteopathic Association (AOA). These groups are among the most powerful and influential medical professional organizations in the United States, representing 330,000 physicians (almost half of all those in America) in the disciplines of family medicine, pediatrics, internal medicine, and osteopathic medicine, respectively.

The following is a thumbnail sketch of the principles underlying the concept of the *medical home*, but you can read much more by visiting the websites of these organizations at http://www.futurefamily med.org, http://aappolicy.aappublications.org/policy_statement/index. dtl#M, http://www.acponline.org/advocacy/?hp, and http://www. osteopathic.org.

Principles of the Patient-Centered Medical Home

1. **Each patient has a personal physician**. The personal physician knows the patient, has access to the medical record, and serves as the source of first access and continuous care.
2. **The physician is the leader of the practice team**. Together, the team takes responsibility for the patient's care.
3. **The personal physician is responsible for delivering comprehensive care**. The personal physician either delivers the necessary care or arranges for specialist physicians or others to provide that care while maintaining knowledge of all aspects of the care delivered. This includes patients at all stages of life, in all health care environments, and at all levels of care: preventive, acute, chronic, and end of life.
4. Care is coordinated, integrated, and delivered in a culturally and linguistically appropriate manner.
5. **The medical home assures quality of care and patient safety**. The care rendered is compassionate and evidence based. It is a partnership between physicians, patients, and patients' families. Patients participate in all decisions, and patient feedback is actively sought to ensure patient beliefs, wishes, and expectations are being met.
6. The medical home uses modern technology and concepts of health care delivery that maximize access to care and communication.

To qualify for designation by the National Committee for Quality Assurance, a patient-centered medical home must meet at least five of the following ten criteria:

1. Has written standards for patient access to care and communication with health care providers
2. Uses paper or electronic charts to organize clinical data
3. Uses clinical data to demonstrate that it meets standards for access and communication
4. Uses data to document diagnoses and clinical conditions in practice
5. Applies evidence-based clinical guidelines for a minimum of three diseases or conditions
6. Demonstrably supports self-management by patients
7. Tracks laboratory tests, imaging studies, and other test data and can identify abnormal test results in a systematic way
8. Tracks referrals in a systematic and organized fashion
9. Measures clinical performance at the level of the individual physician and/or across the entire practice
10. Reports clinical performance at the level of the individual physician and/or across the entire practice

We very briefly touched on the historical, social, and economic circumstances that have evolved into the current U.S. health care system, and we reviewed one plan put forward by organized medicine, the patient-centered medical home, to address our needs, but you're interested in knowing what you can do *starting today* to ensure good health outcomes for you and your family.

To help organize your thinking about your role as an *active* patient, I divide the topic into four areas: 1) before the visit, 2) in the waiting room, 3) during the visit, and 4) between visits. This division is arbitrary, so feel free to exchange these action items in your journey to optimal health.

If I do a good job telling this story, I hope you'll come to see that a well-informed and well-prepared active patient and a good doctor, both working in a patient-centered medical home environment, will blur the somewhat artificial boundaries of these four temporal areas, replacing the brick-and-mortar, visit-driven health care system with one centered around a continuous, open channel of communication and care.

Before the Visit

1. **Spend time searching for the doctor who is right for you and then have confidence in your doctor.** If you haven't read

Chapter One yet, please do so. The cornerstone of quality medical care is a doctor–patient relationship with a physician who is technically competent and makes you feel comfortable. You should be satisfied with your physician's ability to communicate with you and the health care system that supports his or her ability to practice. Appraising the doctor's health care "system" is a step that is often overlooked. To accomplish this goal, a *team* of people and a technologically robust infrastructure are required. One of the most important members of this team is *you*.

2. Spend time researching the health care system in which the physician works:
   a. What hospital does the physician admit to?
   b. Does the physician follow his or her patients in the hospital, or does he or she use a hospitalist?
   c. How is night call handled?
   d. Does the practice offer after-hours or Saturday clinics?
   e. How does the physician handle urgent needs? Does his or her leave appointment spots open for patients' urgent needs?
   f. Who are the other health care providers in the practice, and what are their qualifications?
   g. Is e-mail communication permissible?
   h. How are telephone calls handled?
   i. What if I need to see a specialist or obtain ancillary services (e.g., physical therapy)?

3. **Be prepared for each office visit.** Don't be afraid to think about your visit ahead of time and make notes about what you want to talk to the doctor about. Above all, share that information with your doctor. Feel comfortable giving your doctor your list of concerns; this may enhance efficiency, and your doctor can help prioritize the most important concerns on the list. In most clinical practices, about fifteen minutes will be allotted for your visit; you want to get the most from all fifteen of those minutes. One way to do this is to arrive in clinic with the information you know your doctor will need, legibly prepared ahead of time. If you have received care from one doctor for a long time, and if he or she keeps good medical records (paper or electronic), it may not be necessary to bring this information to every visit. However, early in your relationship with a doctor, or whenever there has been a change in diagnosis or treatment, bringing a written synopsis saves you and the doctor some of the time and effort involved in recounting and recording your history. Keep a diary or log of your symptoms and concerns. Make sure you date and time all entries (or use a personal calendar); the timing of your symptoms may give your doctor important clues as to how to adjust your treatment. Just before your visit, review this diary and prioritize the questions and concerns you have for your doctor. Feel comfortable taking notes on what your doctor tells you, and don't hesitate to bring a friend or family member to help you. The following list will help

your doctor provide care for you and leave more time for one-on-one interaction:

a. Enumerate all your diseases and conditions along with the date of diagnosis (if the doctor uses a standardized form for the health history, you may request one in advance)

b. List all allergies to medications and all other allergens

c. List all medications, including supplements and over-the-counter drugs, as well as dosages and dosing schedules

d. Name all other physicians and health care providers caring for you, and list their addresses, telephone numbers, and e-mail addresses

e. List all family members and friends your physician should know about, including their addresses, telephone numbers, and e-mail addresses

f. List and describe the symptoms and concerns you wish to discuss during your clinic visit. Doctors are taught to characterize symptoms in the following way, so the more you can do to consider and prepare this information, the better:

 i. The character of the symptoms in your own words (e.g., "It's a squeezing pain, doctor – sort of a pressure, like a puppy sitting on my chest.")

 ii. The severity of the symptoms (sometimes it's helpful to characterize the symptoms, especially pain, on a scale from 1 to 10, where 10 is the worst pain you've ever had)

 iii. The location of the symptoms and a description of how they've moved or changed since they began

 iv. When you first noted the symptoms

 v. The setting in which the symptoms occur

 vi. How often the symptoms occur

 vii. Factors that make the symptoms worse

 viii. Factors that make the symptoms better

 ix. Associated symptoms

4. **Be tech-savvy.** Learn to use a computer. The World Wide Web is a vast source of important health information, some of which is good and some not. In general, information found on government or university websites is highly reliable. E-mail communication with your doctor can save time and improve your access to health care. Remember, however, that e-mail is an *asynchronous* form of communication. If your doctor permits e-mail communication, you should use this method only for routine concerns and non-urgent matters. When using e-mail, it may take hours or even days to get a response, so emergencies should never be handled by this method of communication. Keep in mind that e-mail communications between physicians and patients become part of your personal medical record. With regard to medical information you download from the Internet, it's fine to occasionally bring an article to your doctor; however, avoid bringing a large volume of materials and expecting him or her to sift through it and give you an opinion.

5. Unless circumstances dictate otherwise, consider making the first visit with your primary care physician a fifteen-minute "get to know you" session. Much depends on the "chemistry" between patient and physician, which can be determined only by face-to-face contact and communication. If the chemistry is not there, all the time and effort of a complete history and physical examination will be diminished. The complete history and physical examination are not ritual exercises; they are the means by which the patient begins to understand the doctor's thinking, and the doctor begins to understand the patient's thinking, as well as how the patient's heart sounds, skin appears, and so forth.

6. **Appreciate the importance of follow-up.** Make sure you understand what the doctor wants you to do. If concerns remain or there are items still on your list, explore with the doctor how best to follow up on these. Will a telephone call or e-mail communication suffice? Make certain you have a firm understanding of how you will be informed of laboratory tests, consultations, and imaging studies, and know when the doctor wants to see you again.

In the Waiting Room

1. **Germs are an unavoidable part of the world around us, so it's wise to assume all surfaces in a hospital, clinic, or doctor's office are teeming with viruses and bacteria, many of which are pathogenic to human beings.** If you're sick, especially with a respiratory illness with coughing, runny nose, or sneezing, wear a mask, cover your mouth when coughing or sneezing, and carry hand sanitizer and use it frequently. Most viruses and bacteria cannot cause harm through unbroken skin, so keeping your fingers away from mucosal surfaces (your eyes, nose, and mouth are common entry ports) usually is sufficient to avoid contracting disease. Frequent hand washing and hand sanitizer use also are recommended.

2. **Be kind and understanding to your doctor and his or her staff.** Treat your doctor and his or her office staff the way you would like to be treated. You want your doctor to be kind and understanding. If your doctor is technically superb, compassionate, conscientious, and caring, then the likelihood is that he or she is going to run late once in a while. Bring something to read or do, just in case. If your doctor is running late, he or she likely has been practicing the same level of conscientiousness and compassion you may need yourself someday. If long waits are especially bothersome for you, try to get an appointment early in the clinic session. Doctors tend to begin clinics on time, then run late as the clinic session progresses (I certainly do).

3. **Get to know the entire health care team.** Your doctor likely won't be able to provide you with care 100% of the time. Get to know his or her partners, nurse practitioners, physician assistants, nurses, and other co-workers in the practice. You likely will need their help someday, too.

4. **Read the policies on the waiting room wall.** They may provide important information about practice operating procedures, other health care providers in the practice, how to access your physician or his or her representative after hours and on weekends, how to obtain prescription refills, and perhaps other things.

During the Visit

1. **Be knowledgeable.** Don't leave an office visit befuddled. Have your doctor explain your diagnosis and the proposed tests and treatment in language you can understand. If you don't understand the meaning of a word or phrase, say so and ask the doctor for an explanation. Even the most sensitive physicians occasionally fall back on jargon or words doctors use to communicate with one another. Sometimes the doctor may not be certain of your diagnosis or know the best way to proceed. There may be choices that you have to make. In those cases, your doctor should explain the situation and options to the best of his or her ability. You should understand the options, including what they entail and what the risks and benefits are for each. Learn more about the diseases you have and the medicines you take. Whether accessing information at the library or on your home computer, seek reliable sources. Keep a file on your health care – paper, electronic, or both. After each visit, physicians who use electronic health records can give you an "after-visit summary" including your acute symptoms during that visit, the diagnosis, chronic medical conditions, medications and allergies, and everything that was ordered that day.

2. **Adhere to the plan, or tell your doctor if you can't.** When the office visit is finished and you and your doctor have agreed on a plan of investigation and treatment, the doctor reasonably expects you to have the tests performed or to take your medicines as prescribed. You should participate in these decisions, and you have the right to accept or refuse treatment. However, appearing to agree with the diagnostic and/or treatment plan but failing to follow through with it is unwise and sometimes dangerous. If you're uncomfortable with the plan, share your concerns with your doctor.

3. **Be open to new ideas.** Your doctor may suggest that you participate in group visits, or he or she may ask you to consider participating as a subject in a research study. Although no one knows the future, we do know it won't be static. Meeting the challenges of our nation's health and your individual health care will require innovation, imagination, boldness, and a strong partnership between patients and medical professionals.

4. **Turn off your cell phone or put it on mute.** Even while you're waiting for your doctor in the exam room, resist the temptation to make one more phone call. Your doctor, upon entering the exam room, will not feel entirely comfortable interrupting your telephone conversation.

Welcome your doctor with the same enthusiasm and attentiveness you hope to receive from him or her.

5. You'll have your vital signs taken, provide some basic history, and be placed in the exam room by a medical assistant or nurse. Get to know the clinic staff. They serve an important function in every practice and will be part of your health care team going forward.

6. **Make use of your time alone in the exam room.** Hopefully, this time will be short, but doctors and nurses do everything in their power to make this time more enjoyable – invariably by decorating the exam room walls with glossy color prints of diseased coronary arteries or infected nasal sinuses. Somehow, they believe patients will find these illustrations as endlessly delightful as they do. Seriously, though, use this time to review your list of problems and prioritize them in order of importance.

7. **Be concise.** A certain amount of social interaction is appropriate, even desirable, but keep in mind you have fifteen minutes of face time with your doctor, and a full agenda.

8. **Get to know your physician and make it easy for him or her to get to know you.** Among other things, it's reasonable to ask your physician when he or she plans to retire. You have the right to plan a long-term relationship, and if your doctor plans to retire in two years, you have a right to know that.

9. **Immediately after your visit, write down all new diagnoses, planned tests, and treatments.** In some practices with electronic health records, this will happen "automatically," and you'll be given an after-visit summary.

Between Visits

1. **Take more responsibility for your own care.** Know your medical illnesses and your health conditions, including allergies and sensitivities. Know all your medications, their dosages, and how you're supposed to take them. Make certain all of your health care providers are aware of this information. If helpful, keep paper or electronic copies of important medical documents and information, and bring them with you to office visits. The Web-based *personalized health account* is a powerful emerging tool that promises to significantly improve health care outcomes. Examples of personalized health account systems are MyChart® and HealthVault®. Such systems are safe, confidential repositories for your personal health information. The patient controls what information is stored on the site and who else has access to view or change that information. Additionally, some of these systems allow patients to connect various monitors, such as those used to evaluate diabetes, hypertension, heart rhythm disturbances, and asthma, enabling both patient and doctor to have rapid access to information that may improve the control of these chronic diseases. Know what health maintenance and preventive health

care interventions are appropriate for your age, gender, and diseases, and make sure they get done. If you're unsure whether you've had any of these interventions (immunizations, colon cancer screening, eye exam, etc.), feel comfortable accessing your medical record.

2. **Seek information.** The Internet teems with health-related information – some good, some bad. Ask your physician what sites he/she recommends and whether he or she (or his or her group or organization) has a website. In general, the following are reliable sources of health information:

   a. Federal, state, and county governments
   b. Medical and osteopathic schools
   c. The American Medical Association and state and county medical societies
   d. National, state, and local specialty and subspecialty organizations (e.g., AAFP, ACP, AAP)
   e. Nationally recognized charitable organizations (e.g., American Lung Association, American Heart Association)

3. **Discuss compliance issues openly with your doctor.** Follow your doctor's instructions. Take your medications as they're prescribed. If your regimen is complex, use a pill organizer or ask a family member for help. Make sure to obtain your medication refills before your current prescription runs out (not doing so may be dangerous, especially with diseases like coronary artery disease, hypertension, and diabetes mellitus, for which good daily control of the disease is critical). Be certain to have all tests and consultations performed promptly, in accordance with your doctor's wishes. Just as physicians want their patients to be happy and pleased with the care they receive, so too do patients want to please their physicians. In general, this is a good thing, but many times I've seen patients report compliance to their primary care physician when, in reality, they've been unable or unwilling to comply with the recommended treatment. This may be dangerous. Imagine a physician who starts her patient on a drug to treat high blood pressure, but the patient doesn't take the drug because he can't afford it, it's not on his insurance formulary, side effects develop, or some other reason. However, he wants to please his physician, so at the next visit he reports taking the pill and states things are going fine. The doctor likes hearing this but notices his blood pressure is still elevated. The doctor likely would increase the medication dosage or add a second medication, although the problem is really that her patient hasn't been taking the first medication. Studies show that about 50% of prescriptions written by physicians are never filled.

4. **Work with your doctor to overcome clinical inertia.** The term *clinical inertia* was first introduced in the medical literature by Phillips and co-workers in 2001, but the entity itself likely has been around for much longer. The term refers to the tendency to undertreat chronic diseases. In fact, clinical inertia, as reflected in numerous studies documenting woeful

control of hypertension, adult-onset diabetes mellitus, asthma, and other diseases, is nothing short of a national shame. The reasons for clinical inertia are multifactorial, but responsibility lies with patients, physicians, and the health care system itself. Factors known to contribute to the problem of clinical inertia include a history of patient noncompliance with treatment medications, physician ignorance of national target goals for treating chronic diseases, and the total number of chronic diseases the patient has. Undoubtedly, there are more. This problem isn't a parlor game; the national target goals for treating chronic diseases were determined based on decades of research. The following statements are true: If you suffer from adult-onset diabetes mellitus and keep your glycohemoglobin level (a blood test that reflects average blood sugar level over the past two to three months) at 7%, you're less likely, on average, to develop diabetic kidney disease and require transplantation or dialysis than is a diabetic whose glycohemoglobin level hovers around 9%. If you suffer from hypertension and keep your blood pressure at 125/75 mm Hg, you're less likely, on average, to sustain a stroke or heart attack than is a hypertensive patient whose blood pressure is consistently 160/95 mm Hg. However, the question is, What can *you* do to reach target goals for your disease? First, discuss this issue with your doctor. Make certain you understand his or her goals for treatment. Unfortunately, we know that doctors themselves are misinformed or lack knowledge about target goals for chronic diseases. This means you must arm yourself with this information. The good news is that the Internet puts this information at your fingertips, and there is a reputable source of knowledge for every problem. Although it's impossible for me to discuss every chronic disease, adult-onset diabetes mellitus is a common and important public health problem, and there is a superb resource for every patient with the disease: the American Diabetes Association (ADA), whose website is found at http://www.diabetes.org (I encourage all my patients with diabetes to access this website often). The ADA website contains practical information to help patients and doctors alike manage the disease and achieve optimal outcomes.

5. **Practice personal preventive health care.** The road to a long and healthy life is constructed of the lifestyle choices we make, usually early in life, although it's never too late to make good choices. Although the topic of preventive medicine is vast, people who avoid tobacco, eat a healthy diet while maintaining normal body weight, engage in at least thirty minutes of aerobic exercise daily, limit their daily intake of alcohol to the equivalent of two ounces or less, and obtain seven to eight hours of restful sleep each night are well along the path to optimal health. The average American will find a sound dietary plan in the booklet *Your Guide to Lowering Your Cholesterol with TLC*, published by the National Institutes of Health, and the National Heart, Lung, and Blood Institute and available at http://www.nhlbi.nih.gov/health/public/heart/chol/chol_tlc.pdf. Sound guidelines for exercise have been developed jointly by the

American Heart Association (http://www.americanheart.org) and the American College of Sports Medicine (http://www.acsm.org). Recommendations for health maintenance and preventive health care are constantly in evolution and flux, so we all need a reliable, independent source of information. Such a resource is the U.S. Preventive Services Task Force, whose website is found at http://www.ahrq.gov/clinic/uspstfix.htm. Finally, one of the most cost-effective methods of preventing disease is immunization. The resource I recommend for current, up-to-date, reliable information on vaccinations is the Centers for Disease Control and Prevention (http://www.cdc.gov/vaccines).

The future holds challenges and promise for us all, but it will require an active approach and receptivity to novel solutions for you to maximize your health outcomes. If you're comfortable partnering with your physician and his or her health care team; embracing new tools, methodologies, and systems for health-related communication and education; and taking greater responsibility for your own health and that of your family, you're ready for what the twenty-first century has to bring.

THREE

Information That Will Help You with Advance Planning for Your Health Care

– Mark R. Wicclair

At some point in our lives, most of us have to make decisions about our health care. Some of these decisions are relatively simple and straightforward. For example, you probably don't spend much time pondering whether or not to get a flu shot, and you probably would follow your doctor's advice without a second thought if he or she recommended you take an antibiotic for a urinary tract infection or have a biopsy for a suspected skin cancer. None of these decisions would require much reflection or soul-searching.

However, some decisions about health care are neither simple nor straightforward. For women with stage IV breast cancer, deciding whether or not to undergo a combination of mastectomy, chemotherapy, radiation therapy, and bone marrow transplantation may be extremely difficult and stressful. For men with a new diagnosis of prostate cancer, deciding whether to have surgery and risk impotence and/or urinary incontinence is neither simple nor straightforward.

If decision making about our own health care is challenging when we can decide for ourselves, it's bound to be much more so if we try to plan ahead and make decisions today that can be used to guide our health care if we lose our decision-making ability years or decades in the future. If you have to decide today whether to begin dialysis tomorrow, at least you can discuss the pros and cons with your physician and make a decision based on information about your current overall health, the medical condition that has caused kidney failure, the expected benefits and harms, your prognosis, and so forth. However, if you're healthy and your kidneys are functioning today and you try to decide whether you would want dialysis in the future, you would lack such specific information, which can make advance planning about your health care difficult. Nevertheless, there are several reasons for advance planning with the aim of providing guidance for health care decision making if and when you are unable to decide for yourself. This may well be one of those situations in which doing the best you can is better than doing nothing.

Reasons for Advance Planning about Your Health Care

One reason for advance planning is the very real possibility that you may one day lack the capacity to make health care decisions for yourself. The loss of decision-making capacity may come suddenly and unexpectedly as the result of traumatic injury (e.g., a car accident) or a stroke, or it may be the result of a chronic, progressive illness, such as Alzheimer's or Huntington's disease. Although it may strike when people are old, it also may occur when they're still young. This point is illustrated by Terri Schiavo, the Florida woman whose case generated extensive media attention and occasioned the involvement of the governor of Florida, the Florida legislature, the U.S. Congress, the president of the United States, and state and federal courts. Ms. Schiavo was in a permanent vegetative state for thirteen years before she died when medically supplied nutrition and hydration were discontinued. She was only twenty-six years old in 1990 when she experienced the cardiac arrest that caused her severe brain damage. It's natural to hope that we never will lose the ability to make health care decisions for ourselves or develop a serious illness. Sadly, however, whether young or old, none of us is immune from either.

If you care about what kind of health care you will and won't receive if and when you lose your capacity to decide for yourself, you have a good reason to engage in advance planning. Are there certain situations in which you would not want to receive medical interventions that would keep you alive? Conversely, are there certain situations in which you would want those life-prolonging interventions? Do you feel strongly about whom you would want to make decisions about your health care if and when you are unable to do so? Do you have religious beliefs or other values that you would want to be considered when medical decisions are made for you? Do you want to avoid an "undignified" death? Do you want the interests of loved ones to be considered when decisions are made about your health care, or do you want those decisions to be based exclusively on your best interests? If you think these are important questions and you want your answers to guide decision making about your health care if you are unable to decide for yourself, you have a good reason to engage in advance planning.

Another reason for advance planning is to minimize the burden on your loved ones. If you lose the ability to decide for yourself, someone else (usually a family member) may be asked to decide for you. If you haven't given any thought to the kinds of medical interventions you would or wouldn't want – or if you have, but haven't communicated your specific preferences or general goals to your loved ones – they will be placed in the uncomfortable position of having to decide without knowing what *you* would want. The decision will be *theirs* rather than an approximation of the decision you would have made if you could do so. Such responsibility, especially for life-or-death decisions, may produce substantial anxiety, stress, guilt, and remorse.

Designating someone (a surrogate) whom you would like to decide for you when you no longer are able can reduce conflicts and stress on the part of your loved ones. If you haven't designated a pre-ferred surrogate, your loved ones may disagree among themselves. Well-intentioned family members who want you to receive care in accordance with your preferences and/or care that's in your best inter-ests may advocate different decisions. Without guidance from you, it may be difficult to reach agreement about who should be the primary decision maker. Deciding now can prevent future conflicts and spare your loved ones unnecessary emotional trauma.

If you don't select a surrogate, one will be selected for you. The law usually designates a priority order of persons to serve as surrogates. The typical priority order is spouse, adult child, parent, adult sibling, adult grandchild, and close friend. If this priority order doesn't match your own preferences, you have another good reason to plan ahead and identify whom you would like to make health care decisions for you.

Guidance for Advance Planning about Your Health Care

Advance planning about your health care may focus on 1) instructions to guide decision making if and when you can't make decisions for yourself, 2) the selection of a surrogate to make decisions for you if and when you can't make decisions for yourself, or 3) both.

Instructions to Guide Decision Making

If you want to provide instructions to guide decision making about your health care, it's best to begin by thinking about the big picture. One helpful question to consider is whether there's a line beyond which your quality of life would be so poor, unsatisfying, or devoid of meaning that you wouldn't want to be kept alive. If you were to permanently lose consciousness like Terri Schiavo, would you want doctors to prolong your life as long as possible? If you permanently lost your ability to recognize and interact with your loved ones and you developed a treatable illness, such as pneumonia, would you want to receive treatment to prevent your death? Is there some other point beyond which you wouldn't want to be kept alive medically? If so, what's that point? A second question to consider is whether there's a point beyond which the value to you of prolonged life would be outweighed by the pain, suffering, and discomfort you would have to undergo. For example, if you were dying of a disease such as cancer, is there some point at which you would want the primary goal of your care to shift from keeping you alive as long as possible to keeping you comfortable during the dying process? Another question to consider is whether you believe it makes sense to distinguish between a "dignified" and "undignified" death. If you do, how do you understand this distinction, and would you want to forgo medical interventions that likely would result in an undignified death?

As you consider such questions, bear in mind that diminished cognitive capacity also may significantly alter the way we experience our lives. For example, while our cognitive capacities are still intact, it might seem intolerable to live in a nursing home, be dependent on others for our basic bodily needs, spend days sleeping, staring blankly into space or at a television screen, playing bingo, and so forth. We might imagine ourselves in such a person's body, aware of our dependence and boring existence, and think that such a life would be awful. However, if we really were a nursing home resident with diminished cognitive capacities, our awareness of our situation would be significantly affected by those diminished cognitive capacities. Think about your experience as an infant. You were completely dependent on others to satisfy your basic bodily needs (e.g., feeding you, dressing and undressing you, bathing you, changing your diapers, transporting you from place to place). If you had been aware of your total dependence, you might have been deeply troubled and unhappy. However, despite your dependency, because you lacked that awareness, your dependency didn't cause you to experience infancy as unpleasant. Similarly, if you were to become dependent because of diminished cognitive function, you might not experience your life as unpleasant. Still, you currently may have a concern about your future dignity, and you may not want to end your life in a condition similar to how it was at the beginning. Metaphorically speaking, you may not want the last chapter of your biography to depict you as severely demented and totally dependent on others. This is an issue you may want to consider when you think about your health care goals and preferences.

One pitfall to avoid when thinking about instructions to guide decision making about your health care is focusing on types of medical interventions instead of what you'd want the *goals* of your care to be in various circumstances. For example, people have said, "I never want to be on machines." This statement may be an understandable response to seeing an unconscious or semiconscious dying friend or loved one hooked up to various machines in a hospital intensive care unit. However, it's important to keep in mind that mechanical ventilators and dialysis also may be temporary measures to help people regain their ability to enjoy life. You might think that dialysis or medically supplied nutrition and hydration would be pointless if you had advanced Alzheimer's disease, and you might think the primary goal of your care at that point should be to keep you as comfortable as possible. However, you might have a very different response if you suffered a stroke and doctors believed there was a good chance you would recover most if not all of your functioning if you temporarily received mechanical ventilation and medically supplied nutrition and hydration and underwent rehabilitation. Accordingly, it's best to focus on *situations* and corresponding *goals* of health care rather than on types of medical interventions.

Nevertheless, sometimes the kind of medical intervention can make a difference. For example, although antibiotics generally do not cause significant discomfort or diminished quality of life, ventilators and other means of life support may have these effects. When thinking about their future health care, some people might opt for noninvasive measures such as antibiotics in certain situations (e.g., moderate to advanced dementia) and reject more burdensome interventions, such as dialysis or medically supplied nutrition and hydration, if restraints are necessary. What about you?

Some patients, and even some doctors and nurses, think medically supplied nutrition and hydration are "special." That is, they believe that even when it's appropriate to withhold or withdraw mechanical ventilation, dialysis, antibiotics, and so forth, it's not appropriate to withhold or withdraw medically supplied nutrition and hydration. Others disagree. What's your view? If you should wind up in a condition that has crossed your "line" of meaningful quality of life, and you're unable to eat or drink, would you still want to receive nutrition and hydration through a tube inserted into your nose or stomach? Keep in mind that in many cases, when dying patients can no longer eat or drink, they do not experience "hunger," and there are alternative means to keep them comfortable (e.g., by means of sedation and ice chips). Moreover, some studies have reported that in some circumstances, medically supplied nutrition and hydration may cause edema (water retention) and increased discomfort in dying patients. Accordingly, you might consider whether you would want medically supplied nutrition and hydration no matter what, or whether your primary goal is to avoid pain and discomfort.

You might also ask yourself whether there are other considerations that would matter to you besides your own quality of life. For example, if you had to decide whether to have a certain medical procedure today, would you consider the potential impact of your decision on the lives of your loved ones (how it might affect them financially and emotionally and how it might alter their lives)? If your answer is yes, then you might contemplate a similar question when you engage in advance planning.

If you have a primary care physician (e.g., an internist or a family physician), he or she might be able to provide information to help you think about your health care preferences and goals. For example, based on your current health status, he or she might be able to identify some specific decisions you might want to think about. In addition, your doctor can provide you with helpful information about medical conditions and treatments and their likely impact on your quality of life. Above all, your doctor can answer your questions.

Although some physicians may encourage advance planning and initiate discussions of your health care preferences and goals, others may wait for you to do so – either because of time constraints or because they think it's inappropriate to initiate the discussion themselves. Don't be shy. If you have questions that need to be answered before you can make informed decisions, don't hesitate to ask your physician. Your physician also may have brochures and pamphlets providing general information designed to help people think about their health care preferences and goals. The list of Internet resources at the end of this chapter includes websites with useful information about advance planning that you can read online or download. If your physician is unwilling to assist you with advance planning, you might consider finding another doctor who will be more helpful. In addition to clinical competence, a characteristic of a good physician is the willingness and ability to explain and discuss health-related issues with patients, and advance planning is clearly one of those issues.

Selecting Surrogate Decision Makers

If you decide to select a surrogate (someone to make decisions for you when you're no longer able), you should carefully consider who would best serve this function. To make this determination, you first have to determine your goal. Is your primary concern that your designated surrogate will carry out your specific wishes? If so, then you should choose the person who most likely will follow your wishes and put aside his or her wishes and interests, even if he or she isn't the person with whom you have the strongest relationship and emotional bonds. For example, suppose you feel strongly that you don't want to be kept alive by medically supplied nutrition and hydration if you become permanently unconscious. Further, suppose you have good reason to believe your spouse and adult children likely won't be able to carry out your wishes and "let you go," but your sister or cousin likely will insist your wishes are honored. If your primary concern is that your wishes be honored, then even if you're closer to your spouse and children, you should select your sister or cousin as your surrogate. When selecting a surrogate, discussing your wishes with potential candidates may help you identify those willing to carry out your wishes.

On the other hand, your primary concern may not be that the surrogate you select will carry out your specific wishes. You may not have specific wishes; even if you do, you may think that rather than strictly following your current wishes, it makes more sense for your surrogate to decide what's best for you at the time, based on his or her knowledge of you and the specific information about your condition, prognosis, and so forth that will be available when decisions must be made. In that case, you should select someone whom you trust and whose judgment you value. To some people, *who* decides for them is more important than *what* the surrogate decides. Some people's primary concern is that decisions about their health care will be made by a certain person (e.g., a spouse), and they're less concerned about what that person will decide. Your selection of a surrogate decision maker should be guided by what matters most to you.

When selecting a surrogate, you also may want to ask yourself whether the person you're considering has the ability to understand medical information and effectively advocate for you with physicians during the decision-making process. People who tend to be overcome by emotion, do not function well under stress, or are easily intimidated may not be suitable to serve as your surrogate, regardless of the strength and depth of your relationship. Finally, consider selecting at least one backup surrogate in case your first choice is unavailable when decisions must be made.

If you decide to select a surrogate decision maker, it's advisable to inform other loved ones that you've done so. Communicating and explaining your choice may prevent conflicts and hurt feelings if and when your preferred surrogate is called upon to make medical decisions on your behalf.

Advance Directives

Advance directives are instruments by which you can formally specify in writing your preferences regarding health care decision making if and when you lose your ability to decide for yourself. There are three types of advance directives: 1) instruction directives, or living wills; 2) proxy directives, or medical powers of attorney; and 3) combination directives (a combination instruction and proxy directive).

Instruction Directives

Instruction directives give general guidelines and/or specific instructions for decision making about your health care in the event you can't decide for yourself. The primary function of instruction directives is to enable future decision makers (e.g., your family and physicians) to make the decisions you would have made under the same circumstances. If you decide to execute an instruction directive, you must do so while you still have the capacity to make your own health care decisions, but the directive will take effect only if you lose that capacity. Thus, even if you execute a living will, you're still the primary decision maker as long as you have the ability to decide for yourself, and your actual decisions may differ from the instructions in your living will. An instruction directive does *not* authorize anyone to override your actual decisions.

In the United States, as of June 2008, all states (except three: Massachusetts, Michigan, and New York) and the District of Columbia have legislation authorizing individuals to execute living wills. Although New York doesn't have living will legislation, an appellate court decision (*In re Westchester County Medical Center*, 72 N.Y.2d 517 [1988]) provides legal authorization for instruction directives in that state. As will be explained later, even if your state doesn't provide explicit legal authorization for instruction directives, you can execute them with an expectation that they will guide decision making about your health care.

Some states with legislation authorizing living wills provide model forms for their residents. Although there are significant differences among these state model forms, in most states these are only *model* forms, and residents need not use them to execute an instruction directive. Nevertheless, your state's model instrument may suit your needs. A familiarity with a variety of alternatives may help you determine whether your state's model living will meets your needs and, if it doesn't, find or create one that does. The list of Internet resources at the end of this chapter includes websites with links to information about each state's living will as well as its model form. Most websites on this list also provide useful information about living wills and their preparation.

Typically, model living wills specify one or more conditions or scenarios (e.g., a terminal condition) and either order medical treatment to be withheld or withdrawn in that situation (refusal directives) or provide an option to indicate whether or not to withhold or withdraw medical treatment in that situation (option directives). About one third of the model state forms with one of these two formats are refusal directives. Some model living wills specify only one scenario (typically a terminal condition), others specify two scenarios (typically a terminal condition and permanent unconsciousness), and some specify three or more scenarios. These additional scenarios often include one or more of the following: an end-stage condition, advanced progressive illness, an incurable and irreversible condition with severe and worsening physical or mental deterioration, dependency in all activities of daily living, permanent confusion, permanent incompetence, irreversible substantial loss of cognitive ability, advanced Alzheimer's disease, extraordinary suffering, and the likelihood that the risks and burdens of treatment will outweigh the expected benefits.

Typically, "life-sustaining treatments" are the medical measures that are the subject of model instruction directives. Life-sustaining treatments include cardiopulmonary resuscitation (CPR), mechanical ventilation (machine-assisted breathing), dialysis, blood transfusions, antibiotics, and medically supplied nutrition and hydration. Whereas some forms give instructions that apply to life-sustaining treatment in general, others provide separate instructions for specific types of life-sustaining treatment. Many documents, including those that don't otherwise list specific treatments and even some refusal directives, ask people to indicate whether they do or do not want "artificial" (medically provided) nutrition and hydration.

A few states have model living wills with a completely different format. These documents do not feature scenarios and corresponding treatment instructions. Instead, they present several open-ended statements about goals, values, preferences, and so forth for individuals to complete. The following are from the Minnesota and North Dakota health care directives:

- My goals for my health care:
- My fears about my health care:
- My spiritual or religious beliefs and traditions:
- My beliefs about when life no longer would be worth living:
- My thoughts about how my medical condition might affect my family:
- If I had a reasonable chance of recovery and were temporarily unable to decide or speak for myself, I would want:
- If I were dying and unable to decide or speak for myself, I would want:
- If I were permanently unconscious and unable to decide or speak for myself, I would want:
- If I were completely dependent on others for my care and unable to decide or speak for myself, I would want:
- In all circumstances, my doctors will try to keep me comfortable and reduce my pain. This is how I feel about pain relief if it would affect my alertness or if it could shorten my life:

If you want to execute an instruction directive, before you use your state's model form, you should carefully examine it to determine whether it enables you to document *your* goals and preferences and effectively guide decision making about your health care. Obviously, if you think you would want life-sustaining treatment if you were terminally ill and your state's model living will is a refusal directive with instructions to withhold or withdraw treatment, that document is not for you. However, there are less obvious ways in which a model state living will might not be suitable for you. Does your state model instrument give instructions to guide decision making only if you are terminally ill or in a persistent vegetative state? If so, you need to understand its significant limitations. This type of living will does not enable you to provide decision making guidance for a wide variety of possible situations. Generally, a *terminal* condition or illness is understood to be one that is expected to result in death in a relatively short period of time. A typical definition of *terminal* is death expected within six months. This is the definition employed by Medicare to determine eligibility for hospice coverage, and some states have adopted it as well. In any event, whether or not a time frame is specified in your state, someone who has metastatic cancer, advanced Alzheimer's disease, amyotrophic lateral sclerosis (ALS, or Lou Gehrig's disease), multiple sclerosis, or chronic obstructive pulmonary disease (COPD) may not meet the requirements of a living will's terminal condition scenario. *Permanent unconsciousness* refers to the total and irreversible loss of consciousness and the capacity to interact with the environment. Accordingly, a person who is severely demented because of Alzheimer's disease or has suffered severe and irreversible cognitive impairment due to a stroke would not satisfy the requirements of a living will's permanent unconsciousness scenario.

Even if your state's model living will provides several scenarios and gives you the option of indicating whether or not you want various specified treatments, it may not provide you with suitable means to guide future decision making about your health care. For one thing, living wills can't include *all* possible situations. Hence, if you were to experience a condition not included in any of your living will's specified scenarios, the document would fail to provide clear and unambiguous decision-making guidance *in that situation*. You also may find it difficult to anticipate how you would feel if you developed a life-threatening acute illness or a progressive chronic disease. People adapt to a variety of situations, and a life that seems inconceivable to you today may be satisfying enough to you if and when you actually experience it. Moreover, unless you already have firsthand experience (e.g., you've received mechanical ventilation or dialysis), you may not be able to make informed decisions now about specific treatments.

The format of the Minnesota and North Dakota living wills avoids some of these problems by not presenting a list of possible scenarios and treatment options. However, it has another limitation. Your responses to the open-ended questions likely won't provide clear and unambiguous criteria for determining what you would have decided in many situations that might arise. Still, your responses may provide valuable guidance for your family and physicians as they attempt to decide as you would have.

Even if your state doesn't provide explicit legal authorization for instruction directives, or your state's model living will form doesn't meet your needs, you can use a model instrument from another state or one created by an organization. The list of Internet resources at the end of this chapter includes websites of organizations that provide living will forms online. Alternatively, you can write a personal living will, possibly combining features from a variety of model forms. If you decide to write a personal living will, avoid general statements that are vague and ambiguous. The following statement, which was in some earlier model living wills, illustrates this point: "If I am severely disabled mentally and physically and there is no reasonable hope of regaining significant mental functioning, I want no life-extending medical treatment." When is a disability severe? What counts as reasonable hope? How much mental functioning is significant? If you think it's unavoidable to use terms such as these, you should at least try to explain what *you* mean by them and provide concrete examples if possible. For example, what do you consider *reasonable* hope or *significant* mental functioning? If doctors say there is only a 5% chance something will happen, do you consider that grounds for reasonable hope? If not, where do you draw the line? If you can speak and respond to simple commands but can't read novels or recognize friends or family, is that significant mental functioning? If not, where do you draw the line? Although it's not legally required, if you decide to write a personal living will, you may want to seek the advice of a lawyer to make sure your language is unambiguous and effectively communicates your intent. There's no guarantee a living will you create or adapt from somewhere else will be honored, but there's no guarantee a living will written on a state-authorized form will be honored either.

As a general rule, you can execute a living will with the expectation that it will guide decision making about your health care, whether or not your state has authorizing legislation and whether or not you use your state's model living will, if it has one. In the United States, it's generally recognized that individuals have a common law right to accept or refuse medical treatment and can exercise this right by means of advance directives. However, from the perspective of your physician, especially if your living will calls for life-sustaining treatment to be withheld or withdrawn, it may matter whether or not your state has authorizing legislation or whether or not you used your state's model instrument. Living will legislation provides legal immunity to health care providers who withhold or withdraw life-sustaining medical treatment under the specific conditions identified in that legislation and the state's model instrument. Because death is the expected result, physicians rightly or wrongly may fear legal liability if they withhold or withdraw life-sustaining treatment. Accordingly, granting statutory

legal immunity may remove an obstacle to withholding or withdrawing treatment when patients have at least one of the conditions specified in the living will legislation and corresponding model document.
However, physicians who withhold or withdraw life-sustaining measures in conformity with the living will of patients who have other
conditions – or who rely on a living will that doesn't meet the requirements of their state's law – can't count on the immunity offered by
advance directive legislation. For example, suppose your state authorizes living wills that direct life-sustaining treatment to be withheld or
withdrawn if a patient is terminally ill or permanently unconscious,
but you add that you also want treatment withheld or withdrawn if
you can no longer recognize and communicate with your family. If
your physician were to withhold or withdraw life-sustaining treatment
in compliance with your added instructions, he or she couldn't count
on your state's living will legislation for legal immunity. However, even
if physicians can't count on statutory immunity, it's *not* illegal for them
to implement the instructions in a living will that differs significantly
from the state's model document, unless they request an illegal action,
such as active euthanasia (mercy killing).

Although many physicians recognize the moral authority of instruction directives whether or not they conform to the state's model
document, they won't carry out the instructions in a living will if,
in their judgment, doing so would require them to provide medically
inappropriate or ineffective treatment. In addition, some physicians
may have ethical and/or religious objections to carrying out certain
instructions. Thus, whether or not you use your state's model living
will, you should make certain your physician has no objection to carrying out your instructions. If your physician's personal ethical and/or
religious beliefs prevent him or her from respecting your wishes, you
might consider finding one who will.

Proxy and Combination Directives

Whereas an instruction directive provides general guidelines and/or
specific instructions for decision making about your health care, a
proxy directive designates a surrogate to make decisions for you if you
no longer can do so. In the United States, as of June 2008, all states
and the District of Columbia have legislation authorizing individuals
to execute a proxy directive. Proxy directives have various names,
depending on the state. The most common names are *medical power
of attorney*, *health care power of attorney*, *power of attorney for health care*,
and *durable power of attorney for health care*. To avoid confusion, a legally

authorized proxy directive is referred to in this chapter as a medical power of attorney. There also are variations from state to state in what a proxy is called. Common names are *agent, representative, attorney-in-fact,* and *proxy.*

Every state has a model medical power of attorney. Some are independent forms, and others are included in a section of a combination directive; some states provide both options. Significant differences exist among state model medical powers of attorney. However, as in the case of model living wills, these are only *model* forms, and state residents need not use their state's model document to execute a medical power of attorney. Nevertheless, your state's model instrument may suit your needs. A familiarity with a variety of alternatives may help you determine whether your state's model medical power of attorney meets your needs and, if it doesn't, find or create one that does. The list of Internet resources at the end of this chapter includes websites with links to information about each state's medical power of attorney as well as its model form. Most websites on the list also provide useful information about medical powers of attorney and their preparation. Although it isn't necessary, if you decide not to use your state's model medical power of attorney, you may wish to consult an attorney to make sure your document satisfies your state's legal requirements. If conflicts arise, it may be crucial to establish that the person you designated has a legal right to serve as your proxy.

All model medical powers of attorney provide an opportunity to designate one or more alternate proxies in case the primary designee is unable or unwilling to serve. The model medical power of attorney of at least one state (Vermont) provides an opportunity to appoint "co-agents" – two or more people to engage in collaborative decision making. It also provides three options for such collaborative decision making: by agreement of all co-agents; by a majority of those present; or, in an emergency, by the first person available. Even if your state's model form doesn't provide a co-agent option, you might consider whether you want to designate co-agents if you decide to execute a medical power of attorney. An alternative to appointing co-agents is to appoint a single agent and to require that that person consult with other people whom you name. This will assure that your agent takes into account others' views that you wish to be considered, but it avoids the problem of two people who cannot agree.

Model medical powers of attorney in all states provide an opportunity to give guidance (goals and/or specific instructions) to proxies. Model combination forms sometimes provide an opportunity to give instructions to proxies in the living will section as well as the medical power of attorney section. If you execute one of these advance directives, either give instructions to your proxy in only one section or make sure your instructions in both sections are the same, or at least consistent.

If you're uncertain about your health care goals and preferences or you believe you can't communicate them effectively in either a model or personal living will, and you decide not to execute one, you still may want to execute a medical power of attorney. However, keep in mind that your physicians likely will ask your designated proxy to tell them how you would have decided under the circumstances. Accordingly, even if you don't execute an instruction directive, you may want to provide some guidance to your designated proxy. You can provide this guidance in writing in your medical power of attorney or verbally. Discuss your preferences with your designated proxy even if you provide written instructions in your medical power of attorney.

Don't think executing a living will eliminates the need to execute a medical power of attorney. Even the most specific instructions may need to be interpreted to provide a decision in a particular situation. In addition, you might not have anticipated a particular situation, and following your instructions in that situation would harm you. To address such problems, some model living wills provide the option of giving discretion to proxies; some even offer the option of permitting proxies to override instructions in living wills. Some model living wills provide the option of instructing proxies to weigh the expected benefits and burdens of treatment and decide on that basis.

Typically, although model medical powers of attorney authorize proxies to make any decision about health care you can make for yourself, they also provide you with the option of limiting the authority of your proxy. However, some states, such as Louisiana and Montana, authorize the proxy to decide to withhold or withdraw life-sustaining treatments only if the patient is terminally ill. If you live in a state with such a restriction and you want your proxy to be authorized to withhold or withdraw life-sustaining treatments even if you're not terminally ill, you should add a statement to this effect in your medical power of attorney. However, the legal status of such an added statement is unclear, so you may want to consult an attorney. Legal status aside, physicians may recognize the statement's *moral authority*. Nevertheless, if you add statements to your state's model medical power of attorney giving your proxy additional powers, you may want to ask your physician whether he or she is willing to carry out your instructions.

Some model medical powers of attorney enable people to give designated proxies *immediate* authorization to make decisions for them. You may not want anyone to make decisions for you while you still have the capacity to decide for yourself; however, if this option appeals to you and your state's model form doesn't include it, you could add it. Many model forms provide the option of putting a time limit on the proxy's authority. Typically, all types of model advance directives (living wills, medical powers of attorney, and combination directives) require the signature of two witnesses or a notary.

You Executed an Advance Directive; Now What?

If you executed an advance directive, certain steps must be taken to ensure it will effectively guide decision making if you lose your ability to make medical decisions for yourself. If you put the only copy in your safe deposit box, it likely won't be available to guide medical decision making. If you have a medical power of attorney, give copies to your primary and, if you designated one, secondary proxy as well as your primary care physician. If you also have a separate living will, give copies to your proxy or proxies and your primary care physician. However, it's not enough to give them copies of your advance directive; you also should discuss your goals and preferences with them. As helpful as written statements may be, face-to-face discussion and an opportunity to ask questions and hear your answers can facilitate a better understanding of your wishes. Although some physicians and designated proxies may initiate a discussion when you give them a copy of your advance directive, you should take the initiative if they don't. In the absence of such a discussion, your proxy may experience needless stress, discomfort, and misgivings when he or she is called upon to make medical decisions for you. Additionally, those decisions may not reflect your goals and preferences.

If you have a living will but not a medical power of attorney, you should give a copy to your primary care physician and make sure at least one person whom you trust has a copy of or easy access to it. Keep in mind that even if you have a living will, someone who knows and cares for you may be asked to help interpret it and provide guidance to physicians. Accordingly, even if you decide not to execute a medical power of attorney, you may want to think about whom you would want to perform this role. Informing the person or persons you favor gives them an opportunity to accept or decline. It also provides an occasion for a discussion of your goals and wishes that will help prepare them to interpret your living will if the need arises.

If you have only a medical power of attorney, whether or not you included a statement of your goals and preferences, you should discuss your wishes when you give copies to your proxy or proxies and primary care physician. If you are unable or reluctant to identify specific treatment goals and preferences, you should at least explain why you're not disclosing them. You might at least consider providing some general guidance to your proxy or proxies, such as, "I want you to use your judgment and, based on what the doctors tell you about my medical condition and prognosis, make the best decision for me." Keep in mind, however, that to make the best decision *for you*, your proxy has to be familiar with *your* distinctive values and preferences. So even if you don't provide specific health care goals and preferences, you might consider giving some indication of where, if at all, you draw the line between meaningful and unsatisfactory quality of life. In addition, you might want to provide some indication of the kinds of outcomes you would count as *benefits* as well as those you would count as *burdens* or *harms*.

To promote more effective implementation of advance directives in the United States, the Patient Self Determination Act, enacted in 1990, requires hospitals and other health care organizations, such as nursing homes, hospices, and home health agencies, to document in patients' medical records whether or not they have executed an advance directive. In practice, this means you'll be asked whether or not you have an advance directive at admission. In addition, the Joint Commission on Accreditation of Healthcare Organizations (JCAHO) requires health care organizations, as a condition of accreditation, to provide assistance to patients who don't have an advance directive but want to execute one. However, health care organizations are prohibited by law from requiring you to execute an advance directive as a condition of admission or provision of services. Requiring a hospital to ask you or your representative at admission whether you have an advance directive helps ensure that if you have one, it will be included in your medical record. If you have a living will and it's not placed in your medical record, it can't guide physicians when they write medical orders. Also, if no medical order is written to implement your living will, it can't have an effect on the treatment you will and will not receive. Accordingly, if you have an advance directive, it's a good idea to bring a copy with you if you go to a hospital, even if you don't expect to be admitted.

Many states authorize a document called a POLST (physician orders for life-sustaining treatment), which was introduced because of a concern that instructions in living wills sometimes fail to influence actual medical orders. The POLST is a portable physician order, that is, one that follows the patient and is not valid only within a particular institutional setting, such as a specific hospital or nursing home. It indicates whether or not the patient is to receive specified medical interventions, such as CPR, mechanical ventilation, anti-biotics, and medically supplied nutrition and hydration. Instructions in a POLST apply to emergency medical service workers as well as emergency department staff. Unlike a living will, a POLST generally is suitable only if you know you have a serious life-threatening or chronic illness and you want your physician to translate your end-of-life goals and preferences into a portable medical order. Because the POLST must be filled out and signed by a physician, if you want information about this document, you should contact your primary care physician.

It's not uncommon for people's lives to change over time. We may develop new interests, embrace different values, become more or less religious, start new relationships and end old ones, and so forth. Together with either diminished or improved health, such changes in our lives may prompt a reconsideration of what we have written in our advance directive. For example, if you divorce and remarry and your former spouse is your medical power of attorney proxy, you undoubtedly won't want him or her to continue to serve in that role. Similarly, changes in your health or beliefs and attitudes may provide you with concrete information enabling you to think of more specific instructions to add to your living will. Alternately, such changes may lead you to modify or remove instructions in your living will. Even if there are no dramatic changes in your life, if you have an advance directive, especially a living will, you may want to revisit it periodically to make sure it corresponds to your current thinking.

No matter what state you live in, you have the legal right to change or revoke your advance directive at any time while you still have the capacity to make decisions. You can change whom you designate as your medical power of attorney proxy, and you can change the instructions in your living will. You only have to execute a new advance directive and make sure all copies of the previous directive are either destroyed or invalidated. Changing or revoking advance directives of individuals who have lost the capacity to make decisions is more complicated and depends on the state in which that person lives. Some states authorize individuals who have lost decision-making capacity to change or revoke advance directives, others are silent on the issue, and still others authorize only individuals with decision-making capacity to change or revoke advance directives.

Conclusion: Discuss, Discuss, Discuss...

Whether or not you decide to execute an advance directive, it's essential to discuss your general attitudes toward health care and your general goals and preferences with your loved ones and your physicians. Doing so may save them considerable stress, anxiety, and aggravation. It also will make it more likely that, if you lose the ability to decide for yourself, the people you want to make decisions for you will be the ones to do so, and you'll receive the kind of medical treatment you want and won't be subject to medical interventions you don't want.

Internet Resources

California Coalition for Compassionate Care: An organization "dedicated to the advancement of palliative medicine and end of life care." Although it's a California organization, its website provides useful general information about advance directives: http://www.finalchoices.calhealth.org.

Caring Connections: A program of the National Hospice and Palliative Care Organization (NHPCO) whose goal is "to improve care at the end of life." Its website provides useful information about advance directives and links to each state's model advance directive(s): http://www.caringinfo.org.

Health Care Decisions: A program "devoted to educating the community about advance directives." Its website provides useful information about advance directives as well as a model living will and model medical power of attorney: http://www.hcdecisions.org.

NOAH (New York Online Access to Health): A New York–based organization that "provides access to high quality full-text consumer health information." Its website provides links to information and articles about advance directives and to state and other model forms: http://www.noah-health.org/en/rights/endoflife/adforms.html.

University of New Mexico Institute for Ethics: The institute's website has a link to a "values history form" that may be useful if you're considering executing an advance directive: http://hsc.unm.edu/ethics/advdir/vhform_eng.shtml.

U.S. Living Will Registry: Its stated mission is "to promote the use of advance directives through educational programs, and to make people's health care choices available to their caregivers and families whenever and wherever they are needed, while maintaining the confidentiality of their information and documents." Its website includes information about advance directives, links to model state forms, and a service that enables individuals to register – *for a fee* – their advance directives: http://www.uslivingwillregistry.com.

FOUR

Responding to Medical Emergencies

– Kenneth V. Iserson

You're suddenly faced with a medical emergency for yourself or a loved one. What do you do? The real key is to be prepared. Knowing when to "push the alarm button," what to expect, and then how to get the best possible treatment may be the most important elements of your response to an emergency – and preparation is something you can do now.

Preparing for an Emergency

Health care workers are not omniscient. They need accurate information about your medical conditions to give you the best (and fastest) possible treatment. In an emergency, however, you may not recall all the information they need to make good decisions.

Wallet card. Always carry a card in your wallet or purse with the basic information that ambulance and hospital caregivers will need, including:

1. Your name and birth date, for identification purposes
2. The name(s) and contact information of your family (surrogate decision makers) and doctors (include their specialty)
3. List of any allergies to medication and to anything else

46

4. A brief medical history, including the dates, places (hospitals), and types of any operations; the dates and types of any serious medical illnesses; and the dates and reasons for any other hospitalizations. If you don't know the specific diagnosis, contact your doctor for the information.

5. A list of any significant laboratory or x-ray findings. List the values for the tests (e.g., hemoglobin: 18 gm/dL; creatinine: 1.1 mg/dL). One small problem is that the United States, Canada, and some other countries use a gram/deciliter (gm/dL) system, whereas Europe and other countries report values as mole/liter (mol/L). Nevertheless, if you have your current laboratory values in either system, physicians will find this information useful. Copy this information directly from the laboratory results form you receive or get it from your doctor's office.

6. The names of your current medications, as well as their dosages and how often you take them. Include not only prescription medications, but also over-the-counter ones (e.g., aspirin, vitamins, allergy pills) and any herbal supplements.

7. Your medical and dental insurance numbers, and how to contact the insurance companies for authorization. Even better is to carry those companies' cards with you.

A sample wallet card is shown in Figure 4.1. Be sure to update your card when anything changes, including laboratory test results, other medical tests, medications, medical conditions, physicians, contacts, or insurance numbers. The easiest way to make these changes is to create a file with the information on your computer; then you can simply change the card and print out a new version with the updated information.

Note: On the sample card in Figure 4.1, the birth date is needed to make a positive identification and, often, to correctly access medical records. This example uses several common medical abbreviations, however, check with your doctor or his or her nurse to be sure you're providing accurate information on this potentially lifesaving card.

TAH-BSO means total abdominal hysterectomy and bilateral salpingo-oophorectomy (uterus and ovaries removed). Dates next to the medical studies indicate 1) how recent they were and 2) which ones the health care practitioner should be asking for. *H/H* represents the blood counts (hemoglobin/hematocrit); *Creat* means creatinine, frequently needed to determine kidney function. *QD* means once a day, *BID* twice a day, *TID* three times a day, and *QID* four times a day. All physicians and nurses know these abbreviations, and the abbreviations save space. Using a computer, you can easily put this amount of information on a wallet-size card. Smaller type allows for additional information. (Don't worry; emergency personnel can read it.)

Complete medical records. A more extensive medical record including copies of your recent ECGs (electrocardiograms/heart

(Side 1)

Name: **Mary Lou Victoriana, PhD;** Birth date: 5-26-49

Contacts: Spouse: Thomas Victoriana, MD; 415-222-1411

Physician: Kathleen Strong, MD (Cardiologist); San Francisco: 415-855-5111

Daughter: Barbara Stanley; Tucson: 520-987-3555

Medication Allergies: None; **Medical Conditions**: CAD/migraines/
DVT (3/04)/hyperuricemia; TAH-BSO (6/97), appendectomy (8/62)

ECG (1/5/09): 1° A-V block

(Side 2)

Chest x-ray (1/5/09): Perihilar and splenic calcifications

CT scan head (1/5/09): Normal; **H/H:** 13°/37 gm/dL; **BP:** 140/85;

Creat: 1.3 mg/dL. **Medications:** Metoprolol 50 mg BID;

allopurinol 100 mg BID; Plavix 75 mg BID;

Lipitor 80 mg QD; aspirin 81 mg; estradiol 1 mg QD

ODLD Med Insurance: #09-6947-43835AC. Auth: 888-545-5555

DIMD Dental Insurance: #JA83747XXZ. Auth: 800-555-5345

Figure 4.1. Always carry a card in your wallet or purse with the basic information that ambulance and hospital caregivers will need. Be sure to update your card when anything changes, including laboratory test results, other medical tests, medications, medical conditions, physicians, contacts, or insurance numbers.

tracings); x-rays or CT, MRI, or nuclear scans; or recent hospital or clinic records can be kept in a file you've reduced in size using a copier, on microfiche (although some hospitals may have difficulty reading it), or with a readily accessible 24-hour medical information service. These services, the best known of which is MedicAlert® (www.medicalert.org), can keep your information and send it to your health care provider when you give them authorization to do so. They also can copy your records onto a flash drive that can be read on a computer.

You can also copy many of your records into one of several commercially available medical record notebooks. Although these records won't include images from radiographic studies, they can include everything else, such as radiologists' reports describing those images, surgical and pathology reports, and copies of the original ECGs and laboratory reports.

First aid/CPR course. Take a first aid and cardiopulmonary resuscitation (CPR) course. It doesn't take much time. Your loved ones will appreciate your knowing the most basic ways to save a life: how to stop bleeding, open an airway, and do CPR. Maybe the biggest benefit is that you'll be less likely to panic in medical situations when you need to act.

Physician's contact information. Put your doctor's regular and after-hours contact information on bright-colored paper in a prominent place in your home, such as on the refrigerator. That way, you, your relatives, or the ambulance personnel can find it immediately, assuming your refrigerator door isn't too cluttered. If someone in the home has a prehospital advance directive (do-not-resuscitate form) for ambulance personnel to use, the refrigerator door is often where they look.

Where is the emergency department? Know where hospital emergency departments (EDs) are in your city. Which one is the closest? Which one provides specialized (e.g., immediate cardiac or trauma) treatment? Which has the best reputation? If you're visiting another city, it's a good idea to obtain this information in advance. How close are those facilities to where you'll be staying? All this information is available on the Internet. If you don't have a clue, a hospital associated with a medical school generally is your best bet.

Finally, know how to phone for an ambulance in your area. Although most of the United States and Canada uses 911 to call for an ambulance, a few areas still don't use that system.

International travel: special information. If you're traveling internationally, be certain you:

1. Know how to call for an ambulance; this procedure varies among countries. Most *do not* use 911, which generally is used throughout the United States and Canada. Most, but not all, European countries use 112.
2. Have a source for medical assistance and evacuation insurance. One source of assistance is IMAT (International Association for Medical Assistance to Travellers; www.iamat.org; info@imat.org), which makes competent medical care available to travelers by Western-trained doctors who speak English besides their mother tongue. One source for medical evacuation that many frequent international travelers use is the Divers' Alert Network (DAN; www.diversalertnetwork.org).

When Should I Worry about Symptoms?
Is This an Emergency?

How Worried Are You?

For symptoms that have lasted a long time (weeks, months):

1. **Ask a friend, your mother, or your spouse.** They often will have both experience and perspective. If they think it's urgent that you see a

physician, do so. It's been shown that married men live longer than single men. Why? Probably because their wives told them they had to see a physician for something they would otherwise have ignored.

2. **Go online** and read about it – but, be careful! There's good information as well as balderdash on the Web. Go to trusted medical sites such as those of the American Academy of Family Physicians (http://family doctor.org/online/famdocen/home.html), which has symptom-related algorithm pages; the *Merck Manual* (www.merck.com/mmpe/index .html), if you can understand the terminology; and *Up-to-Date Patient Information* (http://patients.uptodate.com), a patient section of a popular physician resource. When you find your symptoms, take in the information with a measure of caution. These websites may list a lot of diseases, but common things occur commonly. Your abdominal pain is much more likely to be a kidney stone (benign and common) than an adrenal hemorrhage (more serious, but rare).

3. **Call a nurse referral line.** As with any health care provider, the advice you get depends on the quality of the person on the other end of the line. If he or she tells you to go to an ED or urgent care center, you probably should do it. If he or she tells you it's okay if you stay home, ask why he or she is saying that.

4. **Contact your physician.** If you think you'll get an answer, call your physician's office and leave your question for the doctor. Increasingly, patients can send their physician an e-mail with questions. If not abused, this method often is an excellent way to get direction about ongoing medical issues. You also may call your physician's office for an appointment if there's hope you'll get one relatively soon.

5. **Call a physician friend/relative.** Okay, so my colleagues won't be thrilled, but many people have friends or relatives who are physicians. I know I get contacted frequently by relatives and friends with various medical questions. If you have that kind of relationship with a physician – and you trust him or her to give you a valid answer – make the call.

6. For a **dental emergency, contact a dentist.** Often there's someone on call who can see you relatively soon, especially if you have an ongoing relationship with that dental practice. Increasingly, patients paying out of pocket have access to emergency dental services that are advertised in the phone book.

If the symptoms are more worrisome or appeared suddenly, but you really think they aren't serious (and your spouse/significant other agrees) and you're pretty certain you're not *underreacting* to the situation:

7. **Call your physician.** This works only if you have a relationship with a physician; calling one "blind" from the yellow pages won't work. If you call and get a nurse, partner, other covering physician, or only the answering machine – okay, you tried. If you do get a physician or nurse on the phone and he or she recommends that you call an ambulance or

go to an ED, ask that person to call ahead and give him or her whatever information you know. This may greatly speed your entry into a crowded ED and accelerate treatment.

8. **Go to an urgent care center.** If the problem is not life threatening, you can go to an urgent care center. These centers are springing up virtually everywhere, even in shopping malls and drugstores, so there's likely one near you. They're usually staffed by a physician, nurse practitioner, or physician assistant who can probably do the initial evaluation. If the urgent care staff thinks it's something more serious, they'll send you to an ED, sometimes by ambulance.

If you think it might be a real emergency:

9. **Go to an ED.** In some instances, driving or taking a taxi to an ED may be better than calling an ambulance. However, if you have chest pain, stroke symptoms, or difficulty breathing, it's probably better to wait for an ambulance. If your symptoms worsen, an ambulance crew will do a better job of helping you en route to the ED than will your friends or relatives accompanying you in an automobile. Depending on the problem and their level of training, the crew also may be able to start evaluation and treatment of your condition before you arrive at the hospital.

10. **Call 911** or the local equivalent.
    a. Tell the ambulance dispatcher that 1) you need an ambulance, and 2) why you need it. **Briefly** tell the dispatcher the **worst** symptoms, such as severe chest pain, shortness of breath, symptoms of a stroke (difficulty moving arms or legs, problems with speech, or decreased consciousness), an accident in which you may have broken your _____, severe pain in your _____, or an accidental overdose.
    b. The ambulance (or non-ambulance) and emergency crew sent to you will depend on how serious the dispatcher thinks the problem is and on what type of units are available. Emergency medical technicians (EMTs) can perform basic first aid and CPR and, of course, take you to the hospital. In some regions, they also have automatic defibrillators.
    c. Paramedics, on the other hand, can start intravenous lines (IVs), check your heart rhythm, give many medications, and, when necessary, insert sophisticated airways. In some regions, they can send ECGs to the hospital and perform surgical airways. In some countries, ambulances are staffed by physicians, although they may have less practical training than many paramedics.
    d. If you're in a rural area, you may be treated by a flight (helicopter or fixed-wing aircraft) team. This often includes a very experienced nurse and a paramedic. They often can do many procedures normally done in an ED, such as put tubes in your chest or do a cricothyrotomy (a surgical hole in the neck through which a breathing tube is placed).
    e. You or your companion should tell the ambulance personnel to which hospital you want to be taken. They generally will honor your request

unless the ED is "on divert," meaning it won't take new ambulance patients (most commonly because of hospital overcrowding), or the ambulance crew believes your condition requires that you go to either the nearest hospital or a specialized center (e.g., the region's trauma or pediatric specialty center).

f. If your companion has no other means of transportation, or if you are with a child, the ambulance can take him or her also. Although your loved one may not want to ride in the ambulance, you should insist. Leaving him or her stranded or being alone in the ED is inappropriate.

Going to the Emergency Department

1. You've arrived.
   - You'll see the "triage" nurse first. Don't play down your symptoms. Tell him or her your worst fears about what's happening. If you or your loved one is in severe pain, say so.
   - If your symptoms change while you're there, tell someone immediately.
   - The waiting time may be very long. People with severe breathing problems, stroke symptoms, chest pain, extreme agitation, severe bleeding, or very abnormal vital signs (pulse, blood pressure, oxygenation); those who are immunocompromised (e.g., cancer and HIV patients); and trauma patients who have – or because of how they were hurt, may have – a serious injury will get priority. You may not see the stream of critical ambulance patients arriving through another entrance, further prolonging your waiting time. Sometimes, however, even some of these patients have to wait to be seen.

2. You're in the patient care area.
   - If you're taken into the ED but you're put in a chair or stretcher in the hallway, understand that this is to get you seen faster. Although it may not be elegant, ED personnel will still place you on a monitor if necessary and will find you a room for any sensitive tests (e.g., pelvic or rectal exam).
   - If you're in the hall, it will be relatively easy to get a staff member's attention if you need something. If you're in a room, ask for a call button.
   - Once in the ED, ask the people who come into the room who they are. A wide variety of personnel work in the ED; you can't tell them apart either by the clothes they wear or by the equipment they use. From time to time, any of these staff members, including orderlies, housekeepers, transporters, laboratory and x-ray technicians, patient care technicians, Licensed Practical Nurses (LPNs), Registered Nurses (RNs), paramedics, nurse practitioners, physician assistants, and physicians (both MD and Doctor of Osteopathy [DO]), may enter your room and interact with you. Identify and be able to recognize – and, if necessary, ask for – your primary clinician (physician, nurse practitioner, physician assistant) and your primary caregiver in the ED, who may be a nurse or paramedic.

- You'll probably have some laboratory tests done. Ask what these tests are, or at least why they've been ordered, when they'll be done, and when the results will be available. Unless you're pretty sophisticated about laboratory tests, be satisfied with a general answer, such as, "We're testing for any heart (or lung/kidney/abdominal) problem." You probably don't want to know what the clinician is considering, that is, the "differential diagnosis." You want to know only what he or she finds. Worrying about what the clinician considered but didn't find isn't beneficial to you.
- Be very nice to your nurse or paramedic. He or she is the one who actually provides most of the care and hands-on treatment in the ED. This person may be your strongest advocate and can make your stay much less onerous.
- If possible, have someone with you in the ED. Especially if you're very ill, that person can be your advocate, contact other people, and generally see that things are done, and done right.
- If you may have trouble communicating with the ED staff – for example, if you speak a different language or have hearing or speech difficulties – try to have someone accompany you who can help with communication.

3. Your medical records:
   - Hospital personnel have legal and administrative barriers to obtaining records from other hospitals or clinics. That's why you're often better off going back to the same hospital where you've had previous care, studies, and hospitalizations. If possible, don't "doctor shop." It will only cost you time, money, and aggravation.
   - Even if you've visited the same hospital repeatedly, bring all your medical records, including a list of your current or recent medications (or the medication bottles), the results of laboratory tests, any x-ray films (or, as is more common now, a disc with the x-rays), the names and phone numbers of your treating physicians, and any written summaries of your prior treatments. Having these records can save you a lot of time and money. It can often shorten the time it takes to determine what will improve your condition, what additional tests you may (or may not) need, what specialists you may need to see, what medications to administer (or not), and whether you need hospitalization.

4. The "nuts and bolts," or needles and machines:
   - If you need special equipment or medication that may not be readily available at the hospital – such as a special adaptor for an airway device, mechanical equipment that goes with a surgically implanted pump or pacer, or a rarely used or investigational medication – bring it with you.
   - If a procedure must be done, ask how much experience the person doing it has. If the procedure is not going well (e.g., two attempts at inserting an IV fail), ask if someone else can do it.

- If you're being given a medication, ask what it is and what it's for. That makes the nurse rethink what he or she is giving you.
- If your IV fluid bag/bottle is about to run dry, tell someone.
- If your pain worsens, tell someone immediately.
- In general, don't be a quiet mouse. Rather, nicely tell people what you need and ask lots of questions about what's happening. Unfortunately, mistakes are made and people are ignored. Try to prevent that.
- Know that if you demand to see a specialist (e.g., a plastic surgeon), you may wait many more hours for something that doesn't need a specialist's involvement. Rather, ask the physician if he or she has experience with and feels comfortable doing that type of procedure.
- If the physician says he or she wants to do a specific procedure, ask if there are alternatives. To give informed consent, you need to know the options – some may be more tolerable or less expensive.

5. You're going to be admitted.
   - If the physician wants to admit you to the hospital, ask the following questions: 1) Why? 2) Specifically, what will that accomplish? 3) If tests will be done, when? (If you're admitted on Friday, tests may not be performed until Monday.)
   - Ask how long you might be in the hospital. Although many diagnoses depend on what's found over the next several hours, the admitting physician often can give you a ballpark idea – assuming nothing unexpected occurs. Knowing this can allow you and your family to plan for your absence from home and work.
   - Once you're admitted to the hospital, you may remain in the ED for many hours – or, in some cases, days – so make yourself as comfortable as possible. Ask for 1) a real hospital bed – ED stretchers are made for resuscitations and are pretty uncomfortable, 2) food and drink if you're not being kept without oral intake (NPO) for a procedure or surgery, 3) the name of the attending admitting physician and to which service (internal medicine, surgery, orthopedics, trauma) you're being admitted.

6. You're being discharged.
   - If the physician wants to discharge you from the ED, make certain you feel safe going home. Speak with the physician before you're discharged to find out about follow-up. The physician should provide you with specific names and telephone numbers to contact, unless you're following up with your own physician or an urgent care center.
   - Be sure to get legible written (preferably typed/printed) instructions before you're discharged. Read them and ask about anything you don't understand. If you don't understand something, this is the time to ask! The purpose of these instructions is to help you and other practitioners you may see later understand what happened to you in the ED. If you really understand the instructions, you'll be better able to explain what was done and what the clinicians found. Make sure you get all the

prescriptions you were told you'd receive. To save (lots of) money, ask for generic medications.

- If you need to obtain medications or other supplies, such as bandages or crutches, at a pharmacy, ask how soon you'll need to have them and which pharmacies are open at that time of day/night. (You may not need some medications immediately, because they may have administered sufficient amounts while you were in the ED.)

- If you're going to follow up with another physician, get copies of all your records, including diagnoses, any x-rays (even if they're only printed copies of a digital image), and laboratory results.

- If you'll need assistance getting home or back to your place of residence (e.g., hotel), ask the hospital staff to help you.

- If you live alone, be sure to let the hospital staff know. It may be unsafe for you to be alone, at least for a day or two.

The Big Picture

In sum, you should be prepared for a medical emergency; eventually, one will happen to you or someone you love. The basic elements of this preparation are carrying a wallet card with basic information and having access to your complete medical records. Know how to access medical information and get answers to your questions about worrisome signs and symptoms. Know the method for accessing the emergency medical system (ambulances) wherever you are in the world. If you're in the ED, know how to optimize your treatment and understand what's going on, any follow-up instructions, and what the physicians think is wrong with you. The key is to, as the Scouts say, "be prepared."

FIVE

What You Need to Know about Medical Errors

– Erica S. Friedman and Rosamond Rhodes

Recent studies have found that errors occur commonly in medical practice. Errors in medical care can be dangerous and may result in permanent damage or death. One study reported that the number of patients who die daily in the United States as a result of medical errors is equivalent to the number who would die if a jumbo jet crashed every day. We are all aware of every crash of a jumbo jet, but few people are aware of the incidence of medical errors. That is because, unlike plane crash deaths, which occur all at once in a horrific drama, bad outcomes from medical errors happen one at a time, often days or weeks after the error occurs, and in the relative privacy of homes and hospitals across the country. This chapter explains how and why errors happen and offers practical advice to help protect you from becoming the victim of a medical error.

The Nature of Medicine

The Uncertainty of Medicine

Humans are biologically complex, and each of us is unique. Although high school biology classes and even medical textbooks present human anatomy and physiology as identical, in fact, no two humans are exactly alike, not even identical twins. We vary in our susceptibility and reactions to disease, as well as in our responses to the environment and to treatment. To the extent that human distinctiveness may have been overlooked in the past, modern genetics has shown in great detail that although we have mapped the human genome, on the genetic level, there is no "normal." Each of us is unique.

Also adding to the uncertainty of medicine is the fact that medical knowledge is limited. Medical science does not completely understand the causes of all disease states or why our physiologic responses to drugs vary. Medicine has limited tools for imaging and identifying the onset of disease conditions, which often are identified only when symptoms occur. Most significantly, medicine has limited resources for responding to illness and very few options for actually curing diseases. Therefore, although doctors know a great deal more than they did in the past, and can now do much more than they used to, there still is a tremendous amount of uncertainty. Their ability to intervene in healing is restricted to a very small domain of treatments that often have only a marginal effect. Although most treatments will not eradicate the disease, it is hoped they will halt or slow its progress. Diseases still have inevitable outcomes that even the most appropriate treatment will not prevent. These are not errors, but consequences of the limitations of medical knowledge and available treatment.

These factors mean that doctors have to make diagnoses with incomplete knowledge, and they have to make treatment decisions based on probabilities. A competent doctor keeps up to date on what is known about the human body; however, even the most informed, carefully thought-out medical decisions reflect only a chance that the specific problem has been correctly identified and that the available treatment will be effective without causing significant unwanted side effects. The best medical practice is based on doctors using their judgment to decipher what is going on and following the odds in their recommendations for diagnostic tests and treatments while being aware they may be mistaken. Whenever anyone follows the odds, there is a chance he or she may be wrong. Medical teaching involves instilling the models of evidence-based practice that apply the best available scientific methods to avoid the worst outcome. This means doctors accept that sometimes their decisions may have unavoidable and unwanted results because of incomplete knowledge.

Medical Complexity

Virtually every medical action, every diagnostic test, and every treatment is associated with some adverse risk to the patient. Unavoidable poor outcomes occur because no result is guaranteed or foolproof. The treatment that works well in most people with a particular condition may not work well in you. A medication well tolerated by most people may have nasty side effects in others. As long as no doctor can predict the outcome for an individual patient, the best guess for most patients with a similar condition may turn out to be the worst choice for that patient.

A patient's condition may deteriorate and result in death because treatments fail, known side effects occur and are unavoidable, or complications occur that cannot be predicted or corrected. People with a single medical problem may be difficult to diagnose or treat, but those with multiple medical problems may be even more difficult to diagnose and treat and more vulnerable to complications. Also, a treatment chosen to help the heart may harm the kidneys, or one that helps the kidneys may cause diabetes. With these interrelated issues in mind, it is important to realize that the best choice for treating an immediate life-threatening problem may involve accepting the risks of causing or exacerbating another problem.

Medical Errors

Understanding the difference between an error and a poor outcome or adverse consequence is important. An *error* indicates that a mistake was made that may have resulted in an undesired consequence. It means that, in those specific circumstances, a different decision or course of action was appropriate and should have been taken. An *adverse event* is defined as an unintended injury caused by faulty medical management rather than the underlying disease or condition. In medical parlance, such an undesired consequence of a medical intervention is called *iatrogenic*. An adverse event might be as simple as delaying or inadequately treating a patient's problem or causing the patient an additional complaint or medical problem. Depending on the error's severity, the resulting additional problem may require more tests, treatments, or hospitalization, or, rarely, may lead to long-term damage or death.

Fortunately, not all errors result in bad outcomes. For instance, a doctor may overlook a lab test showing abnormal liver function requiring a follow-up visit and assessment, but the abnormality spontaneously improves, with no untoward consequence. Another doctor may fail to order an important preventive measure, such as a flu shot or mammogram, but the patient does not get the flu or have a breast mass. Errors that do not result in adverse outcomes are called *near-misses*.

Causes of Errors

Errors may have numerous causes. Some errors result from a failure of equipment or an institutional system; others are consequences of some human deficiency, such as a lack of knowledge, a breakdown in communication, or a failure of professional responsibility. Human error is a consequence of the same mental processes used every day for successful normal daily functioning. Our daily performance requires us to recognize and identify external situations, process information, apply rules, and come up with plans and solutions. These mental processes employ automatic, familiar mental operations and physical response mechanisms and habits, which may be compromised by fatigue, distractions, or physical problems (e.g., illness).

Failures in Knowledge and Professionalism

To be trustworthy, doctors must be knowledgeable and skilled, fully informed of the most recent clinical studies, and able to assess their strengths, weaknesses, and capabilities as to whether they have some required special knowledge or skill. Without professional competence, the physician is not deserving of trust. Competence, therefore, is more than a matter of competitive pride, personal curiosity, ambition, or prudence. Being knowledgeable and skilled is essential to being a trustworthy doctor and, hence, a moral obligation of all physicians. Someone who assumes the title *doctor* and pretends to practice medicine without competence is a charlatan and a quack. Being and remaining competent therefore is a doctor's professional responsibility. Sadly, some doctors fail to acknowledge this core feature of their medical duty.

Other physicians fail to uphold the other profession-endorsed principles of medical ethics and to display the distinctive character we look for in doctors. Physicians who are not caring and respectful, those who are not truthful, and those who put their own interests before the welfare of their patients show failures of professionalism. In itself, any such unprofessional behavior counts as a medical error. Unprofessional behavior also may lead to errors in diagnosis and treatment because of a physician's insufficient commitment, communication, or knowledge in adequately diagnosing and treating his or her patients.

Failures in Communication

The most common cause of medical errors is miscommunication. Communication is a critical component in the care of hospitalized patients because patient information must be shared by many specialists and changing teams of medical professionals. To provide effective treatment, detailed information must be transferred from one professional to another. A lapse in communication may cause a physician responsible for making a critical decision to misunderstand significant details in the patient's medical history or the results of a diagnostic procedure. This lapse may, in turn, lead to a mistaken conclusion about the cause of the patient's problem, what must be done to resolve it, the urgency of treatment, when to reevaluate because the treatment is not working, or how significant a symptom may be for the health of the patient.

Miscommunication may occur between you and your health care providers. It also may occur between health care professionals or teams of health care professionals as the torch of medical responsibility is passed from one shift to another. Important information regarding the medical workup plan, diagnosis, treatment plan, or medications may fail to be passed along; the facts may be misunderstood; the details may go unappreciated; or small points may be misheard, misread, or misremembered.

System Complexity

The complex organization of today's medical systems is another source of medical errors. Today's health care involves many medical professionals, multiple test results, and very limited time for listening, discussing, explaining, and confirming that patients understand the issues and their treatment. With many details requiring attentive action, it is easy for steps to be missed and details to fall through the cracks. Someone inadvertently may skip writing a prescription, someone may forget to order a test or to act on a test result, someone can miss an appointment, and someone may overlook explaining important symptoms for which the patient should be alert. Any of these small errors can lead to a disaster.

Institutional Efforts to Avoid Errors

Patient safety and the prevention of medical errors have received increasing attention from medical institutions, medical organizations, health professionals, physicians, government organizations, insurance carriers, and patients. We all want to improve our understanding of how errors occur so that we can put measures in place to improve the health and safety of patients by decreasing the number and severity of medical errors.

For that reason, medical facilities have instituted specific procedures to avoid certain kinds of errors. Medical institutions and professional groups try to prevent failures of professionalism by maintaining a practice environment that makes the expectation of professional standards explicit. In addition, they monitor the behavior of the health professionals whom they employ and take on the task of discipline or remediation. Lack of knowledge or professionalism also is addressed by regulatory agencies that require accreditation and periodic recertification.

The use of medical record numbers, patient identification bracelets or ID scanners, and repeated requests for you to repeat your name and medical history are all part of the effort to ensure that the wrong patient is not subjected to a treatment or test. The move to electronic medical records is another part of the effort to avoid errors related to miscommunication. Pharmacy measures also are in place to help prevent drug prescribing or dosing errors. Also, many institutions have mechanisms in place for reporting errors and near-misses so that the systems can be modified to prevent future errors of that kind. Yet, although errors typically have to happen in a series before a patient suffers a bad outcome, and despite the number of error-avoiding procedures at many levels, errors continue to occur.

How to Avoid a Medical Error Happening to You

Awareness of the possibility of medical errors and information on how and why they occur allow patients to play an active role in avoiding errors and ensuring their own safety. The remainder of this chapter is devoted to guiding you on what you can do to avoid errors. You – and family members who also are alert to the possibility of medical errors – can help decrease the likelihood of errors caused by miscommunication and systems problems.

Patients who are educated about their illness and treatment are more likely to comply with a treatment plan because they understand why it is important. The greater the involvement of patients and families, the less likely errors will occur. You should have a complete understanding of how to keep yourself healthy, what you should do routinely, and what is required because of your age, family history, or other medical problems. As we age, we are more likely to develop medical conditions. Periodic monitoring is important to detect such conditions early so that medical treatment is effective in preventing serious consequences.

If you have a medical condition, you need to know which symptoms to watch for and when you should contact your doctor or go to an emergency department. If you are being treated for a disease, you need to understand what reactions or side effects are to be expected and which ones require medical attention. If something unexpected happens related to your medical care, you need to ask questions about it and be sure you understand the explanation.

The following lists provide detailed advice on important ways to enhance your knowledge of your illness and treatment and ways in which you can help assure your own safety and decrease the potential for errors. The information is organized in lists of 1) medical records everyone should maintain, 2) what you need to know and do when managing your health in the outpatient setting, and 3) what you need to know and do when you are in the hospital.

Medical Records You Should Keep

Every patient should know about their medical problems, the diagnostic plan, and the treatment plan to help avoid medical errors. To make sure you have all the necessary information and to ensure that the information is also available to your family, you should keep a log or an electronic file. If you store the information on a thumb drive, you can take it with you on doctor visits and even take it along when you travel. Your log or electronic file should include the following information:

- Name, specialty, and contact information of each of your physicians
- Dates of your doctor visits, which doctor you visited, and the reason(s) for your visits (e.g., referred by a doctor, a specific complaint)
- Medications you take, reasons for taking them, dosages, specific start and end dates, and any reactions that may be associated with them
- Every procedure you've had (e.g., skin biopsies, oral procedures such as tooth extraction, colonoscopy) along with the dates, the name of the

person who performed the procedure, and any reports (especially if the results were questionable)
- Dates of lab tests, the type of test (e.g., x-ray, electrocardiogram, mammogram, skin test for tuberculosis, blood work, prostate exam, urine exam, Pap test), and any abnormal results. You may ask your doctors for copies of the results for your personal medical records.
- Medical problems or diseases your doctor has diagnosed, including short-term problems (e.g., bronchitis, stomach virus, allergic reaction, borderline diabetes, urinary tract infection) and long-term ones (e.g., high blood pressure, glaucoma, irritable bowel, osteoporosis); treatments for those conditions; and the treatment dates

In the Outpatient Setting

The following list describes what every outpatient should do:

- Communicate with your health care providers regarding how you learn best.
- Get written instructions for anything you must do (e.g., follow-up appointment, new medication, changes in medication, referral to specialist, future tests).
- Know how to communicate with your doctor to get your questions answered (e.g., call and leave a message, speak with office staff, e-mail), when you should expect a response, and when you should contact the doctor again if you don't get a reply.
- Know which tests and treatments are needed to help keep you healthy and prevent additional medical problems (and why) and the frequency with which they are required (e.g., flu shot; breast exams; stool sample, eye exams; periodic checks of blood pressure, blood glucose, and cholesterol).
- Know when and how you will receive test results.
- Know the medical problems that require follow-up and/or treatment (e.g., borderline elevated cholesterol, family history of cancer, risks for heart attack, stroke, diabetes).
- Know how often you need to follow up with a doctor and why.
- Know which symptoms indicate you should immediately call or see your doctor or go to the emergency room.
- Know when to take each medication, what it's for, which side effects to expect, and what to do if you miss a dose or take too much.
- Before each encounter ends, confirm your understanding of what you should do and what happens next.

In the Hospital

When you or a family member is admitted to a hospital, it is important to understand how hospital care is structured. An overview of who will be involved in your care and their roles will help you avoid unnecessary anxiety, navigate the system, get the best possible care, and avoid errors. Although there are differences among hospitals, the information in this section applies to most.

In addition to providing patient care, many hospitals also teach future physicians and other health care workers. These young people are not only trainees, but also part of the health care team, and they play important roles in delivering your health care. Medical students are college graduates who are studying to become doctors. As part of their learning, they frequently practice taking patient histories. They also perform important jobs for the medical team, such as checking up on patients, performing physical exams, and drawing blood.

Interns and residents are already doctors. They have graduated from medical school. Most medical school graduates, however, take additional years of residency training to become certified in a specific specialty. Before certification in an area such as pediatrics, internal medicine, orthopedic surgery, or neurosurgery, doctors train for an extra three to five years. Most residents are licensed to write prescriptions and certified to perform certain procedures on their own, others under supervision.

After completing residency, some doctors pursue even more specialized training as fellows. This additional training may take another one to three years, for example, to qualify a doctor as a pediatric cardiologist or a transplant surgeon. During their fellowship training, these doctors also are an integral part of the health care team that provides your medical care.

Every patient admitted to the hospital has one doctor – the attending physician – who is ultimately responsible for that patient's care. Which physician becomes your attending physician depends on the problem or disease that leads to your admission to the hospital. You may have a long-term relationship with your primary care physician, but if you are admitted with appendicitis, you will be admitted under the care of a surgeon who will be responsible for your surgery. If you have other medical problems, your primary care physician may also manage part of your care. It is common for an attending physician to ask for a consultation with another specialist to help manage some aspect of your care. For instance, if you have diabetes as well as appendicitis, the surgeon may consult a physician who has expertise with that disease to help in the management of your diabetes. This consultant may make recommendations about specific aspects of your care, but your attending physician is the one who makes the ultimate decision about your treatment and discharge.

If your primary care physician is affiliated with the hospital where you are admitted, you may ask him or her to check in on you to see how you are doing. If the expertise of another of your regular physicians is required, that physician may visit, examine you, and write notes and suggestions in your chart; he or she may send you a bill for the visit. Not all physicians follow their patients when they are hospitalized, and hospitals require that physicians be on staff at that specific hospital for them to assist in your care. Even if your physician is not affiliated with the hospital where you are admitted, the team of doctors caring for you may contact your doctor to update him or her about your progress or ask for more specific information about your health.

Your attending physician usually will see you every day, but other members of the team will follow your progress when he or she is off duty or at another site caring for other patients. Some of the residents from each health care team are present in the hospital all day and all night, whereas the attending physician who is ultimately responsible for your care also takes care of patients in his or her office, in the operating room, or at some other institution.

Typically, the team following your progress includes interns, residents, and Fellows at various stages of training. It also may include medical students, nursing students, nurse practitioners, and physician assistants. Residents are on shifts in the hospital, and their hours are regulated by government rules so that they get sufficient time out of the hospital to sleep. Therefore, several shifts of residents will take care of you during your stay. In general, residents are on specific locations and rotations within the hospital for four weeks at a time before they rotate to another location. Therefore, you may have several teams of residents caring for you during your hospital stay. Others involved in your care may include nurses, nurse's aides, dieticians, physical therapists, social workers, lab technicians, and transporters, who take you from one place to another. All these individuals are responsible for identifying themselves and the role they play in your care.

Hospitalized patients typically undergo numerous tests and procedures. All these involve some degree of risk, which your doctor has considered in light of the information or medical benefits they are expected to provide. You should be aware that the risks involved with some procedures are greater than others. Routine blood work or x-rays do not involve a significant risk and do not require a signed informed consent form. However, procedures involving more than a minimal degree of risk require your signature on an informed consent form. Before you sign, the purpose and risks of the procedure should be explained to you. Feel free to ask questions about what is being done, because you cannot legitimately consent to a procedure you do not understand.

Significant illness brings you into the hospital. When you are seriously ill, you should expect that your mental and psychological faculties might be diminished. Also, any hospital stay may be stressful, frustrating, and confusing. The hospital environment is highly regulated, and being hospitalized involves others controlling your diet, sleep, and activity. People bring your food, wake you up, ask you questions, and examine you. Others decide which tests to administer to you and which medications and procedures you should have. This arrangement encourages patients to become passive.

Therefore, having a family member or friend around may be very helpful and reassuring. A family member or friend can help you sort out who is on your health care team, what your treatment plan is, and what your expectations should be. He or she also may be useful in decreasing the chance of miscommunication and errors.

To avoid mistakes of both omission and commission, and to ensure that you actually receive the right care, you need to know what your recommended care is. The following list describes what you and your family member or friend should be aware of, so you can take an active part in preventing errors:

- Identify the attending physician who oversees all your care and discharge from the hospital, and know the best way to contact him or her (e.g., pager, office phone number).
- Keep a log of the doctors who are caring for you, their names, their specialties, and how to contact them, including the residents on the team and their shifts.
- Know the plan for determining what is wrong and what hopefully will be accomplished in the hospital.
- Know what is to be done each day, the name of each test or procedure, and its purpose.
- Know the name of each medication you are to receive, its purpose, the amount, the frequency, and the potential side effects.
- Understand what is expected of you, which symptoms you should watch for, and what you should do to promote your health (e.g., move your legs frequently to prevent clots, breathe deeply to prevent pneumonia, rotate frequently in the bed to prevent bedsores).
- Know which symptoms (complaints) and findings (e.g., fever, anemia) should be monitored to determine your progress.

If an Error Occurs

As a matter of respect and honesty, you should be informed if there has been an error in your care. You also should be given a complete account of what happened. Most critically, you need to know if there are any short- or long-term consequences from the error and how the error will actually affect you. For instance, if you were given an incorrect medication or an inadequate or excessive dose of a required medication, might there be side effects days or weeks later? Will you need additional tests or medications? Will you have to stay longer in the hospital? Will you be moved to another unit in the hospital? You need to clarify the potential consequences. Is there a risk now that something bad might happen later? Do you require monitoring, or do you have to be aware of signs or symptoms of a problem later on? You also need to be clear about who will pay for any additional tests or treatments you may require.

You may not get a complete explanation of what transpired; however, to the extent the facts are known, it is reasonable to expect to be told what occurred, and how and why it happened. You also have the right to obtain your medical record, which may provide details of the event. You may show the record to others, including your primary doctor or another physician, so they can help you understand what happened and identify any future related health concerns.

When an error occurs, it is reasonable to expect an appropriate response from the physician in charge of your care. As noted earlier, that would involve honest disclosure of precisely what transpired and communication about the likely and foreseeable consequences of the error. It is reasonable to expect an expression of regret for what happened and empathy for the extra burdens you may have to endure. It also is reasonable to expect assurance of what is being done to avoid similar errors befalling you or other patients in the future. Most doctors provide all these responses. Most patients who appreciate the complexity of medical care and the stress on overburdened staff are understanding of how easily errors can occur and are grateful for the thoughtful and caring response of their doctor.

Unfortunately, however, patients sometimes experience an unreasonable response from their doctor. Although there is no excuse for such unprofessional behavior – and, hopefully, it rarely occurs – it nevertheless is useful to understand why physicians sometimes do not meet professional standards after an error. Regardless of who is responsible for the error, those involved likely have feelings of guilt and shame.

Those feelings make people want to evade and avoid dealing with the failure. So, instead of showing professionalism with their presence and communication, they avoid interaction. Also, the physician may fear the anger and accusations of the patient and family. Defensive aggression is the psychological response to a feared attack. So, instead of expressing regret and empathy, the fearful doctor may try to fend off reproach by blaming others, perhaps even the patient who was the victim of the error. Such belligerent behavior clearly is unwarranted and inexcusable, particularly from an individual who is supposed to be dedicated to acting in patients' interests. That said, you must remain focused on your primary goal, which should be to remediate any damage caused by the error and to restore your health. These tasks will require you to look past the unprofessional behavior and address any medical problems that may be consequent to the error.

Ultimately, you will have to come to terms with the error and decide whether you can still trust the individuals responsible for your care. Vigilant and expert physicians make errors, and if you have a good, trusting relationship with your doctor, it should allow you to accept the error and continue the relationship. Often, mistakes prompt individuals to be even more careful and invested in a good relationship and outcome. Ultimately, you are the only one who can decide whether there is sufficient trust in your relationship to allow it to continue.

Conclusion

As in most of life, you are your own best advocate. When it comes to your own medical care, you should be sure you understand your situation. Specifically, you need to know your diagnosis, your prognosis, and your doctor's recommendation for treatment. You need to have a comprehensive understanding of your medical status and to decide whether or not you agree with the specific plans for your care.

The uncertainty and complexity of medicine may result in errors. Medical errors can never be eliminated completely, but each of us can assist in better understanding the factors that have an impact on patient care and the importance of clear communication in minimizing errors. The discussion in this chapter should help you keep informed, aware, and alert. Your attention and vigilance will help improve your safety and diminish the potential for medical errors and adverse consequences.

SIX

Being Informed When You Give Consent to Medical Care

– Ben A. Rich

A little more than a decade ago, an article appeared in a major medical journal on the topic of informed consent. It began with these two very curious sentences: "Informed consent is a foundational concept of medical ethics. Since its enunciation almost four decades ago, it has engendered, and continues to engender, a great deal of debate and opposition among practicing physicians."[1] Neither sentence is particularly remarkable standing alone, but how could both sentences be true? If informed consent truly is foundational to medical ethics, how could it still be the subject of debate and opposition by members of the medical profession? My advice to patients, and to those who care about and sometimes must advocate for them, is to focus your primary attention on the second of the two sentences in the quoted passage and take it as a red flag flapping in the winds of controversy that blow continuously through the landscape of health care. Why this is an appropriate response will, it is hoped, be abundantly clear to everyone who reads this chapter from start to finish.

The organization of this chapter is based on a series of important questions and answers you will need to consider to ensure that your rights and those of your loved ones are protected when seeking or undergoing medical treatment. The questions are as follows:

- What is informed consent, and why is it important?
- How did informed consent come to be recognized, and what do its origins indicate about its acceptance by health care professionals?
- What are the major limiting or qualifying factors associated with informed consent?
- What can you reasonably expect with regard to informed consent, and how does that differ from what you can properly demand?
- What relevance, if any, does informed consent have to advance directives and advance care planning?

In the following pages, we will address each of these questions in turn. As you will see, the answers may be controversial, and reasonable people may differ on some points. To the extent possible, I will note when a statement is arguably an objective fact and when it is a matter of informed opinion. In the final analysis, the goal of this chapter is to empower you to advocate more effectively for yourself or your loved ones in making decisions about medical care and treatment.

What Is Informed Consent, and Why Is It Important?

The distinguished U.S. Supreme Court justice Benjamin Cardozo wrote in the very early years of the twentieth century (before assuming a seat on the highest court), "Every person of adult years and sound mind has the right to determine what shall be done with his own body."[2] This pithy statement goes to the very essence of what informed consent is intended to protect in the context of medical treatment and medical practice – the right of individuals to make decisions for themselves. Unfortunately, in the nearly 100 years since its enunciation, it has died the death of a thousand qualifications. An underlying presupposition of informed consent is that to truly be a matter of personal choice, such decisions must be informed. Stated in the negative, an uninformed consent (as well as a coerced or manipulated consent) is no consent at all. In fact, there is another term that more accurately describes such circumstances: *assent*. In pediatrics, physicians seek the "assent" of the minor child to treatment because the law presumes that children, as minors, do not have the capacity to give a truly informed consent.

The nature and extent of the concept of informed consent can be understood more fully by listing its essential features. Following is my preferred list, which may be more extensive than what appears in other treatments of the subject. I believe in erring on the side of more, rather than fewer, elements in achieving understanding when patients are being asked to give their consent.

Diagnosis or Differential Diagnosis

There are two broad categories of medical interventions: diagnostic and therapeutic. When a physician is attempting to determine the nature of a patient's ailment, he or she may order one or more tests or diagnostic procedures. The purpose is to rule in or rule out a range of possible conditions that fit with the medical history and description of the symptoms provided by the patient, as well as the physician's findings on physical examination. This process is what is meant by the term *differential diagnosis*, a range of possible conditions the physician must refine to ultimately arrive at a diagnosis for which to formulate an appropriate treatment plan. Patients are entitled to know what conditions are in the differential diagnosis before being asked to consent to any tests or procedures. Of course, if your physician has confirmed a diagnosis, this should be disclosed and fully explained to your satisfaction.

Nature of the Diagnostic Procedure or Treatment

As the statement by Justice Cardozo indicates, you are entitled to dominion and control over your own body. When a health care professional proposes to do something that in any way invades the province of your person, consent is required. Even the few narrow exceptions to that general principle, which we discuss later, do not suggest that consent is unnecessary, but rather only establish conditions in which consent may reasonably be presumed. Part of the prevailing mythology concerning informed consent, about which I will say much more later, is that informed consent is required only for major, invasive, and risky procedures. Technically, that is not correct. For example, often it is thought that a simple blood test is virtually devoid of risk when properly performed, except for a slight bit of pain when the skin is pricked or infection if the skin is not properly cleaned before the blood is drawn. The risk in such "minor" diagnostic procedures is not so much in the blood drawing but rather in what the test may reveal and the cascade of events that may follow. To take only one example, a prostate-specific antigen, or PSA, test is routinely administered to men over fifty as screening for prostate cancer. Many men with an elevated PSA do not have cancer. Furthermore, even among those who do, many have a very slowly developing form that may never actually become life threatening. Nevertheless, once the PSA test results come back "positive," meaning the level is above whatever is considered normal (which has been a consistently moving target), the primary care physician likely will refer the patient to a urologist for a prostate biopsy. Undergoing this diagnostic procedure may be painful, is not without risk, and may lead to stress and anxiety in the patient, even when the results are "negative," meaning no cancer was found. Men should never be subjected to a PSA test without their prior informed consent – yet, it happens! Furthermore, the discussion of risks should include the cascade of events that may follow (the PSA "juggernaut").

Another example that illustrates this point is magnetic resonance imaging (MRI), a high-tech process for obtaining very elaborate images of the inside of the body. Some physicians, in recommending this sophisticated form of diagnostic imaging, say dismissively that it is completely noninvasive and painless. Although it is true that no part of the procedure involves touching the body, it is not without the potential for serious discomfort or distress if the patient has any tendencies toward claustrophobia. Depending on the part of the body being studied, the patient may be placed in a long tube not much larger than the circumference of his or her body for more than thirty minutes, during which there is a very loud (some would say deafening) noise (which may be somewhat muffled if earplugs or headphones are provided) much of the time as images are taken. These patients need to know in advance what it may be like for them to experience the procedure and be offered sedatives to help them endure it without unnecessary discomfort.

Benefits and Risks of the Procedure

It is reasonable to assume that no ethical health care professional would recommend any procedure or treatment (diagnostic or therapeutic) unless he or she had a good-faith basis for believing it has a reasonable chance of benefiting the patient, and that the benefits outweigh the risks. To do otherwise would be unethical and violate the professional's fiduciary duty to the patient. The critical point, however, is that the professional should not be the final arbiter of what constitutes a benefit or a reasonable risk, or how the balance of benefits and risks is assessed – because it is the patient, not the professional, whose health, safety, or even life may be at stake. These assessments are not entirely objective; they have subjective and value-laden dimensions, which must be viewed from the patient's perspective. Although the professional's knowledge, insights, and perspectives are important and worthy of consideration, it is ultimately the patient's decision.

We already considered how even simple diagnostic procedures have risks. Major treatment interventions such as open heart surgery and chemotherapy for cancer present much more significant risks. One reasonably can argue for a more expansive interpretation of the term *risk* that might aptly be characterized as the "burdens of treatment." These burdens may include not only the patient's pain and discomfort during treatment or in the days, weeks, or months afterward, but also his or her temporary or longer-term inability to resume work or engage in activities of daily living. Although there is great variability among patients, experienced professionals have seen many patients and can make reasonably accurate generalizations that may be instructive to those who are facing such decisions.

Alternatives and Their Risks and Benefits

For every proposed medical intervention (diagnostic or therapeutic), there is always at least one alternative – *not* doing it. In some situations, the risks of doing nothing instead of the only available intervention may be significant and perhaps unacceptably high, but professionals who declare there is no option but to do as they say have not made an accurate statement. What they probably intend to convey is the message that there are no "reasonable" options from their perspective. That is an opinion to which they are entitled but not one they are at liberty to foist upon the patient.

In many other situations, there is a range of acceptable options for treatment. It is important to be aware that physicians tend to develop expertise in and, to some extent, a natural bias toward one form of treatment over other equally acceptable options. You certainly would want to know of such a bias so that, if need be, you can seek a referral to another physician who has more experience with and presumably a greater affinity for one of the other possible approaches to the same condition. If there are reliable clinical studies comparing the effectiveness of the options for treating a condition, you should be provided with that information and any questions about it should be fully and objectively answered. The same is true when different prescription medications exist for treating the same illness. In choosing one medication over another, informed consent involves a basic discussion of the benefits, risks, relative effectiveness, and side effects of each.

Often risk and benefit are measured through statistics. Although this information may be complex and technical, your physician should be able to distill it into accurate statements that can be presented in a way the average person can understand and use in making an informed choice. The use of terms such as *slight* or *negligible* when referring to the possibility of a particular risk is not very informative because it involves a value judgment by the physician. If a number can be attached to the level of risk – for example, a 1 in 100 chance of death – then patients can make their own determination as to whether or not that is "slight." In general, the greater the consequence should the risk occur, the lower the level of risk a reasonable patient would be willing to accept.

Identity and Qualifications of the Key Professionals Involved

For some patients, knowing the identity, credentials, and qualifications of the professionals primarily responsible for their care is of major significance. These patients have an absolute right to this information before they consent to undergoing any procedure or initiating any form of treatment. Identity issues may be particularly complicated (and important) when receiving treatment at an academic medical center, where there are many Fellows, residents (novice physicians undergoing graduate medical education), and even medical students on clinical rotations who may be involved in patient care. The old saying that "you can't tell the players without a program" is true with a vengeance in academic medicine. If you are assertive about obtaining this information, to which you are entitled, you may encounter someone who suggests that seeking care at an academic medical center means you waive the right to object to the involvement of trainees in your care. That is not correct. Although many patients assume such involvement and actually do not mind it, others do object and let that be known. There are still a few old-school faculty physicians who introduce medical students to their patient as "Doctor" in what they consider to be a little white lie that is of no moral consequence. Quite the contrary, it is a material misrepresentation of fact and verges on fraudulent deception. There is no valid informed consent to anything the student does to you as a patient in such a case.

Even outside of academic medical centers, there may be situations in which the professional whom the patient believes will be primarily responsible for performing a procedure in fact is not; indeed, he or she may not be anywhere in the vicinity when the procedure takes place. Sometimes this approach is addressed by vague consent documents that state the following: "the patient consents to the performance of the identified procedure by Dr. William Jones and/or his colleagues." This is why it is important to read consent documents carefully before you sign them and insist on your questions being answered to your satisfaction. If it is important to you that Dr. Jones performs all important aspects of the procedure, then the consent form should make that expectation clear.

Costs and Insurance Coverage of the Procedure or Treatment

Once upon a time in the United States, when most patients had some form of health insurance that paid whatever the health care institution or professional charged, patients had little or no reason to need or want to know the associated cost. Today, in the era of managed care – with its deductibles, co-payments, prior approval requirements, and many exclusions from coverage – no reasonable patient can afford to cultivate ignorance regarding the cost of health care. Even seemingly minor procedures or routine medications may be very costly in today's health care environment if you ultimately must pay the medical bill. Nevertheless, you should not be surprised if your physician does not immediately know what the actual cost is likely to be. However, with a reasonable effort, an accurate cost estimate can be determined and provided to you.

Cost is probably the most controversial item on this list of essential elements of an informed consent. There is a prevailing perception among health care professionals that a medical procedure, even an elective one, is not like, for example, a tune-up on your car, which you may or may not choose to have performed depending on what it will cost. However, not all medical decisions are matters of life or death, and the location and timing of many interventions may reasonably be adjusted to take into account the cost that must ultimately be borne by you.

From the patient's perspective, how health care professionals *think* about informed consent is as important, if not more so, than whether they understand and acknowledge the essential elements listed previously. The following are key points to help you think about or understand informed consent in clinical practice:

1. Consent is a process, not an event. Informed consent is an ongoing dialogue between professional and patient. Although there are a few situations in which a patient gives consent to an intervention that is performed immediately, more typically, a patient gives consent to a treatment plan, not a single intervention. For this reason, the patient's situation and attitudes about treatment will change over time. Under no circumstances should you be led to believe that once consent has been given it cannot be revoked, except in the case of a single intervention once it has been completed.

2. Consent is not merely the signing of a form. Documenting the informed consent process involves the review and execution of a consent form that, when properly drafted, includes a recitation of the essential information about the procedure or treatment and is signed by you or your representative. However, properly considered, informed consent is the dialogue between you and the professional that the signed form simply confirms by documenting its essential details.

3. The use of medical jargon or complex terminology is never acceptable during the consent process or in the language of the form itself. Any time a health care professional uses terminology in discussions with you or your family member that a nonprofessional would not understand, he or she promptly and forthrightly should be asked to rephrase the statement in nontechnical terms. No one should ever be reluctant or self-conscious about making such a request. It is not an admission of ignorance. Quite the contrary, it is the professional who is demonstrating ignorance of the nature and purpose of the informed consent process, which is to convey important information to another person in language he or she can reasonably be expected to understand. No layperson can be reasonably expected to understand complex medical terminology. Professionals who are not comfortable with the informed consent process or who resent having to meet this obligation to patients often cite an individual's failure to understand jargon-filled statements as "proof" that informed consent is completely impractical, because patients cannot reasonably be expected to understand complex medical concepts and principles. However, a truly knowledgeable, articulate, and conscientious professional should be perfectly capable of distilling complex medical or scientific concepts and principles into statements that anyone with a high school education can understand.

4. The manner in which the professional gives information essential to an informed consent discussion is at least as important as the information itself. Health care professionals reveal a great deal about themselves and their attitude toward informed consent's role in patient care by the manner

in which they conduct these discussions. Their manner includes things such as:

a. The physical setting in which the discussion takes place. Is it quiet and private or in a hallway or a room with other people not involved in the patient's care?

b. The professional's demeanor. Is it hurried and abrupt or patient and methodical, conveying a willingness to take the time necessary to ensure that effective communication has taken place?

c. The professional's attitude about consent. Does it seem to be one of simply getting the patient's signature on a form or acceptance of whatever is proposed, or is there a sincere effort to ascertain that the patient really understands what is being recommended and why? Is the patient asked if there are further questions? Is the patient asked to restate in his or her own words what has been conveyed?

5. Finally, and perhaps most importantly, the ultimate goal of the informed consent process is not your consent but your *understanding*. It must always be within the realm of possibility for you to say no to what is being proposed. If "no" is not considered an option in the mind of the professional, then he or she has not grasped or refuses to accept the patient's autonomy. "No" may not be a wise choice; it may not be the choice most patients in that situation would make, but that does not nullify your right as a patient to make it. Patients, and those who support them in their decisions, need to understand they may encounter frustration, perhaps even anger and resentment, on the part of very determined professionals when their recommended treatment is refused; however, this in no way negates patients' rights to decide and to have their decisions respected.

How Did Informed Consent Come to Be Recognized, and What Do Its Origins Indicate about Its Acceptance by Health Care Professionals?

To understand the role of informed consent in the medical profession and the various settings in which health care is provided, it is critical to have at least a rudimentary sense of when and how the concept originated. The original Hippocratic Oath included nothing about respect for individual patient autonomy or the duty to disclose accurate information to patients. Indeed, key texts throughout the history of medicine admonished physicians not to trouble patients with detailed information about their conditions or prospects for recovery. The operative philosophy of patient management was that of beneficent paternalism.

The language quoted earlier from Justice Cardozo speaks of consent, but not of *informed* consent. As a general principle, patients could not be treated over their express refusal; however, the consent was not required to be truly informed because medical professionals did not consider that kind of detailed disclosure to be in their patients' interest. The first use of the term *consent* that presumed that relevant information would be conveyed to the patient was the Nuremberg Code in 1946; however, the code pertained to research on human subjects, not to patient care. It was in the context of a medical malpractice suit against Stanford University in 1957 that the term *informed consent* was first used to identify such a duty on the part of a physician to a patient. This event is highly significant for at least two reasons. First, it indicates how recently the principle of informed consent was formulated. Second, it came to be recognized in the courts (Nuremberg tribunal, California Court of Appeals) as a legal duty of medical researchers and physicians decades before it was recognized as an ethical duty and a matter of professional responsibility.

Within barely more than a ten-year span in the middle of the twentieth century, the courts, by judicial fiat, insisted that medical researchers and practitioners radically alter their rules of engagement with research subjects and patients. These rules of engagement were not merely routines, but rather were informed by the very ethos of the medical profession. The long-reigning paradigm of that ethos was paternalism. The heart and soul of paternalism is the basic belief that the professional – whether in the role of a medical scientist doing research on human subjects or of a physician in patient care settings – knows what is in the patient's best interest or will meet his or her basic needs. The concept makes no room for the contrary proposition that is operative in virtually every other form of human endeavor: that individuals are best situated to know how their needs or priorities might best be met. This historical background helps explain the initially confusing second sentence of the passage quoted at the beginning of this chapter, that informed consent continues to engender much debate and opposition from the medical profession. Implicit in the informed consent concept, which in turn is grounded in respect for individual autonomy, is the basic presupposition that the professional, no matter how knowledgeable and experienced, does not necessarily know what is best for another person.

Simply stated, paternalism is inconsistent with respect for individual autonomy and a duty of full disclosure of pertinent information. If the courts were going to insist that the medical profession adhere to these new principles and practices, an alternative paradigm would have to replace paternalism. That new paradigm, and the grudging way in which it has been adopted in fits and starts over the past fifty years, has come to be known as "shared decision making." In the patient care setting, this concept presupposes that the physician and patient come together in a kind of joint venture with mutual responsibilities in pursuit of a common goal, most generally characterized as the restoration or maintenance of the patient's well-being or, in the face of terminal illness, in the pursuit of a peaceful death consistent with the patient's core values. In the unlikely event of irreconcilable conflict between the values or goals of the physician and those of the patient, the physician's duty is not to insist on dictating the course of treatment, as might have been the case under the paternalistic paradigm, but rather to disengage from the professional relationship in a manner that ensures continuity of care during the transition.

To this very day, attitudes about respect for patient autonomy, informed consent, and the shared-decision-making model of patient care run across a broad continuum. The patient or surrogate decision maker's reluctance or outright unwillingness to go along with the physician's recommendations for treatment sometimes may spark frustration, at times even indignation on the part of old-school physicians (some of whom actually may be quite young). The take-home (or take-to-the-clinic) message for you, or those who may be called upon to make decisions for you, is to not be shamed or intimidated into consenting to approaches to care with which you, or they, are uncomfortable. Insist on continuing the informed consent dialogue following the approach suggested previously. It is entirely possible the discomfort and disagreement are products of misunderstanding that can be eliminated with a clearer explanation of the goals of care and the means proposed to achieve those goals. If the disagreement appears irresolvable, the alternative is to pursue a change in professional. Think of informed consent as a coin, which of course has two sides. The flip side of informed consent to treatment is informed refusal of treatment. Sometimes physicians seem to forget there is another side.

What Are the Major Limiting or Qualifying Factors Associated with Informed Consent?

As courts (and, in some cases, legislatures) in various jurisdictions addressed informed consent for the first time, they considered three different approaches to the standard by which the adequacy of information disclosure might be determined. The first, and the one ultimately adopted by a slight majority of states, is the physician-based standard. The fundamental question asked when a challenge is made to the adequacy of disclosure is whether the information provided to the patient or surrogate decision maker was sufficient for an informed consent or refusal. If the physician-based standard is applied, the focus of the inquiry becomes what a reasonable physician would disclose to such a patient in similar circumstances. When this approach originally was considered, the strongest argument against it was that in the long history of medical paternalism, there was no routine custom and practice of disclosure by physicians to patients; therefore, there was no legitimate basis on which to ground a notion of what a reasonable physician might choose to disclose to a patient. Furthermore, the major reason for creating the duty to disclose information sufficient for a patient's informed consent (or refusal) was to respect the patient's autonomy. Therefore, the focus should be on patients and their informational needs and not on the physician's proclivities to disclose. Many who opposed the physician-based standard argued for an alternative approach.

The second approach is characterized as the patient-based standard. Importantly, the "patient" in this approach is not the actual patient whose care is in question, but a "reasonable" patient in a similar situation. If the information is deemed sufficient to meet the needs of a typical patient whose medical circumstances are similar to those of the patient in question, the physician is deemed to have fulfilled his or her duty. Of course, this approach leads to a challenging question: What kind of evidence is necessary or sufficient to establish that the information disclosed would meet the needs of a reasonable patient? This difficulty led some patients' rights advocates to demand the adoption of yet a third standard, one based not on the needs of some hypothetical patient, but rather on those of the actual patient. Only this standard, its proponents have argued – unfortunately, with very little success – truly has the potential to achieve the purpose of the informed consent doctrine, which is to ensure respect for each patient's autonomy. Because only a handful of jurisdictions have actually adopted this third subjective, or "actual patient," standard of disclosure, the best hope for patients, or those who must speak for them, is to ask the professionals responsible for their care to provide them, as clearly as possible, with all the details they need to know to make an informed decision. When these expectations are clearly articulated, the professionals are put on notice that if they err, it should be on the side of providing too much rather than too little information until the patient or spokesperson indicates he or she is satisfied.

There are three generally recognized exceptions to the professional's duty to obtain an informed consent/refusal for a proposed treatment or intervention. The first, and least problematic for those who advocate respect for patient autonomy, is a patient who waives his or her right to pertinent information. Some patients simply do not wish to be burdened with the information necessary for a truly informed consent or trust their physician implicitly and want to place their medical fate entirely in his or her hands. A basic misunderstanding that persists among some medical professionals is that the doctrine of informed consent requires them to provide, and that patients agree to receive, whatever information is necessary to ensure an informed consent. That simply is not true. A patient who genuinely wishes to decline this information may do so, and the professional who respects his or her decision (assuming the patient has the mental capacity to make a decision in the first place) may not subsequently be held liable for failure to disclose.

A second exception to the duty to obtain informed consent arises during a genuine medical emergency in which a patient is critically ill and incapable of processing information and making a decision (perhaps because of unconsciousness), no one in a position to speak for the patient is readily available, and the failure to act immediately to treat the patient's medical problems may result in death or grave injury. In such circumstances, the patient's consent to the measures necessary to deal with the medical emergency is "presumed," that is, a reasonable person in that situation would want all reasonable measures to be taken without delay and consistent with good medical practice.

The third exception, potentially the most problematic, has come to be known as "therapeutic privilege." When, in the exercise of sound clinical judgment, a physician concludes that disclosing certain information to a patient would pose a serious risk of harm (physical or mental), he or she may exercise professional discretion and withhold that information until the threat to the patient's well-being from such a disclosure passes. Some authorities have suggested that in invoking therapeutic privilege, the physician may – or perhaps should – disclose the information withheld from the patient to someone closely related to the patient. However, this approach is problematic because it may constitute a breach of patient confidentiality unless the patient previously agreed that disclosure of confidential medical information to that person would be acceptable.

The major flaw in therapeutic privilege is that it assumes physicians have a level of insight into the mental state of their patients that very few actually do. Considering the nature of our health care system, it is highly unlikely that a physician knows his or her patients well enough to conclude, in good faith, that disclosing certain information to a patient likely will result in significant harm. The continual recognition of therapeutic privilege, as the courts that originally articulated it acknowledged, creates an exception to the duty to disclose that has the potential, if abused, to undermine the duty itself. Patients should be aware of this exception, and if they suspect their physician might have a propensity to invoke it, particularly as a means to avoid difficult discussions in the face of serious illness, they should state in no uncertain terms that they expect complete and accurate information about the diagnosis, the prognosis, and the potential risks and side effects of treatment.

Before we conclude this section, you should understand the major underlying premise of informed consent/refusal: you possess decisional capacity. Decisional capacity is your ability to 1) understand the pertinent medical information, 2) appreciate the surrounding circumstances in which the decision must be made, 3) evaluate the available options, and 4) communicate a choice or decision. In situations in which you do not have decisional capacity, an appropriate spokesperson (proxy or surrogate) must be identified to speak on your behalf.

Every adult is presumed to have decisional capacity, and the burden of persuasion lies with anyone who claims otherwise. Except for patients in extreme situations such as coma or severe psychosis, decisional capacity is task or issue specific and may wax and wane. Valid decisions a patient made during a period of lucidity are binding in later circumstances when he or she has lost decisional capacity. Just because a patient has a psychiatric or psychological condition does not preclude his or her having capacity; it merely raises a concern that must then be assessed carefully. Finally, and perhaps most importantly, the mere inclination or propensity of an individual to make a decision about treatment that goes against a physician's recommendation does not constitute conclusive evidence of incapacity.

What Can You Reasonably Expect with Regard to Informed Consent, and How Does that Differ from What You Can Properly Demand?

Patients or their spokespersons have a right to expect not only complete disclosure but all information they consider necessary for an informed consent or refusal. If at any time you sense you have not received this, or you simply are unsatisfied with the level of detail of information provided, you can – and should – insist that more information be provided or that it be offered in a different way or by a different person. As noted previously, the ultimate objective of the informed consent process is not to secure your signature on a consent-to-treatment form, but rather to achieve your, or your spokesperson's, understanding of all clinically relevant factors, even if the result is a refusal to consent. It would never be acceptable, for example, for a physician or other health care professional to declare, "I have told you all I am required to tell you or all I think you need to know." Even in jurisdictions that have adopted the physician-based consent standard of disclosure, you have the right to have your informational needs satisfied or to replace a physician unwilling to do so with another one who will.

What Relevance, If Any, Does Informed Consent Have to Advance Directives and Advance Care Planning?

Chapter Three addresses advance directives and advance care planning in detail. The only point to be made here is that informed consent involves respecting the real-time autonomy of the patient. However, courts in all jurisdictions have recognized that patients who lose their capacity to make decisions, either temporarily or permanently, still have a right to have their autonomy respected. The best way for you to insure this happens is to exercise what is known as "prospective autonomy" through the drafting and execution of an advance directive. The best directives not only designate someone (and ideally an alternate as well) who will be your spokesperson (health care proxy/surrogate), but also provide some indication of the level of care you would wish if you become personally incapacitated and gravely disabled. In the absence of such declarations by you in anticipation of potential future disability, it becomes increasingly difficult for caregivers and courts to accept that a surrogate actually is making the decisions you would make if you could.

Conclusion

Many settings in which patient care is provided today are not conducive to fully informed decision making. Even in the primary care clinic, managed care has seriously limited the amount of time physicians are supposed to spend with patients and still meet the prevailing expectations for the number of patients they will see each day. When the site of care shifts to the hospital – or worse yet, the emergency room or intensive care unit – patients and their families have entered an environment that is truly hostile to thoughtful, deliberate, and fully informed consent. The only way to increase the chance you will be provided all the information you need or may wish to receive is to be persistent and assertive in pursuing it.

Once they realize patients have a high level of need for accurate information, most health care professionals will seek to meet that need. Usually, it is not necessary to escalate from a diplomatically presented request to a much more insistent demand. However, when and if that becomes necessary, patients and their families should understand that there is nothing unreasonable about maintaining such expectations. If answers to some questions are not available at the time, you are entitled to know when the information will be available and what needs to be done to secure it, and to receive assurances that it will be forthcoming as soon as reasonably available. Particularly when it comes to questions regarding prognosis or statistical probabilities of success or likelihood of risk, beware of a professional tendency to dismissively declare that all patients are different, so there is no way to know the answers. For virtually every major clinical intervention, there are studies and other sources of reliable information upon which the professional can draw to answer such questions. If a care provider is not currently knowledgeable about the up-to-date information pertinent to your clinical situation, he or she must take the time to become familiar with the material and synthesize it in a manner that satisfactorily answers your questions. As in most other situations, knowledge is power in patient care. To be deprived of information that will make you a knowledgeable (informed) patient is to be disempowered and made vulnerable unnecessarily. No responsible and caring professional should ever allow you to be treated that way.

REFERENCES

[1] Meisel A, Kuczewski M: Legal and ethical myths about informed consent. *Arc Int Med* 2006, 156:2521–3536.
[2] *Schloendorff v. Society of New York Hospital*, 105 N.E. 92 (1914).

SEVEN

Beware of Scorecards

– James J. Strain and Rosamond Rhodes

In this age of quick and easy mass communication, we have come to rely on published rankings to make our selections of things to purchase, places to vacation, and services to employ. The Internet makes advice especially accessible, and we have all become accustomed to searching out recommendations to guide our decisions about all sorts of choices, from the exhibits we should visit to the beaches that are best for snorkeling. Now, scorecards have even been introduced into the world of medicine.

Relying on public advice often is an improvement over mere guess-work and shooting in the dark. We now look to published performance data in the form of "report cards," for example, on airline departure time records. Tourist guides have become a standard resource for travelers, with some authors developing a following because of their track record of reliably steering readers toward desirable restaurants, hotels, and resorts. Reports from the Consumers Union uphold high standards for testing products by objective and carefully constructed standards, so many of us consult their recommendations and rely on their assessments before we purchase a new car or vacuum cleaner.

Medicine certainly is an area in which expert advice is valuable. Decisions regarding what treatments to pursue and which to avoid,

85

what sort of specialist is needed and when, which institutions to visit and which physician to consult all may be critical, and their consequences may be significant and enduring. The information that must be processed and synthesized often is complex and difficult to comprehend and evaluate without extensive medical training. Frequently, patients who have to make medical decisions are incapacitated by illness, overwhelmed by a serious diagnosis, or so far out of their depth that they do not even know which questions they should ask. What's more, the recommendations of untrained friends and family members, who often may be useful guides in evaluating hair salons and supermarkets, hardly constitute the expert advice needed to make important health care decisions. Opinions of those who are outside the medical establishment may amount to no more than anecdotal comments on bedside manner and the rather superficial factors the average consumer can assess competently.

To fill the void and respond to the need, medical establishments such as hospitals, medical practices, and drug manufacturers recently have taken to advertising to promote their expertise. In addition, would-be evaluators have been offering their advice, and medical raters have been publishing performance scorecards.

Scorecard Rationale

Scorecards are presented as reliable measures of medical outcomes. They are used as a means for measuring the quality of care provided and as a tool for negotiating fees for medical services. The existence of scorecards reflects our society's desire for openness and transparency in public affairs. Scorecards also respond to recognition of the wide variability in standards of medical practice, dramatized by public evidence of deficiencies in quality of care. In theory, scorecards can provide us with measurements of health care quality and serve as benchmarks that inform us about who is doing what best. In doing so, scorecards might allow us to look and learn how to make health care better. As public policy information, these reports are supposed to allow patients, referring physicians, and health care purchasers to select high-quality physicians.

Scorecards are now featured in advertisements, posted on websites, and published in the form of short brochures. They typically encompass three areas:

1. Structural qualities, such as the number of specialists in a facility, their qualifications, or complaints about individual doctors or medical institutions

2. Process measures, such as a doctor's rate of performing preventive screening or how frequently a doctor provides recommended vaccinations
3. Outcome measures, such as how often patients have complications after an operation or how satisfied patients are with a doctor's service

Scorecards may be useful tools for patients like you, for regulatory agencies, for managed care organizations, and even for physicians. When you are making health care decisions, scorecards can provide you with valuable information on the costs of treatments or services, as well as the availability and the quality of service. You can use such information to guide patient decisions for yourself or other members of your family. Scorecards also can help state and local governments regulate medical practice and assure public accountability by providing standards for assessing quality of care. Hospitals do appear to respond to the public release of performance data and use that information as a basis for instituting changes. Furthermore, scorecards may encourage market competition between physicians and hospitals based on quality, by either driving out low-quality providers or stimulating them to improve the quality of the care they provide. Finally, ratings can influence health care professionals to improve their practice by making expectations about the standards they should meet explicit and by using public embarrassment as a tool for reforming their behavior.

An Example

In New York State, section 501(b) of the Medicare Prescription Drug, Improvement, and Modernization Act (MMA) of 2003 establishes a financial incentive for all hospitals to report quality-of-care information voluntarily as a public service. To receive this incentive payment, hospitals must submit data for specific quality measures related to three medical conditions: heart attack, heart failure, and pneumonia. Specifically, hospitals are required to report three kinds of quality data related to these medical conditions: the treatments they recommend, facts about the patients' medical conditions as composite scores, and information on the outcomes of the treatments, that is, how the patients did after the treatment. The rating scores for each hospital are calculated by dividing the number of cases in which recommendations were provided (the numerator) by the total number of eligible cases (the denominator) in each reporting period.

In addition, ratings are risk adjusted, meaning that the rating formula accounts for the fact that patients who are sicker or are more fragile to begin with are less likely to have a good outcome and more likely to have a medical complication or to die. The mortality rate indicates the percentage of patients who die in the hospital after a procedure. For example, some heart surgery patients face a greater risk than others of dying during heart surgery because of their age or other underlying medical conditions. Because the risk level of patients treated at each hospital varies, the New York State Department of Health identifies risk factors and uses a statistical model to estimate what a hospital's mortality rate would have been if each hospital had identical patients. The result is a risk-adjusted mortality rate that accounts for the differences in illness severity. In addition, the Department of Health provides volume data on the number of times a particular procedure was performed and facility data on the number of beds and services available in the hospital. In these ways, the system compares not only the number of patients who underwent each kind of procedure, but also how much the patients were at risk of having a poor result. Together, the outcome measures are designed to indicate each hospital's performance rate in relation to the statewide average for each procedure. For instance, the reports of the New York State Department of Health Cardiac Services Program include risk-adjusted mortality rates for isolated coronary artery bypass graft surgeries, valve surgeries, percutaneous coronary interventions, and pediatric congenital surgeries. The program's website (http://www.health.state.ny.us/nysdoh/heart/heart_disease.htm) publishes each institution's overall number of mortalities and compares that with the total number of procedures.

People who are interested can now go online and access the program's reports to find out how one New York hospital compares with another with regard to these four conditions. There is no similar information available on other conditions and few similar programs in other states.

Scorecard Hazards

The problem with scorecards and other publicly accessible ratings is that some of the recommendations they issue do not warrant the reliance of the public. In other words, scorecards that present ratings of medical professionals and medical institutions may themselves be untrustworthy. Even when rating systems are available, few are constructed as carefully as the New York State Department of Health Cardiac Services Program. In general, you should exercise caution when examining these ratings. In what follows, we explain some of the potential hazards inherent in these evaluations.

We often place our trust in numbers because they appear to be objective reports and we associate them with scientific standards.

Numbers can certainly be informative, but they also may be misleading. Sometimes relevant information is reported, and sometimes the data offered lead to false conclusions. Data-collection methods for scorecards are not standardized. Reports that rely on inadequate data collection may provide incomplete or inconsistent information on health care. Besides these general concerns, several more specific problems deserve attention.

Risk Adjustment

Consider, for example, reports on complications after bariatric stomach reduction surgery. We are inclined to assume that the best programs would have the lowest rate of complications. In leaping to that conclusion, we overlook the fact that high-risk patients for bariatric surgery are expected to have more complications. If a report lists the complication rate of a practice that never accepts high-risk patients and compares it with the complication rate of a practice that does, it may appear that the less-skilled surgeons are better because they have fewer complications. In fact, the practice that actually has the expertise to manage high-risk patients and does so with outstanding success may be the more skilled and experienced one, but an uninformed potential patient may reach the opposite conclusion simply by looking at complication rates.

Most data are not risk adjusted to reflect differences among patients who undergo a procedure. As we explained, this can make the most skilled practitioners who accept high-risk patients appear less competent than practitioners who know their skills are not up to the difficult task of managing high-risk patients and who refer such patients to facilities with more-skilled practitioners. The point here is that knowing which factors are relevant, how they are being reported, and what is being compared requires a good deal of medical sophistication. The selection and inclusion of appropriate risk adjustors has a significant impact on ranking profiles. Yet, it is difficult for nonexperts to identify whether risk adjustment is used or reasonably employed in the construction of a scorecard.

The Zero Mortality Paradox

Every story has a beginning, a middle, and an end. Frequently, the choice of where to start and end the telling will make the conclusion look very different. Consider this example: A study by J. B. Dimick and H. G. Welch, published in the *Journal of the American*

College of Surgery[1] in 2008, reports on the operative mortality – that is, the number of deaths – associated with four procedures: abdominal aortic aneurysm bypass, lobectomy for lung cancer, colon cancer resection, and coronary artery bypass surgery. During a three-year period, the operative mortality in certain hospitals was zero. In the subsequent year, the operative mortality rate was no different than the mortality rates in other hospitals. Clearly, the hospital that reported no deaths following these major surgeries would appear to be the safer choice. However, based solely on the report of zero mortality, it is hard to know whether the hospital with zero mortality truly had superior performance, whether the three-year track record was a matter of chance, or whether the reported operative mortality of zero was only a function of the careful selection of only low-risk patients or the small number of procedures performed. A reported mortality of zero by itself is not a reliable indicator of future performance.

A sign in one hospital declares, "We have no deaths from our cardiac surgery." You reasonably might conclude this is the place for you to have your cardiac surgery. However, the sign does not tell you the relevant information you need to know to reliably draw that conclusion. For example, you may not know that all seriously ill patients with additional medical conditions have been sent to other institutions, or that the volume of cardiac procedures at this institution is low, or that a hospital with a higher mortality rate, but serving a sicker patient group, may actually give you a better chance for a good outcome with a lower chance of a serious complication (i.e., less morbidity) and a greater chance for survival.

Sample Size

Studies show that a good report may be made on a bad hospital when the volume and mortality, or rate of death, for the reported procedure is low. To have a valid and reliable measure of quality, the procedure must be performed frequently enough, and with a sufficient number of complications or deaths, to accurately assess the quality of care at a hospital. It may be surprising, but it is a fact that small samples and low rates of untoward events are flaws in the research design that make it impossible to justify any conclusion. A related point that should raise suspicion about good reports based on small sample size is the fact that studies of all sorts of medical procedures repeatedly have shown that institutions that perform a procedure often tend to do it better. In other words, high volume is associated with better outcomes across a wide range of procedures and conditions, although the degree of success may vary greatly.

Data Reporting

In most rating programs, the participation of a doctor or hospital is voluntary. Participation involves an investment of time and effort in data collection and transmission. When a medical practice or program anticipates that the findings reported will not be favorable, it has no incentive to participate. This means only practices and programs that expect the data to show they have an above-average performance rate will provide information. Moreover, if a program or practice is surprised by a reported score that is lower than expected, it likely will stop disclosing its quality data and will withdraw from the study.

Clearly, voluntary reporting of quality data by medical professionals or health care institutions fails to provide accurate and useful ratings. When survey participants are allowed to selectively disclose or not disclose information about their performance, the studies are undermined and the results cannot be relied on for either informed consumer decisions or public accountability. Again, it would be very hard for you to recognize when a report is based on only voluntary submissions.

Significance

Aside from the problems associated with making sense of the numbers, it also is difficult to tell whether a scorecard provides information that is actually useful. For a study reporting which physicians or institutions are providing good care, it is important to know whether the factors being counted and reported actually are meaningful. In multiple studies of physician report cards for the care of patients with diabetes, one of the highest-prevalence conditions in medical practice, the studies could not detect reliable practice differences. This suggests it is hard to know which differences in medical practice matter or which outcomes of medical practice are significant. It may turn out that scorecards cannot distinguish good from marginal clinician performance. When ratings cannot discriminate between high- and low-quality performance by institutions and professionals, the rating system is not helpful for consumers to use in making choices about where to receive care.

Complexity

Health care delivery is a complex system involving numerous interdependent factors, including medical professionals, facilities, payments, and patients. The ratio of staff members to patients, the rapport among the medical team, the team's level of effort and commitment, and its continuity over time all are contributing factors to overall success. Similarly, health care organizations are complex and adaptive systems, involving many interdependent facilities, caregivers, processes, and leaders. These observations point to the need to assess many dimensions simultaneously as well as the fact that the practice being assessed is a moving target. Care that was excellent at a particular institution yesterday may not be nearly as good today, after the team leader moved to another institution, a new head nurse came on board, or cost containment led the institution to lay off some of the staff.

Furthermore, numerous studies have shown that geography and the educational and socioeconomic status of patients also are factors contributing to outcomes. For example, studies have shown that mortality rates are significantly higher among patients of lower income and education. Perhaps this difference arises because patients who are poorer cannot afford their prescribed medication or other recommended medical interventions. This group may not be able to make lifestyle changes; perhaps they do not fully understand the prescribed treatments or why they are important, or perhaps they do not fully trust their doctors or believe what their doctors tell them. Regardless of the causes, this finding demonstrates the need for a risk-adjusted variable reflecting differences in patients' social and economic status and education. Similarly, significant differences in insurance reimbursement contribute to health outcomes. Variables associated with the pressure of seeing a large volume of patients, the level of physician training, and even where physicians were trained may have a significant impact on medical outcomes, yet no scorecard takes these differences into account.

When these variables are ignored and bundled into a rank of individual doctors, the result likely will be a misleading evaluation of the doctor's ability. At the same time, reporting only on a physician's performance fails to assess the system in which he or she works, which also has significant consequences for patients. Scorecards should account for this complexity, yet it also is true that the more factors that are taken into account, the more difficult it is to produce a meaningful rating.

Unintended Consequences of Publicly Reporting Quality Information

The aforementioned issues all speak to the reliability of scorecards. Aside from the problems inherent in figuring out just how useful a particular report may be, you should be aware that making the reports public actually raises additional concerns.

Deselecting Patients

When information about the quality of a physician's performance is made available to the public, it can be expected to have an impact on the physician's behavior. Obviously, every physician wants to appear highly competent and to be reported as providing high-quality care. Those who initiated these reports hoped that providing feedback would help physicians identify areas for quality improvement and thereby improve their performance. To date, however, the value of publicly reporting quality information has not been demonstrated. Indeed, public reports on physician performance invite physicians to adopt strategies that may be contrary to patient interests.

Because outcomes of studies assessing the quality of physician performance are related to the fragility and compliance of patients, doctors who want high ratings are encouraged to select their patients accordingly. Therefore, they tend to avoid sick patients and those unlikely to adhere to medical regimens. They select patients with higher education who are motivated to maintain their physical health, and they are inclined not to accept as patients smokers, couch potatoes, the obese, the less educated, the poor, and the elderly, precisely because they have been shown to have worse health outcomes. Although the ethics of medicine espouse a commitment to nonjudgmental regard and the physician's responsibility to respond to the needs of every patient, if the penalties for doing so are significant – and the incentives for not taking on those patients who will damage a doctor's ranking also are significant – it is hard to imagine that doctors would not be tempted to protect themselves by discriminating against the patients who would make them score poorly.

Patient Preferences

Scorecards are designed to encourage physicians to achieve "target rates" for health care interventions. If given the option, because of cost, inconvenience, or personal aversion, some patients may choose an intervention other than the one targeted by the ranking. Knowing that a patient's preference could deviate from a scorecard ranking, some physicians may be reluctant to disclose treatment options other than the target choice. In this way, rankings could interfere with doctor–patient communication and undermine physician respect for patient autonomy.

Clinical Judgment

Reports on physician performance also may undermine doctors' clinical judgment. Treatment guidelines or scoring criteria employ standards and recommendations that are best for most people, most of the time. These standards are general in nature; they are intended to apply to everyone. However, patients are individuals. Doctors should deviate from the standard of care only when they feel they must based on the patient's particular medical condition or values, and if they can justify this deviation to colleagues in their field. Scorecards, however, have no tolerance for treatments that differ from those recommended by the guidelines, and this intolerance might interfere with a doctor's clinical judgment in the service of his or her patients.

Payments

Payment schemes that are tied to scorecards also are likely to have an impact on physician behavior. Financial incentives already have been shown to affect physician decisions regarding medical treatment and diagnostic testing. For example, angiography as a diagnostic tool reportedly is underused in the Veterans Affairs Health care system,[2] in which physicians are encouraged to contain costs, as compared with a fee-for-service system, in which doctors are paid for each procedure they perform. As payment schemes are increasingly linked to physician performance ratings, financial incentives likely are reflected in physicians' treatment and diagnostic recommendations. The Institute of Medicine already has suggested[3] that government payers increase payments to health care providers who deliver high-quality care. Similarly, John Rowe, the former head of Aetna Insurance Company, has postulated[4] that pay-for-performance and accountability are related themes in improving health care, whereas other authors discuss paying physicians for high-quality care. Payment schemes always have an impact on physician behavior; this one will too. You need to be aware of how these arrangements might affect your health care.

Conclusions

Scorecards have been touted as a mechanism to improve patient care, advance patient decision making, and hopefully improve health outcomes. It now is recognized that the goals of improving the quality of health care and controlling its costs must be considered simultaneously. We need tools to address both interrelated agendas, and rating the performance of physicians and hospitals certainly will have a role in that effort. Public reporting, however, has not been demonstrated to improve health care or to contain costs in a desirable way.

That said, as a patient or family member, you may be eager to consult rankings and ratings because you have little else to guide your critical health care decisions and because such scorecards appear to provide objective and reliable information. If you do consult scorecards, you need to be aware of the hazards of relying on them. Because reporting is not mandatory, because the rankings often omit critical factors such as risk adjustment, and because the factors measured may not actually reflect outcomes, scorecards can be misleading and steer you to options that oppose your interests.

Furthermore, you need to be aware of how ratings of physician performance may affect your physician's clinical judgment, recommendations, and communication. In an age when we are aware of how incentives from drug companies can affect physician prescribing patterns, we also must consider how glory, shame, and payments may be involved in the options physicians disclose and the treatments they recommend.

Awareness will not make you immune to the impact of scorecards. In the absence of other guides, it still may be useful for you to consult them. This chapter merely is a guide to the hazards of this uncharted road.

REFERENCES

[1] Dimick JB, Welch HG: The zero mortality in surgery. *J Am Coll Surg* 2008, 206:13–16.
[2] Peterson LA et al. Regionalization and the Underuse of Angiography in the Veterans Affairs Health Care System as Compared with a Fee for Service System. *N Eng J Med* 2003, 348 (22):2209–17.
[3] Rowe, JW. Pay-for-performance and accountability: related themes in improving health care. *Ann Intern Med* 2006, 145 (9):695–699.
[4] Ibid

EIGHT

Transplantation 101

Negotiating the System

– Aaron Spital and Steven Smith

Kidney (or renal) transplantation involves removing a healthy kidney from either a deceased or living person and implanting it in a patient whose kidneys have failed, in the hope of restoring lost renal function. Transplantation is a complex process that begins with a detailed evaluation of a person with irreversible kidney failure to determine whether he or she is eligible for a transplant. For qualified candidates, the next step is to find a suitable kidney donor. Once this is accomplished, the transplant is performed, after which the recipient will need regular medical check-ups for the life of the transplanted organ (which is also called a "graft").

Despite its complexity, transplantation generally is very beneficial, but it also poses risks. This chapter is designed to educate you about renal transplantation in the hope of reducing anxiety, developing realistic expectations, avoiding unpleasant surprises, and enhancing understanding so that you will be able to make informed choices at the many decision points along the way. We strongly believe that the more informed you are, the more you will advocate for yourself, and that the more responsibility you take for your own care, the more likely your transplant will succeed and the smoother will be the road to success.

The chapter uses a question-and-answer format, addressing what we believe are the most common and important concerns faced by people considering kidney transplantation. We note two caveats before we begin. First, most of our discussion is based on experience in the United States and may not be applicable to transplant programs in other parts of the world, although practice in developed countries likely is similar. Second, our goals are to provide a broad overview of transplantation and offer general guidance to help you navigate the process; you may encounter unusual situations that are not covered here.

Should I Opt for a Kidney Transplant?

Although transplantation is now considered the treatment of choice for patients with end-stage renal disease (ESRD; i.e., irreversible loss of all or nearly all kidney function), it is not for everyone. As you think about pursuing this option, several considerations are relevant, including exclusion criteria, the chances of success, survival rates, quality of life, duration of graft function, and the costs and dangers of transplantation.

Exclusion Criteria

Not everyone with kidney disease is eligible for a transplant. Only patients with irreversible kidney failure are considered. Even if you fall into this group, you still may not be eligible. Reasons for exclusion include recent cancer; untreated active infection; severe incurable nonrenal diseases, such as intractable heart failure; nonadherence to prescribed medical regimens; active recreational drug use; and morbid obesity. Advanced age does not automatically preclude transplantation – physiological age is more important than chronological age. HIV infection used to be an absolute contraindication to transplantation, but some transplant centers now consider HIV-infected people if the infection is under excellent control.

It is important to keep in mind that many exclusion criteria are relative rather than absolute and that centers may vary in their approach to affected patients. Therefore, unless you have one of a few incontrovertible exclusionary conditions, such as terminal liver disease, incurable cancer, or AIDS, you should be evaluated by a transplant professional before concluding that you would not be considered. Also, remember that if one transplant program says no, another may say yes, and you are entitled to a second opinion.

What Are the Chances That a Kidney Transplant Will Work, and If It Does, How Long Will It Last?

Although almost all living donor kidney transplants start functioning immediately, function is delayed in about 20% to 40% of kidneys transplanted from deceased donors. This is known as delayed graft function (DGF). Although the great majority of kidneys affected by DGF eventually work, dialysis often is required until the transplant starts functioning.

Long-term success in kidney transplantation generally is measured by "graft survival" rates, defined as the percentage of transplants working after a certain period. These rates are higher among recipients of living donor kidneys than among recipients of deceased donor kidneys. Overall, about 90% to 95% of kidney grafts are functioning one year after transplantation, 67% to 80% at 5 years, and 40% to 55% at 10 years. This means that although most kidney transplants function early and last for years, there is a significant rate of attrition such that by 10 years, about half of all grafts have failed. In general, if you opt for a transplant, the sooner you undergo transplantation, the better. A kidney transplant performed before you need to start dialysis (preemptive transplantation) usually lasts longer than one performed after dialysis has been initiated, and longer times on dialysis before transplantation correlate with shorter graft survival.

Why Are Kidney Grafts Lost?

The body sees the transplant as something foreign and therefore as potentially harmful, like bacteria. Not surprisingly, the body acts to rid itself of the invading kidney by mounting an immunological attack against it, a process known as rejection. There are two main types of rejection: acute and chronic. Whereas acute rejection (i.e., rejection that starts suddenly and usually soon after transplantation) often can be treated successfully, chronic rejection progresses slowly and is difficult to treat. Chronic rejection is one of the most common causes of graft loss (see "What If My Transplanted Kidney Never Works or Stops Working?")

Does Kidney Transplantation Affect Length and Quality of Life?

Evidence strongly suggests that kidney transplantation provides an important survival benefit compared with dialysis. More than 95% of transplanted patients are alive one year after transplantation, and 80% to 90% are alive five years later. This survival rate is significantly better than that of patients who remain on conventional (thrice-weekly) dialysis, even those considered well enough to be listed for transplantation.

In general, patients who have a functioning kidney transplant have a better quality of life than do patients who remain on dialysis. After successful transplantation, dietary restrictions usually are relaxed, travel becomes easier because there is no need to arrange for or perform dialysis, and there is more time and freedom to return to structured activities, such as work and school. Transplantation can restore independence and allow people to resume their prior position in the family. Perception of general health, physical and social functioning, energy level, and stamina all are better in transplant recipients than in dialysis patients. This is not surprising, because a successful kidney transplant may replace all lost kidney functions, whereas dialysis never does.

What Are the Risks of Kidney Transplantation?

Complications may occur at any time following transplantation. This section considers those that develop soon after surgery. (Long-term complications are discussed later in the chapter.) Because the rate at which these occur may vary among transplant centers, we recommend asking your transplant center for its own surgical mortality and complication rate. Here we provide some ballpark figures.

The combined operative and perioperative mortality of renal transplantation is very low, about 1%. This rate likely correlates inversely with the surgeon's and the center's experience, but even among less experienced programs, average mortality rates are much less than 2%. Patient-related factors such as obesity and cardiovascular health usually are much more important determinants of outcome than the center you choose. A thorough pre-transplant evaluation (see later), which all centers require, will identify potential problems and allow the center to gauge your risk before transplantation.

Many other complications may occur soon after renal transplantation. The most common surgical ones include wound infection (about 5%) and an incisional hernia (about 5%), which is a weakness of the abdominal wall at the surgical site. Obesity is a major risk factor for these complications, meaning that if you are overweight, you can reduce your risk by losing weight before surgery. To minimize the risk of serious bleeding during and after surgery, you must inform your physician if you are taking blood thinners such as Coumadin

Kidney Transplantation Procedure

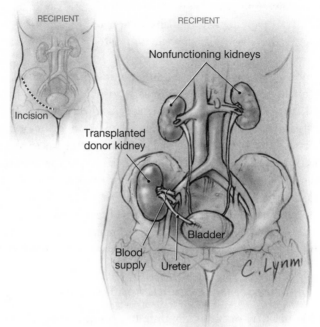

Figure 8.1. A diagram showing a typical location and connections of a transplanted kidney in relation to native kidneys. Reprinted with permission from *JAMA* 2009, 301:1730.

(warfarin), Plavix (clopidogrel), or aspirin. If the indications for these medications permit, you may be asked to stop them for a brief period before your surgery. Failure to follow this advice may result in cancellation of your transplant. Other possible surgical complications include blockage of or leakage from blood vessels, lymph vessels, and the ureter (the tube that carries urine from the kidney to the bladder; see Figure 8.1).

Before and after surgery, you will receive many new medications designed to prevent certain common infections and to prevent rejection of your transplant. These medications may cause serious side effects, and you should review these with your physician before surgery.

Taking good care of yourself (by not smoking and by following your physician's recommendations regarding diet, medication, exercise, dialysis, office visits, and laboratory tests) before as well as after transplantation is very important. The healthier you are at the time of transplantation, the less likely you will experience complications and the more likely your transplant will be successful.

If I Pursue a Renal Transplant, What Costs Will I Incur?

Kidney transplantation is expensive. Fortunately, there are several financial assistance programs that usually cover most of the costs. The most important of these is Medicare, a federal health insurance program available to people 65 and older, those with certain disabilities, and all ESRD patients who have worked and contributed enough to social security to meet eligibility requirements. A useful review of Medicare coverage of dialysis and kidney transplant services may be found at http://www.medicare.gov/Publications/Pubs/pdf/10128 .pdf.

All the direct costs related to your pre-transplant evaluation are covered, and you should not receive a bill for them. Your transplant program will make sure you have insurance to cover most, if not all, of the costs of surgery and hospitalization, but deductibles may apply. In rare instances, your insurance plan may consider your transplant center out of network. This will be addressed by your center before transplantation, and if this is the case, you may wish to transfer to an in-network center.

The greatest financial burden faced by recipients occurs after surgery and is posed by the great expense of essential medications. Although insurance covers much of these costs, many patients discover that high co-payments and yearly caps on medication costs apply, depending on the type of coverage they have. If Medicare is your primary insurance and if you have part B or are eligible for it, Medicare will cover 80% of the cost of your immunosuppressive medications, which may exceed 15,000 dollars per year, for at least thirty-six months. Medicare part D coverage may pick up the cost of other medications as well. If you are eligible for Medicare only because of having ESRD, immunosuppressive drug coverage will end after three years; however, if you are eligible for Medicare because of age or disability, coverage will continue for the life of the transplant. If you are not eligible for Medicare, you may be eligible for Medicaid. Also, many private insurance companies cover many of the costs of transplantation, including those not covered by Medicare. Incidental costs for food, travel, and lodging are not covered, and you will not be reimbursed for time off from work. However, you may be entitled to up to 12 weeks of job-protected, but unpaid, time off under the

federal Family and Medical Leave Act (for more information, go to
http://www.dol.gov/esa/whd/fmla). Finding insurance coverage for
transplant surgery and immunosuppressive (and other) medications
(which must be taken for the life of your transplant) may be challenging but rarely is an insurmountable barrier. Your transplant center has
counselors who will work with you to develop a financial plan. It is
important to develop such a plan very early in the process.

If I Opt for a Transplant, Which Donor Source Is Best, Who May Serve as a Living Donor, and What Are the Different Types of Deceased Donors?

As previously mentioned, transplanted kidneys may come from
deceased or living donors. If a potential living donor is available,
then you will have to make a choice. This decision may be difficult.
To help you decide, we review the advantages and disadvantages of
each donor type.

Living Donor versus Deceased Donor Kidney Transplantation

Living donor (LD) kidney transplantation offers several advantages
compared with deceased donor (DD) transplantation. LD kidneys are
less likely to be damaged during recovery and, as previously mentioned, usually function immediately – many DD kidneys do not.
LD transplantation may be scheduled electively when the recipient's
condition is optimal. LD transplantation avoids the long waiting time
experienced by most recipients of DD kidney transplants and sometimes may be performed even before the recipient has started dialysis.
The health history of an LD is almost always better known than that
of a DD (which is relevant to the risk of transmitting infectious or
malignant disease via the donated kidney). In addition, the function
of LD kidneys is evaluated more carefully, and often they come from
donors who are younger than those of DD kidneys. All these factors
contribute to the superior outcome seen after LD versus DD renal
transplantation: about 90% of LD kidney grafts are functioning after
three years versus slightly fewer than 80% of DD grafts – and this
discrepancy in graft survival continues to widen over time.

The major disadvantage of LD transplantation is the risk to the
donor. Fortunately, the risk of removing one kidney from a healthy
person is very low. After laparoscopic nephrectomy (i.e., kidney
removal by a minimally invasive technique requiring only a few small

incisions), donors usually are discharged within two days and generally return to normal activities in two to four weeks. Complications occur in fewer than 10% of donors, and most of these are minor. The mortality rate of the donor surgery is about 0.03% (3 in 10,000). As you would expect, after donating a kidney, overall kidney function initially goes down by 50%, but the function of the remaining kidney increases to compensate so that it quickly reaches about 75% of the pre-donation level within days. This "residual" kidney function is sufficient to maintain good health, and the survival of healthy kidney donors is at least as good as that of the general population.

Besides posing risk of physical harm, kidney donation also disrupts one's normal routine. This is a special problem for caregivers, such as parents of young children, and for people who work or attend school. Thus, it is not surprising that many potential recipients are hesitant to accept a kidney from a living donor, not only because of the medical risk of donating but also because of concern about the inconvenience and disruption of the donor's ability to fulfill his or her normal responsibilities. Some potential recipients also are fearful of damaging relationships by incurring a debt they can never repay and feeling permanently beholden to the donor. These issues may be difficult to resolve, and there are no easy answers. If you have such feelings, it may help to ask yourself what you would want to do if the situation were reversed? That is, what if you were healthy and the person volunteering to help you needed a kidney? It also may be helpful to speak to actual recipients and donors of LD kidneys. Your center may be able to provide contact information for some who are willing to share their experiences.

Who Can Be a Living Kidney Donor?

Living kidney donors once were restricted to biologically related family members, but this no longer is the case. Today, any healthy adult with two normal kidneys, a compatible blood type, and a negative "crossmatch" (a test that, if positive, makes rapid severe rejection likely) may donate a kidney to you. Although blood relatives of the recipient are still the most common type of LD, spouses and friends now contribute importantly to the donor pool. Some transplant centers are even willing to consider strangers who offer to donate a kidney anonymously to someone on the transplant waiting list. According to the United Network for Organ Sharing (UNOS), of the 6,039 LD kidney transplants performed in the United States in 2007, about a third of the kidneys came from genetically unrelated donors, 752 of whom were spouses. The message here is that you should assume any healthy adult who offers to donate a kidney to you without expectation of financial reward is eligible to donate until proven otherwise. Paying for organs is illegal in the United States under the directives of the National Organ Transplant Act (NOTA).

If you decide to pursue LD transplantation and are fortunate enough to have several willing suitable volunteers, you will have to choose among them. Donors whose human leukocyte antigen (HLA) pattern is very closely matched to that of their recipients provide superior long-term results compared with donors who are less well matched. However, matching is less important today than it was in the past, and many experts believe transplants from spouses do just as well as those from parents or most siblings. Still, there are two situations in which close HLA matching affords clearly superior results: transplantation between identical twins – which provides excellent long-term results without immunosuppression – and between HLA-identical non-twin siblings. There is a 25% chance any sibling pair (with the same two parents) inherited the same sets of HLA genes from each parent and are thus HLA identical. Donor age also may affect outcome. Transplants from donors older than 55 to 60 may not last as long as those from younger donors, but older kidneys still provide results superior to those provided by dialysis.

When choosing among several potential living donors, nonmedical issues also may be very important. For example, you may wish to consider the potential donors' ages (even when younger than 60), responsibilities (e.g., to dependent children, school, work) that would be interrupted by donating, your past and anticipated future relationships with these volunteers, and their level of commitment. Missed appointments at the transplantation center are a strong sign that the volunteer is at least ambivalent about donating; in general, such people should be eliminated from your pool of potential donors.

Living Donor Paired Kidney Exchanges

If your potential donor is incompatible with you based on blood type or a positive crossmatch, you may wish to consider entering an LD exchange program. Under this program, two or more incompatible donor–recipient pairs exchange donors and recipients, thereby creating compatible pairs and utilizing volunteers who previously would have been excluded from the donor pool. Figure 8.2 provides an example of how this works. In this scenario, the wife of recipient 1 cannot donate to her husband because of a positive crossmatch, but

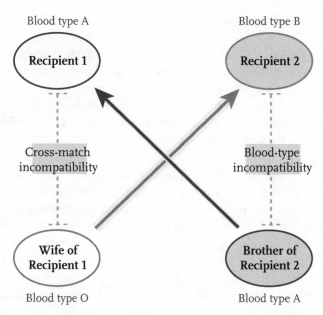

Figure 8.2. How living donor paired kidney exchanges work. Reproduced with permission from *N Engl J Med* 2004, 350:1812.

she can donate to recipient 2 because blood group O is the "universal donor." The brother (blood type A) of recipient 2 is blood group incompatible with his sibling (blood type B) but blood group compatible and crossmatch negative with recipient 1; therefore, he can donate to him.

Categories of Deceased Kidney Donors

There are three types of deceased kidney donors: standard criteria donors (SCD), expanded criteria donors (ECD), and donors after cardiac death (DCD). SCD kidneys may be thought of as ideal kidneys and are the benchmark against which other deceased donor (DD) kidneys are judged. ECD kidneys are not ideal because of donor characteristics that increase the likelihood of graft failure (age 60 or older, hypertension, reduced renal function, and/or death from a stroke): their one-year graft survival is about 84%, versus 91% for SCD kidneys.

Most DD kidneys are recovered from "heart–beating donors": those declared dead based on the loss of all brain function (brain death) but whose hearts continue to beat and in whom lung function is maintained by a mechanical ventilator. In contrast, DCD kidneys are recovered from individuals minutes after their hearts have stopped beating. DCD donors are people who are near death and on a ventilator; they – or much more commonly, their health care surrogates – decide to have the ventilator removed and agree to have this withdrawal of support take place in the operating room to facilitate organ recovery. After the ventilator is removed, if the patient fails to breathe and the heart stops for at least two minutes, the patient is declared dead on the basis of permanent loss of heart and lung function, and the organs are recovered.

Because the results of transplants with ECD kidneys on average are not as good as those with SCD kidneys, according to UNOS (see http://www.unos.org), you will be asked by your transplant center if you would accept a kidney from an ECD donor. The following considerations should help you decide. The waiting time for an ECD kidney may be considerably shorter than for an SCD kidney. Therefore, accepting an ECD kidney may provide advantages compared with waiting the extra time it may take to locate an SCD kidney. However, recent data show that only certain groups derive a survival benefit from this approach, including recipients older than 39 years who live in areas where the waiting time for a DD kidney exceeds 3.5 years, especially if they are diabetic. Although some centers consider DCD kidneys to be less than ideal, graft survival after DCD kidney transplants, at least from donors younger than 50 years, is similar to that following SCD transplants, despite an increased rate of delayed graft function (DGF). Based on the near equivalency of outcome, UNOS policy does not require transplant centers to ask potential recipients if they would be willing to accept DCD kidneys, as it does for ECD kidneys. If you are offered an ECD kidney, before deciding, you should discuss this with your nephrologist (kidney doctor) and transplant team. Many patients obtain excellent results with ECD kidneys despite their lower quality compared with SCD kidneys.

If I Choose to Pursue Deceased Donor Transplantation, When and How Do I Get on the Waiting List and How Long Must I Wait?

UNOS maintains and manages the recipient waiting list, which is nationwide, matching organs from deceased donors to potential recipients. Only patients who have permanently lost most of their kidney function and have a glomerular filtration rate (GFR – the rate at which the kidneys filter fluid from the blood) less than 20 mL/min or are receiving chronic dialysis are eligible to be listed. Some UNOS regions only allow listing once you are on dialysis, and new rules are being proposed that would make the date of your first dialysis your listing date (which determines when you start receiving credit for time on the list – see later). If you have chronic kidney disease but have not yet started dialysis, your nephrologist can tell you if your GFR is less than 20 mL/min. Even if your GFR is above this level, it is a good idea to learn about transplantation so that you will be prepared if you ever need it. In addition to discussions with your physician, helpful printed and video educational resources are available.

To get on the waiting list, you must be seen and evaluated at a UNOS-approved transplant center. Your nephrologist will probably refer you, but you can also self-refer (schedule your own appointment), which is common practice among people who register at more than one center. If your kidneys are failing and your physician has not raised the possibility of transplantation, don't hesitate to ask about it. Remember, it is important to advocate for yourself and not assume that if your nephrologist has not mentioned transplantation, then it must not be appropriate. After the referral is made, the center will invite you to come in for education about transplantation and a detailed medical and psychosocial evaluation (which often requires several visits). If the center finds you to be an acceptable candidate, it will add your name to the national waiting list.

Once on the waiting list, you are eligible to receive kidney offers. While you are waiting, it is very important to notify your transplant center, which may or may not be the hospital at which you receive your other medical care, of changes in your medical status. This will reduce the possibility of your being called in for a transplant at a time when you are not suitable for transplantation – for example, during an active infection or after a recent heart attack.

Because there are not enough kidneys for everyone on the ever-growing national waiting list, which now contains about 75,000 names, an approach to equitable distribution is necessary. In the United States, deceased donor kidneys are procured and distributed by organ procurement organizations (OPOs) according to UNOS policies. Currently, allocation of deceased donor kidneys is based on several factors, including the location of recovery (recovered kidneys are offered first to local patients), blood type, and a point system. The point system is based on three factors: time on the list, the degree of recipient and donor tissue matching, and the presence (or absence) of high levels of antibodies that greatly limit the chance of finding a compatible kidney. How long you will have to wait for a kidney depends on the number of points assigned to you, your blood type (people with blood types O and B wait the longest), where you live, and whether you are willing to accept an ECD kidney. Your transplant center can tell you what the average waiting time is for people with similar characteristics listed at that center.

If I Choose to Pursue Deceased Donor Transplantation, May I Be Listed at More Than One Transplant Center?

Under UNOS policy, you may register at more than one transplant center. This is called "multiple listing." Some potential recipients choose to do this in the hope of shortening the waiting time for a transplant. For this approach to be effective, you must register at transplant centers in different OPO regions, because all patients registered at centers served by the same OPO are listed on a single local waiting list (a subdivision of the national list). In the United States, waiting times vary (sometimes dramatically) from region to region.

Each center requires its own evaluation to determine acceptability. Therefore, if you choose to multiple list, it is important to check that your insurance will cover the cost of nonemergency medical care outside your area of residence. You also should consider the added cost and inconvenience of travel and lodging, not only for yourself but also for family members and friends who will want to visit you during your hospitalization.

Unconventional Approaches to Donor Recruitment

Two new approaches to donor recruitment are being used: transplant tourism and living donor solicitation via the Internet.

Transplant Tourism

Transplant tourism refers to travel to a foreign country, most often China, India, or the Philippines, to obtain a kidney transplant. After transplantation, the recipient returns home and seeks follow-up care at a local transplant center. The source of the transplanted organ may be a living or deceased donor native to the country where the transplant is performed; alternatively, the recipient may bring a person from his or her country of origin to serve as a living donor.

We discourage this practice for several reasons. The most important one is that when transplantation is performed in countries without stringent regulation of this complex process, the risks for the recipient (and the donor) may be greatly increased. Although some recipients of these transplants have done well, others have experienced complications resulting from poor surgical technique; inadequate infection control practices, leading to serious and even life-threatening infections; over- or under-immunosuppression; poor postoperative care; or insufficient or absent communication from the transplanting to the receiving center. In addition to presenting these serious medical concerns, transplant tourism is ethically troubling, at least when deceased donor kidneys are involved, because this practice diverts a precious resource to wealthy people and away from the local population.

Living Donor Solicitation via the Internet

MatchingDonors.com is the Internet address of a nonprofit organization founded in 2004 whose stated mission is to find altruistic unrelated living kidney donors for renal transplant candidates. For a fee ($595 for a lifetime membership, $295 for one month, no fee if you are indigent), you can register as a potential recipient. Registered volunteers can search the personal information you choose to post on the website, after which they may contact you (by e-mail) and offer to donate a kidney. If you accept an offer, the potential donor contacts your transplant center and the living donor process proceeds normally. Free air transportation for testing and surgery is available for patients and donors through the MatchingDonors program. Although the program has some appeal and is legal, it has yet to reach its full potential. At the time of this writing (December 2009) 7,394 potential donors and 505 potential recipients were registered on the MatchingDonors site. Given this high ratio of potential donors to recipients one would expect that most of the registered recipients would soon undergo transplantation. However, as of December 29, 2009, only 106 kidney transplants had been arranged. Part of the explanation may lie in the number of people who register as potential donors but who do not follow through. Furthermore, the program is controversial because of concern about fairness (some potential recipients may be more computer savvy and appealing than others) and the possibility that some of the volunteers have ulterior motives (which is supported by our own experience). Not surprisingly, many transplant centers are unwilling to transplant donor–recipient pairs matched on the Internet.

How Do I Choose a Transplant Center?

If you live in an area that has several transplant centers (or you have the means to travel frequently), you will have to choose a center. Deciding which transplant center is "best" for you depends on personal preferences as well as center characteristics. One way to compare centers is to examine their results. Each transplant center is required to maintain and report statistical information such as its percentage of kidney transplants that last one year and longer (i.e., one- and three-year graft survival). These results can be found on the Scientific Registry of Transplant Recipients website: www.ustransplant.org.

It is important to understand that these data are averages and give the expected results for most recipients; the outcome for any individual may differ greatly. Furthermore, most centers' overall results are similar (see "What Are the Chances That a Kidney Transplant Will Work, and If It Does, How Long Will It Last?"). It is unlikely that differences of a few percentage points in these averages are meaningful for any given patient. Moreover, variations in center acceptance criteria affect the results. For example, some centers may accept very sick potential recipients that other centers would refuse. Such a liberal selection policy may have a negative impact on a center's results, even if it delivers excellent care. Another caution is that the reported data often are several years old. The bottom line is that for a standard kidney transplant, most U.S. centers are comparable; most use similar surgical procedures and immunosuppressive medications, and most offer excellent care. Thus, which center is performing the procedure generally is not a major determinant of outcome. The quality of the transplanted organ and the health of the recipient are much more important.

Before and after your kidney transplant, you will form and maintain a close relationship with a team of transplant professionals. It is important that you feel comfortable with them and they are responsive to your needs. You can assess this during the evaluation process (discussed later) and by talking to other patients who have received transplants at the center you are considering.

When choosing a center, your nephrologist can be very helpful. Usually, but not always, he or she will be aware of the quality of care provided and the level of satisfaction among patients who have received transplants at centers in your area. If your hospital and/or dialysis center are affiliated with a transplant program, there are advantages to listing with that program, including physicians who know you, a familiar environment and staff, easy access to your medical records, and better continuity of care.

Another issue that may be important to you is which physicians will provide your long-term care. Will it be your nephrologist, the transplant center, or a combination of both? You should inquire about this during your pre-transplant evaluation. After discharge from the hospital, the transplant center will follow up with you closely, but after a certain period, the center likely will transfer your care back to your original nephrologist. If you undergo transplantation at a center far from your home, most if not all of your long-term follow-up care will be provided by your primary nephrologist with the help of a local transplant center (if there is one – some rural communities do not have local centers).

There may be medical reasons to choose a center other than the one closest to your home. For example, not all centers perform combined organ transplants (e.g., kidney and heart); if you need such a procedure, your choice of centers is limited. Also, if your blood group is incompatible or you have a positive crossmatch with your potential donor, transplantation still may be possible if you can find a center willing to proceed in the face of these immunological barriers. Not all do, because of the increased risk and complexity of such transplants.

If you do not have a living donor, you may decide to be listed for a deceased donor transplant at several centers (see previous discussion on multiple listing) in the hope of reducing your waiting time for a kidney. A final issue you may wish to consider is the size of the transplant program. Although outcome is not clearly related to center size, some people may find smaller programs more personal and easier to navigate, whereas others may find the greater experience of larger centers comforting.

What Should I Expect during the Evaluation Process, the Surgery, and the Postoperative Period?

The Evaluation

During the pre-transplant evaluation, you will receive information about kidney transplantation, become familiar with the transplant staff, and experience the facility where much of your care will take place. This is the time to decide if you are comfortable with the center. You will have the opportunity to ask questions, and it is a good idea to write them down before, during, and after your evaluation. Patient education is crucial to successful transplantation, and the quality of communication and the level of connection are important indicators of your compatibility with the program.

Although the evaluation affords you the opportunity to evaluate the transplant center, its main purpose is to determine whether you are an appropriate candidate for transplantation. Three major areas will be explored during this process: medical, psychosocial, and financial/insurance.

Medical

The transplant team will assess your overall health, focusing on medical conditions that affect the risk of surgery, your ability to tolerate immunosuppressive medication, and the likely outcome of a kidney transplant. Major active infections, severe heart disease, and recent cancers are examples of conditions that preclude transplantation, at least until those conditions are resolved (see "Exclusion Criteria"). Don't assume you are too sick or unfit to receive a transplant – if you are interested, consult your transplant center. Your nephrologist may be very helpful here, but the final decision rests with the center. Also, exclusion criteria may vary from center to center, which are more liberal than in the past. For example, many centers now consider potential recipients over 70 years old, and some will even consider HIV-infected patients whose infection is well controlled.

You will be required to undergo a detailed medical evaluation. Although centers vary in their required testing, some tests are common to all programs. Simple blood tests will determine your blood type, whether you have antibodies against your potential donor, and whether you have been infected by a harmful agent (e.g., HIV or hepatitis) that may be activated by immunosuppression. Other necessary blood tests include a complete blood count, a "chemistry panel," and blood clotting studies. Your heart's function and blood supply will be assessed by a stress test, an echocardiogram, and perhaps a coronary angiogram (cardiac catheterization). Pre-transplant cancer screening also is important; required tests include a Pap smear, a mammogram, and a colonoscopy, as recommended for the general population based on age, sex, and family history of cancer. If you have had some of these tests recently, and the results are available, most centers will not ask you to repeat them. Depending on your history, you may be asked to undergo other studies as well. This detailed evaluation may uncover unsuspected health problems, and although these tests may be beneficial, some have inherent risks. Moreover, the discovery of some conditions (e.g., cancer) may be disturbing and affect insurability. As a result, most centers require written consent for the evaluation.

Psychosocial

As part of the evaluation, you will meet with a social worker and possibly a psychiatrist. Mental health problems and substance abuse may adversely affect outcome and must be addressed and managed before transplantation. The social worker also will assess your home situation to ensure that you will have adequate care and support after leaving the hospital.

Financial/Insurance

Kidney transplantation (like dialysis) is expensive. Although most recipients can obtain coverage for the costs of surgery, hospitalization, and follow-up care, long-term coverage for immunosuppressive and other essential medications may not always be available (see "If I Pursue a Renal Transplant, What Costs Will I Incur?"). Sadly, some patients lose their transplanted kidneys because of an inability to obtain medications. For this reason, inability to obtain coverage or pay for medications is a contraindication to kidney transplantation. During your evaluation, the social worker and/or financial coordinator will review your financial and insurance situation to be sure that the transplant procedure, as well as essential post-transplant medications, will be covered. If not, they will help you find necessary funding.

Getting and Staying on the Waiting List

It is a common misconception that simply appearing for the pre-transplant evaluation automatically places you on the waiting list for a deceased donor kidney transplant. In fact, only after your evaluation has been completed, which could take several weeks or even months, will the medical team decide whether you are an acceptable transplant candidate. You can expedite this process by keeping appointments, knowing which tests are needed, and making sure results of tests performed outside the center are forwarded to your transplant team. If the team finds you acceptable, you will be placed on the waiting list and notified in writing. If you have not received an acceptance letter within a few weeks of completing your evaluation, we recommend you call the center to check your status.

Once you have been placed on the waiting list, the transplant center will request periodic blood samples (usually sent from your dialysis center), which are tested for compatibility (crossmatched) with kidneys that may be offered to you. The transplant center also may require periodic health updates, because your medical condition may change. Furthermore, it is important for you to inform the center of any intercurrent illnesses or other changes in your health (see "If I Choose to Pursue Deceased Donor Transplantation, When and How Do I Get on the Waiting List and How Long Must I Wait?").

The Surgery and Postoperative Period

Your new kidney will be inserted through an incision (typically four to five inches long) just above your right or left groin. The artery and vein of the kidney will be connected to one of your arteries and one of your veins, and the donor ureter (the tube that carries the urine from the kidney) will be connected to your bladder so that after transplantation you will urinate normally (see Figure 8.1). Unless your kidneys are extremely large (as may happen in polycystic disease) or chronically infected, they will not be removed. The transplant procedure takes about two to three hours and is performed under general anesthesia.

Assuming all goes well – which usually is the case – after surgery you likely will go to a room on a transplant floor. You should be awake and talking soon after surgery. Although postoperative pain is unavoidable, it usually is managed easily with patient-controlled anesthesia (PCA). PCA allows patients to self-administer small amounts of morphine or similar medication with the push of a button. By the first day after surgery, assuming postoperative pain has decreased significantly – as it usually does – you will be encouraged to start walking. Early ambulation helps reduce the risk of serious postoperative complications.

Your hospitalization may be as short as four days, but lengths of stay vary depending on the center and your medical condition. Several problems can delay discharge. Some transplants (particularly those from deceased donors) may not function immediately (see "What Are the Chances That a Kidney Transplant Will Work, and If It Does, How Long Will It Last?"). When this happens, dialysis will be provided until the transplanted kidney starts to work. Other kidneys function "too well," and for a short time produce so much urine that intravenous fluids are needed to prevent water and electrolyte depletion.

Before discharge, it is essential that you have all your medicines and that you are able and know how to take them according to the prescribed schedule. After discharge, it is a good idea to carry a list of your medications at all times and to wear a medical alert bracelet indicating you have received a transplant.

In the absence of complications, the surgical wound will heal rapidly and the convalescent period may be surprisingly rapid. After a successful kidney transplant, there often is an immediate sense of improved well-being, and many patients are functioning almost normally within one to two weeks. Although the vast majority of kidney transplants are successful, postoperative problems can delay recovery.

These problems include slow wound healing and infection, which are more common in patients who are diabetic or overweight (see "What Are the Risks of Kidney Transplantation?"). Medication side effects, such as diarrhea and low white blood cell counts, are not uncommon (see later). Most postoperative complications can be treated successfully.

How Much Help Will I Need after the Transplant?

How much help you will require after the transplantation depends on your pre-transplant health and independence. Highly functional patients whose transplants proceed without major complications can care for themselves and perform activities of daily living by the time of discharge. Before leaving the hospital, the transplant team will assess your needs and make sure an adequate home support system is in place.

What If My Transplanted Kidney Never Works or Stops Working?

Although most transplanted kidneys function for years, a few do not. Permanent failure of transplanted kidneys may occur in three ways:

1. *The kidney never functions* – A very small number of kidney transplants (less than 2%) never work. This rare situation, called primary nonfunction, is more likely to occur with deceased donor transplants.
2. *The kidney works initially but then stops working abruptly because of severe rejection or some other complication* – Acute rejection is a condition in which the recipient's immune system attacks the transplanted kidney as if it were a foreign invader (see "Why Are Kidney Grafts Lost?"). There are several types of acute rejection, and each type may vary in severity. Up to 20% of all kidney transplant patients experience acute rejection during the first post-transplant year. However, because of improvements in immunosuppressive regimens, many centers now report acute rejection rates of 10% or less. Fortunately, most acute rejections (about 90%) can be partially or completely reversed if treated early, which is one reason for careful monitoring during the first year after transplantation, when acute rejections are most likely to occur. Less common causes of early transplant failure include viral infections (especially BK polyomavirus) and clotting within small blood vessels (hemolytic uremic syndrome).
3. *The kidney works at first, then slowly loses function over months to years* – This is a common problem and has many causes, including episodes of incompletely reversed acute rejection, chronic rejection, drug-induced injury, high blood pressure, and diabetes. Although very few of the many kidney

diseases that cause ESRD present contraindications to transplantation, some may recur in the graft and contribute to loss of kidney function. Recurrent disease does not necessarily lead to graft loss, but in some cases, it does.

If your kidney transplant fails, you will have to return to dialysis unless a living donor is available, in which case you may be able to undergo a second transplantation before dialysis becomes necessary. If you still are an acceptable candidate, you also may be placed on the deceased donor waiting list for a second kidney transplant. In general, second (and third) transplants have a higher risk of rejection, but the long-term results still may be excellent. As with first transplants, outcome depends largely on the quality of the organ being transplanted and the general health of the recipient.

What If I Don't Like the Physician or Another Member of the Team Caring for Me?

Conflicts between health care providers on the transplant team and patients can usually be resolved. However, if resolution is not possible, you have the right to transfer your care to another member of the team or to another center.

What If I Am Invited to Participate in a Research Study?

Either before or after receiving a kidney transplant, your doctors may invite you to participate in a research study. This is entirely up to you. Lack of participation will not affect the quality of your care or your waiting time for a kidney. On the other hand, participation in the study might afford you the benefits of a new drug or protocol that turns out to be superior to current therapy. Before you decide whether or not to participate, you should learn all the known risks, purposes, and potential benefits of the study. If you choose to partici-pate, you may withdraw at any time. However, if you think you might withdraw before the study is completed, you should discuss this with the transplant team before you sign on.

How Often Will I Need to Be Seen by My Doctor? How Important Are Follow-Up Visits?

Careful follow-up is critical to the success of kidney transplantation. After discharge, medication dosages must be adjusted, side effects must be dealt with, kidney function has to be monitored, and infections must be prevented, and treated if they occur. Rejection and infection are two of the most important dangers after transplantation, and the period of highest risk is the first few postoperative months. These risks never disappear entirely, but they gradually diminish over time. For this reason, close follow-up is particularly important during the early post-transplant period.

For about the first month after surgery, transplant clinic visits and blood tests to monitor graft function and levels of certain medications will be scheduled two or more times each week. Gradually, your medications will be reduced to "maintenance" doses, and if you are doing well, the frequency of office visits will be reduced to every two to four weeks. If after six months your transplant course remains uncomplicated, office visits and blood tests will be required about every two to three months.

It is important to realize that no matter how smooth your post-transplant course, regular follow-up is essential for the life of the graft. Although less common than in the early post-transplant period (defined as the first six months after transplantation), acute rejections and other transplant-specific problems may occur many years after a successful kidney transplant. Some patients mistakenly believe that because their early transplant course went well, regular follow-up is not important or is necessary only when they feel ill.

What Medications Will I Have to Take and for How Long?

Transplant-specific medications fall into two general categories: antimicrobial agents designed to prevent opportunistic infections (infections that occur primarily in people with weakened immune systems) and immunosuppressive agents designed to prevent transplant rejection. Immunosuppressive agents must be taken for the life of the graft. The only exceptions to this rule are transplants between identical twins and patients enrolled in research protocols designed to achieve "tolerance," a state in which the body no longer sees a transplant as a foreign invader. Additional medications may be required to treat high blood pressure, diabetes, and elevated cholesterol, as well as any other medical problems. It is apparent that the general issues of medication can be quite complex and will require patients to follow through on their medications and careful monitoring by the medical team.

What Are the Common Side Effects of Transplant Medications?

Any drug may cause unwanted side effects, and transplant medications are no exception. How many side effects you will experience, if any, cannot be predicted. Transplant professionals are trained to look for adverse effects and adjust the medications to avoid or minimize them, which is another reason regular follow-up is so important.

How Much Do the Medications Cost, and Who Pays for Them?

Transplant medications cost thousands of dollars per month, and most patients need insurance coverage to pay for them. Even when you have such coverage, large co-payments may apply and maximum yearly allowances for medicines, which are easily exceeded, may be imposed. The transplant social worker and financial coordinator may be invaluable in finding solutions to help pay for medications (see "Financial/Insurance" under "The Evaluation").

Will There Be Physical or Dietary Restrictions after Transplantation?

Successful transplantation lifts many of the dietary restrictions imposed on patients with chronic kidney disease. However, diabetics still must limit carbohydrate and caloric intake and may experience drug-induced exacerbation of glucose intolerance. A heart-healthy diet (i.e., one low in saturated and trans-fats) should be followed, because cardiovascular disease is very common among transplant patients and some immunosuppressive medications may elevate fat levels. Weight gain is a problem for some patients and contributes to elevated blood pressure and lipid levels, as well as to the development or worsening of diabetes. Prednisone contributes to weight gain because it stimulates appetite.

In general, no physical limitations are imposed on kidney transplant recipients. Professional athletes have returned to their sport after successful transplantation. However, you should not engage in strenuous physical activity until your wound has healed completely and you have obtained approval from your transplant physician. Aggressive contact sports that might injure your transplanted kidney (such as tackle football) are discouraged.

Will I Need to Limit Contact with Ill People?

Exposure to crowds, groups of young children in a school or day care setting, and other pools of potentially sick contacts may increase your risk of infection with respiratory and gastrointestinal viruses. It is best to avoid these exposures during the first month after your transplant, but you do not need to be quarantined. If you anticipate exposure to crowded spaces (e.g., traveling on a subway), it is advisable to wear a simple facemask during the first post-transplant month. If a child or other person in your home has contracted an infectious disease (e.g., chickenpox), you should inform your transplant physician immediately. He or she may recommend that you avoid contact with the infected person, especially if you have undergone transplantation recently (within the past month) and are not immune. For the first few months after transplantation, you will be prescribed medications that can prevent some, but not all, infections. However, it is important to understand that these medications will not protect you against common viruses you may be exposed to in crowds and through sick contacts. After the doses of your immunosuppressive medications have been lowered to maintenance levels, your risk of infection will become similar to that of the general population, and you will no longer need to take special precautions.

May I Travel after Transplantation, and Must I Always Be Near a Transplant Center?

Compared with dialysis, successful transplantation provides much greater freedom to travel. However, you should not travel until the frequency of your medical visits has decreased and your doses of medication and kidney function are stable (generally by two to three months after transplantation). At that point, it is not necessary to be near a transplant center, but it is essential that you take your medications and be able to get blood tests at the appropriate interval (see "How Often Will I Need to Be Seen by My Doctor? How Important Are Follow-Up Visits?"). Extended travel to a rural area or a long vacation in a remote location without sophisticated medical services should be delayed for at least six months after transplantation. Even then, you should consider such a trip only if you are stable, with good graft function, and can return for blood tests or have them performed remotely on a schedule acceptable to your transplant team. Most rural and foreign locations have access to e-mail, by which you can contact your transplant program for advice in case of an emergency. It is crucial that you do not run out of medications; some insurance companies allow a "vacation override" that can provide you with coverage for up to six months of medicine.

Travel to undeveloped parts of the world poses a risk of contracting endemic infections not encountered in the developed world (e.g., malaria and certain diarrheal illnesses) for healthy persons as well as those with well-functioning kidney transplants; preventive behavior (e.g., insect repellant, protective clothing, avoidance of contaminated food and water), prophylactic medicines, and vaccines are advised for both groups. Consultation with your transplant physician and a travel medicine specialist is strongly suggested when visiting such locations. For those traveling outside the United States, we also recommend obtaining evacuation and comprehensive medical insurance and carrying medical alert bracelets and cards.

What If I Lose My Medications? Must I Replace Them Immediately, or Can I Skip a Day?

You should always take your medications as prescribed. Although some patients have missed doses without a problem, others have developed acute rejection. However, the fear of losing your pills should not prevent you from traveling. If you lose your medicines, the risk of missing one or two doses, until you can secure replacements, is very small.

Pregnancy after Transplantation

The ability to conceive and carry a pregnancy to term usually is lost in women with advanced kidney failure. Successful kidney transplantation generally restores these functions. However, pregnancy is strongly discouraged during the first several months after transplantation, when kidney function may not yet be stable, doses of medications are being adjusted frequently, and the risk of rejection and infection is greatest. During this early post-transplant period, sexually active premenopausal women should use contraception. In women with good kidney function (serum creatinine less than 1.5 mg/dL) one year after transplantation and without recent rejections, there is little risk pregnancy will damage the transplanted kidney. Under these circumstances, if managed by experienced obstetricians and transplant physicians, most pregnancies (90%) are successful, although they still are considered at increased risk for complications such as premature birth, elevated blood pressure, preeclampsia, and worsening kidney function. During pregnancy, increased monitoring is necessary and medications that might be harmful to the fetus must be discontinued or changed (especially angiotensin-converting enzyme inhibitors and mycophenolate mofetil). An excellent resource for physicians and their transplant patients who want to become pregnant is the National

Transplantation Pregnancy Registry in Philadelphia: (877) 955-6877 or www.temple.edu/ntpr.

Conclusions

Renal transplantation is a complicated, expensive, time-consuming, and hazardous process. Nevertheless, because transplantation is so successful and the only treatment that can fully restore kidney function, generally the benefits far outweigh the risks. Indeed, in the absence of contraindications, transplantation usually is the treatment of choice for patients with advanced, irreversible kidney failure, and private and public funding makes it affordable for most. If you have this condition, we strongly recommend you consider transplantation, and we hope this chapter presents a clear picture of what to expect and what questions to ask. As you explore this subject, you may find UNOS (http://unos.org/SharedContentDocuments/WEPNTK2008.pdf) and the National Kidney Foundation (http://www.kidney.org/atoz/atozItem.cfm?id=86) to be helpful additional resources.

Glossary

Acute rejection – a type of transplant rejection that starts suddenly and usually soon (within the first months) after transplantation; it often is treatable.

Chronic rejection – a type of transplant rejection that occurs slowly and insidiously (over months to years) and is difficult to treat; in contrast to acute rejection, chronic rejection rarely is reversible.

Contraindication – something to make a treatment or procedure inadvisable.

Crossmatch – a test used to predict whether a person's immune system is likely to attack a kidney being offered for transplantation; a positive crossmatch indicates that the risk of rejection is high and may be a reason to decline the offered kidney.

Deceased donor – a recently deceased person from whom organs are removed for transplantation with consent.

DGF – an abbreviation for delayed graft function; this term refers to situations in which kidney grafts do not start functioning very soon after transplantation.

Donation after cardiac death (DCD) – organ recovery from individuals who have been declared dead on the basis of traditional cardiopulmonary (rather than neurological or brain) criteria; at the time of this writing, the great majority of deceased donor organs were recovered from individuals declared dead based on loss of all brain function (i.e., brain death).

ESRD – an abbreviation for end-stage renal disease; this term refers to the irreversible loss of so much kidney function that some form of kidney replacement (either dialysis or a transplant) is necessary to maintain health.

Expanded criteria donor (ECD) – a deceased donor who has one or more risk factors for a transplant outcome that is not as good as that expected with a standard criteria donor.

GFR – an abbreviation for glomerular filtration rate; this term refers to the rate at which the kidneys filter water from the blood, which is the first step in urine formation.

Graft – an organ or tissue transplanted from one person to another.

HLA – an abbreviation for human leukocyte antigen, a series of proteins found on the surface of most cells that allow a person's immune system to recognize a foreign invader when its HLA proteins do not match those of the host. In transplantation, the degree of matching is determined by the number of these proteins (antigens) the recipient has in common with the donor.

Immunosuppressive medications – medicines designed to weaken the immune system and prevent transplant rejection; they also increase the chances of infection.

Laparoscopic nephrectomy – a widely performed surgical technique for removing a kidney from a living donor through a few small holes rather than through a large incision (an "open nephrectomy"); this facilitates rapid recovery.

Multiple listing – the process by which a transplant candidate goes on the waiting list at more than one center (each of which is served by a different organ procurement organization – see text).

Nephrologist – a nonsurgical physician who specializes in the care of people with kidney disease.

Opportunistic infection – an infection usually seen only in people with weakened immune systems (e.g., transplant patients taking immunosuppressive medications).

Preemptive transplantation – kidney transplantation performed before a patient starts dialysis.

Rejection – a complex process by which a recipient's immune system attacks and injures a transplanted organ because it is seen as foreign.

Renal – an adjective meaning "related to kidney"; for example, a renal graft is a kidney that has been transplanted.

Standard criteria donor (SCD) – a deceased donor who has no known risk factors that may compromise transplant outcome; also known as an ideal donor. The waiting times for SCD kidneys often are considerably longer than those for ECD (expanded criteria donor) kidneys.

Tolerance – a poorly understood process by which a transplant (graft) no longer is viewed by the recipient's immune system as foreign and thus no longer is attacked and injured by it; when tolerance develops, which is rare, immunosuppressive medications may be decreased greatly or even eliminated.

UNOS – an abbreviation for the United Network for Organ Sharing; it is a nonprofit organization that manages the nationwide U.S. organ procurement and transplantation network. UNOS collects data on all organ transplants performed in the United States, helps allocate all organs recovered from deceased donors, and develops organ transplantation policy.

Ureter – the tube that carries urine from the kidney to the bladder. Kidney transplant recipients receive both the donor kidney and its ureter.

NINE

When the Illness Is Psychiatric

– Leonard C. Groopman

Medical illnesses target our bodies. Psychiatric illnesses target our selves. Psychiatric disorders, even when understood as disorders of the brain, strike us directly where we live – where we think, feel, and make decisions. Although in recent decades psychiatry has moved further into the mainstream of general medicine, the fact that psychiatric diseases go to the heart of who we are has a profound impact on how these disorders are experienced both by the affected persons and by those around them. Moreover, psychiatric practice differs in significant ways from general medical practice and likely is unfamiliar to many people. For these reasons, psychiatric illness remains a special case, with its own particular features, warranting separate consideration.

Recognizing Psychiatric Disorders

Many psychiatric diagnoses have entered into everyday language and daily use. We now commonly speak of our own – or someone else's – "ADD" or "OCD" or "mania" or "narcissistic personality" or "panic attacks." Our culture has become saturated with popular psychiatry, and we have become a self-diagnosing people. It is important not to jump to conclusions that you or someone else has a psychiatric illness based on a single symptom or a unique experience, or on what you hear on radio or TV, or what you read in a magazine or on the Internet.

For example, everyone experiences difficulty with concentration and attention at times. That does not mean they have attention deficit disorder. Even if a person is distracted often, it does not mean he or she has attention deficit disorder (ADD). Similarly, just about everyone worries excessively at times, or gets excited and agitated, or behaves in a cold and selfish way, or feels panicked. That does not mean they are suffering from obsessive-compulsive disorder, or mania, or narcissistic personality disorder, or panic disorder.

This tendency toward the fast and loose usage of psychiatric vocabulary, fed by the popular media, may lead us unnecessarily to fear we are suffering from psychiatric illness. Paradoxically, it also may lead us in the opposite direction, toward taking psychiatric problems less seriously than other medical problems, because they seem so much a part of everyday life. When we refer casually to our ADD or obsessive-compulsive disorder (OCD), we may not be giving these problems in ourselves or in others the seriousness they deserve.

The popular media are not solely responsible for this paradoxical situation of simultaneously exaggerating the prevalence of psychiatric symptoms and underestimating them. Medical practitioners and psychiatrists themselves also must share the blame. Unlike most other medical specialties, psychiatry lacks diagnostic data such as radiographic findings, blood test abnormalities, or biopsy results. Psychiatric diagnoses, for the most part, are based on the information reported by the patient (and sometimes by third parties, such as family and friends) and on the observations made by an examining psychiatrist. There is no blood test to diagnose bipolar disorder, no x-ray for schizophrenia, and no tissue diagnosis for anorexia nervosa. Yet psychiatric syndromes, like other medical diseases, do represent specific constellations of signs and symptoms that allow trained professionals to identify them as illnesses. Moreover, anyone who has ever suffered from a psychiatric illness, or has been close to someone who has, knows that psychiatric illness is as real as any other medical disease in its impact on the life of the individual and his or her family.

The psychiatric profession itself is partially responsible for the recent tendency toward overdiagnosis as well as some of the consequent skepticism toward psychiatry and psychiatric illnesses. Some psychiatrists unjustifiably have expanded the boundaries of certain diagnostic categories to the point of overinclusiveness. In my view, this has been true in recent years for ADD, OCD, PTSD (post-traumatic stress disorder), and bipolar disorder, among others. These diagnoses represent valid illnesses, but the loosening of the criteria for diagnosis has led to their excessive diagnosis and treatment, and, unfortunately, to cultural skepticism about the validity of psychiatric diagnoses in general.

Fear and stigma still surround psychiatry and psychiatric illness, further complicating the recognition and treatment of psychiatric disorders. Psychiatric illness may conjure up images of losing one's mind and of losing control over one's behavior and oneself. Despite considerable progress in recent decades in attitudes toward mental illness, fear, shame, and worry about stigma lead many people to delay seeking professional help.

Therefore, if you are concerned that you or someone close to you may be suffering from a psychiatric illness, it is especially important that you seek diagnostic consultation from a trusted physician. I recommend that you consult your primary care physician first, rather than going directly to a psychiatrist or other mental health professional. I make this suggestion for several reasons. First, if you have a relationship with a general physician, you already will feel comfortable talking to him or her about your concerns. Second, sometimes medical problems manifest themselves as mental symptoms (e.g., disorders of the thyroid gland may first present as depression), so it is worth having a general medical evaluation before assuming, or concluding, that your problem is psychiatric. Third, most general physicians have psychiatrist colleagues whom they know and trust and to whom they refer their patients. This relationship provides you with a reliable method of finding a treating psychiatrist or other mental health professional.

The Psychiatric Consultation

Let us assume you have been referred by your internist – or in some other way, such as through a friend or a colleague, or by calling your local hospital – to a psychiatrist for a consultation. What should you expect?

Most psychiatric consultations involve one or two meetings, each lasting anywhere from forty-five minutes to an hour and a half. Sometimes the psychiatrist will extend the consultation process beyond two sessions. As with other medical consultations, the psychiatrist will ask why you have come or let you know what your internist, who has referred you, has said about the reason for the consultation. During the course of the consultation process, the psychiatrist will ask you about your current symptoms and concerns; your prior relevant history, if any; and your family history. He or she likely will ask about any medical problems and medications you take as well as your use of alcohol, tobacco, and other drugs. The psychiatrist probably will spend some time asking you about your past, "the story of your life," your work, and your relationships. He or she likely will have a set of questions regarding thoughts, feelings, and behaviors that might be relevant in diagnosing a psychiatric syndrome. For example, if the therapist thinks you might be depressed, he or she likely will ask you questions not only about your mood, but also about your ability to concentrate and your feelings of self-worth, as well as any thoughts you have had about taking your life or harming anyone else. Part of a psychiatric consultation usually involves assessing whether someone is a danger to him- or herself or to others. Finally, whether through a series of formal questions or as part of the ongoing conversation, the psychiatrist will perform what is known as a mental status examination. The mental status examination is the psychiatric equivalent of the physical exam other doctors perform when they see a patient. However, instead of listening to your heart and lungs with a stethoscope or tapping on your knees with a reflex hammer, the psychiatrist, by listening, observing, and questioning, assesses your mental state, including your speech, thought process and content, mood, judgment, insight, and other cognitive abilities.

Toward the end of the consultation, which may last one, two, or more sessions (if the psychiatrist doesn't make clear how long the consultation process likely will last, don't hesitate to ask), the doctor probably will give you his or her sense of what is going on. In other words, like other medical specialists, the therapist will tell you what, based on the time you have spent together, he or she considers to be the likely diagnosis and will offer you some opinions and recommendations. The psychiatrist might remain uncertain about your situation and recommend further assessment, which might include anything from blood tests to psychological tests to a neurological consultation to gathering more history from you or other sources. He or she may conclude you are not suffering from a psychiatric illness and perhaps recommend no treatment, or suggest you wait and see how things evolve over time and return later if you do not feel better. The therapist may offer to treat you personally, or suggest you might be treated more appropriately by another professional if he or she believes the best treatment for you would take place in another setting or be given by someone with skills he or she does not have. Because most psychiatric illnesses can be treated more than one way, upon completing the consultation, you should have a sense of your treatment options. At the same time, because most psychiatrists have preferences with regard to treatment for each of their patients, you also should leave the consultation clearly knowing the psychiatrist's treatment recommendations for you.

What if, at the end of the consultation, you are uncertain about the "chemistry" between you and the psychiatrist? What if you are uncomfortable with or have negative feelings about the doctor? Should you begin treatment nonetheless in the hope that the rapport and your feelings will improve over time? Should you seek consultation with another psychiatrist?

It may, of course, take time to feel comfortable in psychotherapy in general and with any given therapist in particular. However, if you are feeling very uncertain about the doctor, I recommend you seek a second consultation with a different psychiatrist. The relationship with the therapist is an important feature of psychiatric treatment – perhaps more important than the relationship with nonpsychiatric physicians when being treated for strictly medical disorders – and therefore, it is worth trying at the outset to find a therapist with whom the chemistry feels right. Moreover, after you have seen two different psychiatrists, you will have a means of comparison and can make an active choice for yourself. This alone may be valuable therapeutically.

Psychiatric Treatments

What kinds of treatment is the psychiatrist likely to recommend? Psychiatric treatments can be divided broadly into three categories: biological treatments, psychological treatments, and social treatments.

Biological treatments, also known as somatic treatments, directly affect the brain with chemical or electrical means. The most common form of biological treatment is medication, including antidepressants (e.g., fluoxetine, or Prozac), antipsychotics (e.g., risperidone, or Risperdal), antianxiety medications (e.g., diazepam, or Valium), stimulants (e.g., methylphenidate, or Ritalin), and mood stabilizers (e.g., lithium and valproate, or Depakote), as well as other so-called psychotropic medications that affect psychiatric symptoms. In addition to their therapeutic benefits, all psychiatric medications – like medications of any kind – have potential unwanted side effects. If you are placed on a medication as part of your treatment, inquire about the side effects beforehand so you will be prepared if you experience one or more of them.

Pharmaceuticals are not the only form of somatic treatment. Electroconvulsive therapy, known as ECT, also is an important biological treatment for some clinical conditions, especially severe depression and a form of depression known as delusional or psychotic depression. ECT involves electrically inducing a seizure in the patient while the patient is anesthetized and asleep. It has been portrayed in popular culture – most notably in *One Flew over the Cuckoo's Nest* – as cruel and barbaric and continues to generate opposition among some individuals and groups in the general population. However, within the psychiatric profession, ECT is recognized as an effective, safe, and at times lifesaving treatment. I have seen many patients with debilitating depression who did not respond to several courses of antidepressant medication improve dramatically as a result of a course of ECT. A course of ECT usually involves a total of six to ten treatments administered over the course of two to three weeks in the hospital. Psychiatrists who specialize in biological treatments often are called psychopharmacologists.

Whereas somatic therapies work directly on the body, psychological treatments work directly on the mind. There is a wide – sometimes confusing – variety of psychologically based therapies, known collectively as psychotherapies. All of them involve some aspect of talking – hence, they often are called "talking cures" – and some use other treatment methods, such as behavioral exercises or homework, to change cognition, or how a person conceptualizes or gives meaning to his or her experience. Although there are many schools of psychotherapy, broadly speaking, they can be divided into two types: psychodynamic psychotherapies and cognitive-behavioral psychotherapies.

Psychodynamic psychotherapies approach the mind as a field of interacting forces that, under certain conditions – such as trauma, loss, disappointment, or aging – lead to emotional distress and mental disorder (much the same way an internist sees the body as a system of physiological forces that, under certain circumstances – such as infection, vascular blockage, toxic exposure, or immunological failure – lead to physical illness). The therapeutic goal of psychodynamic therapies is the same as the goal of all therapies – relief of suffering. Its therapeutic instrument is insight – the enhancement of one's understanding of one's own emotional and mental life. The exploration of one's inner life usually includes an exploration of one's personal past.

Cognitive-behavioral therapies, also called CBT, approach the mind as a system of beliefs, which, under certain circumstances, lead the person astray, again down the road of emotional distress and mental disorder. CBT tends to focus on changing mistaken beliefs and their resulting behaviors. Like other therapies, CBT's therapeutic goal is relief of suffering, and its main instrument is the correction of pathological beliefs and patterns of thought and behavior. CBT might include a program of testing one's beliefs through guided homework assignments, or changing one's pathological behaviors through a structured program of gradual desensitization. These therapies are more likely to focus on one's present life and are unlikely to involve an extensive exploration of the past, although in the service of understanding the sources of mistaken beliefs, some attention may be paid to the past.

Psychotherapy may involve an individual, a couple, a family, or a group of unrelated people. The consulting psychiatrist usually recommends one of three modes of therapy depending on the problem: individual psychotherapy, if the problem is seen as an individual issue; couples or family therapy, if the problem involves more than the individual; or group therapy, if the person's difficulties are believed best addressed in the context of interactions with others.

In some cases, the duration of psychotherapy is determined at the outset of treatment, in others it is not. The former approach is known as brief or time-limited therapy and the latter as long-term or open-ended psychotherapy.

Although biological and psychological treatments are the most common options, psychiatrists sometimes recommend social therapy or a change in environment. Day programs, which offer a wide complement of therapies for individuals, families, or groups (e.g., those focusing on occupational issues, anger management, eating disorders, or drug abuse), provide a fuller social context for those who may require more regular and intensive treatment for their problem. Also, psychiatrists sometimes recommend a change in social environment, such as a change of job, school, or living situation, as a therapeutic option.

Hospitalization plays an important role in the psychiatric treatment of some patients. Although most patients will never need it, psychiatric hospitalization is strongly indicated for certain situations. The hospital provides a protective environment for suicidal people – those who, in the considered clinical judgment of a doctor, are at sufficient risk for self-harm. The same applies to dangerous or homicidal patients. Hospitalization also can protect patients in a manic state from harming themselves or others by preventing promiscuous sexual behavior or ruinous spending sprees. People engaged in other self-destructive behaviors they cannot control by themselves in their everyday environment – such as drug abuse or self-starvation – also may require a protective and controlled environment such as a hospital or in-patient rehabilitation program.

Some treatments are better performed inside rather than outside a hospital. A course of ECT frequently requires hospitalization, and changes in medication regimen are sometimes done more safely in the monitored environment of a hospital.

Hospitalization is either voluntary or involuntary – that is, the patient consents to it (voluntary) or, under certain circumstances, the patient is hospitalized against his or her will (involuntary). Involuntary hospitalization, or commitment, is reserved for circumstances in which it is determined that the patient, after being examined by two doctors, is dangerous to him- or herself or to others. This generally means the patient is considered imminently suicidal or homicidal or is likely, in some other way, to endanger his or her life or that of another. Involuntary hospitalization cannot continue indefinitely. After a certain period, varying from state to state but generally forty-eight to seventy-two hours, the patient may request to be discharged. The hospital must discharge the patient unless the doctors in the hospital believe he or she remains an imminent danger, in which case the hospital must go to court and argue the case for continued hospitalization before a judge. The patient, with the assistance of legal counsel, provided by the state if necessary, is represented before the judge and can argue for discharge. Depending on the outcome of such a hearing, either the patient is free to leave the hospital or the hospital is allowed to hold the patient for another fixed period.

The optimal treatment of a psychiatric disorder may involve more than one form of therapy, used in combination or in sequence. For example, pharmacological therapy – the use of a medication – may be combined with psychotherapy, or one form of treatment, such as medication, may be initiated and another, such as psychotherapy, added later, depending on the response to the first treatment.

What Causes Psychiatric Illness?

Recent decades have witnessed an explosion of research on the brain and the biology of psychiatric illness, including a search for genetic causes of mental diseases. However, despite many advances in understanding the biology of these disorders, we still do not know what causes them. Our best understanding is that mental illnesses are heterogeneous disorders caused by a variety of factors, from genes and the intrauterine environment of the developing fetus, to the family milieu and wider social world of the developing child, to biological, psychological, and social experiences throughout life.

To illustrate with one example: If one of a pair of identical twins develops schizophrenia, the chance of the other twin having schizophrenia is approximately 50%. This is much higher than the random chance of having schizophrenia, which is 1% in the population at large. However, it is not 100%, despite the fact that the twins are genetically identical. So, in the case of schizophrenia, genetics seems to account for 50% of the cause, whereas other, nongenetic factors contribute the other 50%.

In all likelihood, other psychiatric disorders also result from more than one cause, although the proportions of the sources that make up a particular condition will vary, for the most part these contributing factors are not clear. In their approach to each of their patients, psychiatrists consider different causal factors. Sophisticated psychiatrists think about a patient's illness in terms of three dimensions – biological, psychological, and social – and develop a treatment strategy based on these three factors. They try to take all three variables into account and not become too wedded to any one way of thinking about or seeing their patient and his or her difficulties.

Understanding and Evaluating Psychiatric Treatment

Somatic treatment by a psychiatrist resembles medical treatment by other specialists. A person with a heart condition sees a cardiologist; reports his or her symptoms; answers the cardiologist's questions; is examined; perhaps gets an electrocardiogram, blood test, or scan; and then sits down with the cardiologist to talk about his or her condition and receive the doctor's ongoing recommendations (e.g., increase one medication or decrease another, exercise more, eat less). Similarly, the psychopharmacologist listens to the patient, asks questions, performs (formally or informally) a mental status exam, perhaps orders blood tests (e.g., blood levels of medications or screening tests for medication side effects), and then discusses his or her findings and recommendations with the patient (e.g., increase or decrease the dosage of one medication or another, sleep more, or sleep less).

In contrast, psychological treatments differ significantly from most other medical treatments and therefore may be more difficult for the patient to understand and evaluate. Psychotherapy is an ongoing process, often but not always open ended in terms of duration and content, conducted during regularly scheduled appointments that last a fixed period of time. For example, a typical psychotherapy program might involve one or more weekly sessions of forty-five minutes each in which whatever the patient raises is discussed. The treatment might last anywhere from weeks to months to years.

The material that emerges during therapy sessions often is deeply personal, and the patient's relationship to his or her therapist may become emotionally intense. Given the emotional content of the material – and often of the relationship – for the therapeutic work to take place, the doctor must maintain the framework of therapy. This framework consists of a safe, predictable, and confidential environment; a specific treatment location; appointments of defined duration; and an agreed-upon fee and method of payment. It also includes an asymmetry of self-disclosure between patient and therapist; that is, patients talk about themselves, whereas therapists, for the most part, do not. The therapist's role is to help resolve the problems that brought the patient to treatment, and this is achieved best by creating a safe and secure environment in which this process can take place.

Although a consistent frame is necessary for therapeutic effectiveness, too rigid a frame can impede or stifle therapy. Some flexibility is necessary to respond to the needs of the individual patient. Extending a session by a few minutes because of the emergence of particularly charged content represents therapeutic common sense, just as answering a patient's question about why the therapist unexpectedly had to be out of the office for a week might represent sound clinical judgment. However, repeated extensions of appointment times are a sign of a therapeutic issue that merits discussion (e.g., the patient may feel unsatisfied at the end of the session or anxious about separation). Similarly, a therapist's explaining his or her personal problems without a triggering event constitutes a breach in the therapeutic frame. A handshake at the end of the session might be reassuring to some patients (although worthy of exploration), and an occasional encouraging pat on the back or sympathetic hand on the shoulder might be appropriate at the end of a particularly difficult session. However, other physical contact violates the frame. Although the line between maintaining a flexible frame and violating a therapeutic boundary may not always be clear, as a general principle, if a therapist exploits his or her position for personal gratification, he or she is violating the therapeutic boundaries necessary for treatment to take place.

A secure yet not too rigid frame allows therapist and patient to work together as allies on the patient's behalf. Besides listening and understanding, the therapist likely will probe, confront, or challenge you, at times raising your anxiety or otherwise making you uncomfortable. If this is done in the service of therapy, it is not a boundary violation but a necessary part of treatment. Moreover, most therapists encourage their patients to discuss their feelings about the therapy and the therapist, and it is valuable to do so, whether or not you are uncomfortable with something the therapist is doing. Often, we feel and act with a therapist in a manner similar to how we feel and act with others in our life. This is known as transference. (Therapists also must be sensitive to their own reaction to relationships with patients and deal with it appropriately. This is known as counter-transference.) Recognizing and exploring transference may be a very fruitful aspect of treatment. Whereas in most of our life we cannot explore how and why we feel and act the way we do, in therapy we can explore these questions. Therapy can be a laboratory for observing, understanding, and, yes, changing ourselves, and the exploration of transference may be an important aspect of this process.

It is important, then, to be able to discuss your feelings about therapy and the therapist with the therapist. It also is important to be able to ask questions of the therapist. Given the asymmetry of self-disclosure that is part of the therapeutic frame, the therapist may choose not to answer your question if it concerns him or her directly but rather to explore it in the interest of understanding and helping you. Questions regarding the therapy, such as how long it might continue or how the therapist feels it is progressing, also can initiate valuable conversations in treatment.

Confidentiality is an important aspect of the therapeutic frame because it contributes to the safety of the therapeutic environment and frees the patient to speak openly. However, there are both clinical and legal limits to confidentiality. In clinical situations in which the therapist believes the patient is an imminent suicide risk, confidentiality may be violated to protect the patient's life. The therapist may conclude that revealing the suicide risk to a member of the patient's family or to a close friend is in the patient's best interest. Of course, in cases of hospitalization, the therapist will communicate to other mental health professionals clinical information obtained in the confidence of treatment. If the therapist believes the patient is likely to act on homicidal ideas, he or she is legally obligated to inform the potential victim. The therapist also is likely to seek hospitalization of the patient. Therapists are obligated to report child abuse or suspected child abuse to the state, even if they learn of this abuse in the context of a confidential therapeutic relationship.

If you have questions about the confidentiality of what you reveal in the course of psychotherapy, discuss them with your therapist. In fact, if you are uncomfortable about any part of the therapy – whether about an issue of confidentiality or another matter – it is important to talk with your therapist. If you feel your therapist is exploiting his or her relationship with you, it is important to talk about your concerns with your therapist and others whom you trust. In cases of flagrant boundary violations, such as sexual transgression, it is best to interrupt treatment (because it no longer is therapy but has become something else) and to seek consultation with another mental health professional.

Consultation or a second opinion may be indicated, not only in situations of boundary violation – sexual or otherwise – but also in cases of therapeutic stalemate. The pace and rhythm of psychotherapy vary. Sometimes there is a sense of progress and forward motion, whereas other times there may be a feeling of spinning one's wheels or stagnation. At any given time, it is not always easy to see where the treatment is going, or if it is going anywhere. On one hand, seemingly stagnant periods may later prove to have been fallow times, preparing the patient and therapist for an impending fruitful phase of therapy. On the other hand, some treatments become bogged down or stalemated, and neither patient nor therapist can move forward. If you experience the latter situation, you should try to address it with your therapist first. A consultation with another therapist on the psychotherapy itself also may be very valuable. The consulting therapist will probably speak with your therapist and meet with you one or more times in an effort to understand the problem and recommend a solution. The consulting therapist's recommendation might include changing the focus or approach of the current therapy, exploring a problematic issue, or terminating the current treatment and changing therapists.

Because they hit us where we live, psychiatric disorders may be very frightening. Psychiatric therapies often are unfamiliar and confusing, because they differ in some respects from other medical treatments. However, with a better sense of what to expect and a better understanding of the rationale behind psychiatric treatments, you can find the help you need and benefit from the wide range of effective therapies available today. From the pharmacological relief of difficulties in thought and mood to the psychotherapeutic untangling of self-defeating relationship patterns, psychiatry offers the possibility of living a healthier, more fulfilling life.

TEN

On the Horizon

Genetic Testing

– Robyn S. Shapiro

Scientific developments in the field of genetics are being referred to as a "revolution." One demonstration of that revolution is the recent dramatic growth in the number and availability of genetic tests. Today, more than 1,500 clinically applicable genetic tests are available. Many experts tout our developing genetic testing capability as the dawning of a new age in medicine's ability to diagnose, treat, and prevent illness, whereas others fear its abuse. This chapter discusses basic concepts in genetics, addresses more focused questions relating to genetic testing, and makes recommendations about whether genetic testing is right for you and, if so, how to proceed.

The Basics

Genetic testing has both benefits and limitations, and the decision whether to be tested is personal and complex. It is important to start with an understanding of the basics.

- *Cells* are basic building blocks of all living things. The human body is composed of trillions of cells, which provide structure for the body, take in nutrients and convert these to energy, carry out specialized functions, and contain the body's hereditary materials.

- *DNA* (deoxyribonucleic acid) residing within the nucleus of each cell constructs the blueprint for making proteins that build cells, tissues, and enzymes that trigger biochemical reactions in cells. The structure of DNA is a two-stranded, spiraled double-helix. Every cell in your body (except for mature red blood cells, which have no nucleus) contains the same DNA.
- *RNA*, or ribonucleic acid, receives instructions from DNA and carries them to the ribosome, the site of protein synthesis in the cell.
- *Chromosomes* are structures in the nucleus of the cell that contain the DNA. Humans receive twenty-three chromosomes from each parent. A complete set of forty-six chromosomes is found in almost every cell, except for sperm and egg cells, which contain twenty-three chromosomes.
- *Genes* are subunits of DNA. Each gene contains a special set of instructions for building a specific protein. Through the proteins they encode, genes determine all body processes, including how the body responds to environmental challenges, how efficiently it processes foods, and how vigorously it responds to infections.
- *Proteins* are large complex molecules that play critical roles in the body. They do most of the work in the cells and are required for the structure, function, and regulation of the body's cells, tissues, and organs.
- The *human genome* is the entire collection of genetic information for a human being. It may be thought of as a complete instruction book, with each gene a single instruction. A copy of the instruction book is in almost every one of the trillions of cells in the body.
- *Genetic testing* identifies changes in chromosomes, genes, or proteins. Most often, genetic testing is done to find changes that are associated with inherited diseases or disorders.

All these components fit together as follows:

Each cell contains information that directs it to function in a particular way. For instance, a liver cell does not do the same thing a nerve cell does, and a nerve cell does not do the same thing a heart cell does. The control center of each cell is the material contained in packets called chromosomes. Each chromosome comprises long paired strands of DNA that twist around each other. There are more than three billion base pairs of DNA in each cell in the body (with a few exceptions). Segments of these strands, called genes, transfer messages to a messenger (messenger RNA), which informs another group of molecules (called RNA) to actually construct the proteins and other biological markers that keep the cell functioning in its particular way. A change in the sequence or basic structure of the DNA, or a change in the construction of the RNA, may disrupt a cell's proper functioning and, therefore, the function of the tissue or organ with which it is associated. Genetic testing is the search for those and related changes.

Following is a discussion of some commonly asked questions about genetic testing.

How Are Genes Linked to Disease?

It is estimated that 4,000 rare diseases are the result of a single mutated gene inherited from one's parents, which, in turn, causes proteins encoded by that gene to be abnormal. Because healthy bodies depend on the continuous interplay of thousands of properly functioning proteins acting together, gene mutations can cause a protein to malfunction or be missing entirely, and this can trigger disease.

The nature and effects of gene mutations are complicated. Sometimes one gene mutation causes a person to have a disease, as is the case with the most common form of sickle cell anemia. In many other cases, disorders arise from interplay among several genes, or between genes and environmental factors such as diet or exposure to toxins. Many times, gene mutations have no impact on health or development. Often, gene mutations that could cause a genetic disorder are repaired by certain enzymes before the gene is used to make a protein. In other cases, altered proteins are normal enough to function, but not well (e.g., in sickle cell trait, which involves flawed hemoglobin – the blood's oxygen-carrying protein). In still other cases, the protein is totally disabled. Also, different mutations in the same gene can produce a wide range of effects. For example, in cystic fibrosis, the gene that controls mucus production may have several hundred different mutations, some of which cause severe symptoms, some none at all. Better understanding of how genes influence health eventually will lead to more effective ways to treat, cure, and prevent disease.

What Is Genetic Testing Used For?

There are several types of genetic testing, which are used in health care for a number of purposes.

- *Newborn screening* is widely performed throughout the United States. Each year, blood samples from millions of newborns are tested for abnormal genes or missing gene products. One commonly used newborn genetic screen is the test for phenylketonuria (PKU), a genetic disorder occurring in about 1 of every 10,000 Caucasian or Asian births that involves the body's inability to utilize an essential amino acid (amino acids are the building blocks of protein). This causes severe brain problems, including retarded mental development, if left untreated. Another example of a common newborn screen is the test for congenital hypothyroidism, a disorder of the thyroid gland. Other newborn screening programs test for disorders that can cause infectious disease, premature death, hearing disorders, and heart problems.

- *Carrier testing* evaluates whether individuals carry a gene alteration for a type of inherited disorder called an autosomal recessive disorder. A person who has only one altered copy of a gene for this type of disorder is called a "carrier." Although carriers will not be affected by the disorder themselves, they can pass on the alteration to their children; if both parents are carriers, their children might inherit the alteration from each parent and get the disorder.

- *Prenatal genetic testing* is available to pregnant women for diagnosis of conditions such as Down syndrome in the fetus. Often prenatal testing is offered to women who are 35 or older (because they are at a higher risk for having a child with a chromosomal abnormality), women whose ancestry or ethnic background suggests they have a higher risk of an inherited disorder such as thalassemia or Tay-Sachs disease, and women who have a family history of an inherited condition such as Duchenne muscular dystrophy. Prenatal genetic tests cannot identify all possible inherited disorders.

- *Preimplantation genetic testing* is used to detect genetic changes in embryos that were created using assisted reproductive techniques such as in vitro fertilization – in which egg cells are removed from a woman's ovaries and fertilized with sperm outside her body. When preimplantation genetic testing is done, a small number of cells are taken from the embryos and tested for certain genetic changes that can cause disease (e.g., cystic fibrosis, Tay-Sachs, sickle cell anemia). In most cases, only embryos without genetic changes are implanted in the woman's uterus.

- *Predictive gene testing* identifies individuals who have no symptoms of disease but have a higher chance of getting a particular disease. For instance, one type of predictive test screens for an inherited disposition to certain cancers, such as colon and breast cancer.

- *Diagnostic genetic testing* is used to confirm or rule out a diagnosis when a person has signs or symptoms of a genetic disease or chromosomal condition. Diagnostic testing may be performed before birth or any time during a person's life, but it is not available for all genetic conditions.

- *Pharmacogenetic testing* examines a person's genes to evaluate how drugs would move through the body and break down. For example, a test used in patients who have chronic myelogenous leukemia can show which patients would benefit from a medicine called Gleevec (also called imatinib mesylate). Another pharmacogenetic test looks at a liver enzyme called cytochrome P450, which breaks down certain types of drugs. People with gene alterations that cause their liver cells to produce a less active form of this enzyme might metabolize certain drugs differently.

How Are Genetic Tests Done?

If you decide to go ahead with genetic testing, and your primary care doctor, specialist, or nurse practitioner orders the test, it will be performed on a sample of blood, hair, skin, amniotic fluid, or other tissue. For example, sometimes a buccal smear is done, which involves use of a small brush or cotton swab to collect cells from the inner surface of the cheek. The sample is sent to a laboratory, and technicians look for changes in DNA, chromosomes, RNA, or proteins; the test results are then reported in writing. Before having a genetic test, it is important for you to understand the benefits and limitations of the test and the possible consequences of the test results.

What Do Genetic Test Results Mean?

Genetic test results often are difficult to interpret and understand. A positive test result means there is a change in a particular gene, chromosome, or protein, which may confirm a diagnosis, identify an increased risk of developing a disease, or indicate you are a carrier of a certain genetic mutation. Usually, a positive result of a predictive genetic test cannot establish the exact risk of developing a disorder.

A negative test result means no change can be detected in the gene, chromosome, or protein under consideration; this may indicate you are not a carrier of a specific genetic mutation, are not affected by a specific genetic condition, or do not have an increased risk of developing a specific disease.

However, it also is possible for a test result to be uninformative or inconclusive. Because there are several natural DNA variations (called polymorphisms) that do not affect health, when genetic testing reveals a change in DNA that has not been associated with a disorder in others, it is difficult to tell whether it is a natural polymorphism or a disease-causing mutation.

What Is Direct-to-Consumer Genetic Testing?

Direct-to-consumer genetic tests are those marketed directly through television, print, or Web-based advertisements, without explicit authorization from or involvement of the individual's health care provider. This process often involves being sent a genetic test kit, collecting a DNA sample at home (often by swabbing the inside of your cheek), and sending the sample to a lab. Notification of your test results arrives by mail, by phone, or online. Issues that have been raised about direct-to-consumer genetic testing include concerns about access to such testing and the potential of individuals to be misinformed about the purpose of the test and the meaning of the results.

What Is Gene Therapy?

Gene therapy refers to the potential for using genes themselves to treat disease – for example, by using normal genes to replace or supplement defective ones or to bolster a normal function such as immunity. Currently, gene transfer research is in early stages – aiming to establish whether gene transfer procedures are safe, not whether they work to treat disease. Eventually, gene transfer technologies may be able not only to prevent or treat disease, but also to enhance or replace genes that affect traits such as height, strength, stamina, and intelligence.

What Are the Benefits and Risks of Genetic Testing? How Should I Decide?

The various forms of genetic testing described earlier may provide important benefits. For example:

- A newborn who tests positive for PKU may be put on dietary restrictions to promote maximal development and cognitive abilities.
- A child whose parent is affected by multiple endocrine neoplasia type 2 (MEN-2), a medical disorder associated with tumors of the endocrine system, has a 50% chance of inheriting this condition. The child can be tested and, if test results are positive, undergo a prophylactic thyroidectomy (removal of the thyroid gland) before clinical complications occur, to prevent medullary thyroid carcinoma (thyroid cancer).
- An adult who tests positive for hereditary hemochromatosis, a genetic disease that causes the body to absorb and store too much iron, may be spared complications of iron overload (e.g., diabetes, gallbladder disease, liver disease, heart attack, cancer, and failure of other organs) by the early initiation of phlebotomy treatment (regularly drawing blood).
- A woman who tests positive for BRCA-1 gene mutation, which is associated with an increased risk of breast cancer, may consider a prophylactic mastectomy to reduce the possibility of developing the disease.
- An adult who tests positive for a gene for familial adenomatous polyposis, an inherited disorder characterized by cancer of the large intestine and rectum, can be monitored aggressively to detect and remove colon growths.
- A woman with family members affected by Duchenne muscular dystrophy can undergo a test to detect a deletion in the dystrophin gene – the cause of the disease – and if the test results are positive, she may decide to avoid pregnancy.

Despite the important benefits genetic testing offers, the gathering of genetic information may present significant challenges and risks, which should be understood fully before you consider genetic testing.

Some people who have a fundamental objection to genetic testing believe it constitutes or leads to an unacceptable degree of interference with the natural order. Such concerns are most strongly voiced with respect to genetic testing of embryos and fetuses, which raises the possibility of terminating pregnancies or discarding embryos that test positive for gene mutations. However, even beyond this fundamental objection, if you are considering genetic testing, you need to think carefully about the following issues.

Limited Information, Limited Options

As briefly noted earlier, in many cases a positive genetic test result will not provide clear-cut information regarding whether you will get or show symptoms of a disease or condition, how severe the symptoms will be, or whether the disorder will progress over time. Rather, a genetic predisposition may indicate only an increased likelihood of disease manifestation – and the likelihood may be significantly affected by lifestyle choices (e.g., nutrition, exercise, smoking) and environmental factors (e.g., exposure to toxins, radiation). Moreover, a genetic test may fail to identify a genetic mutation because of a false-negative result (i.e., when a test incorrectly gives a negative result), or it may erroneously identify a genetic mutation because of a false-positive result (i.e., when a test incorrectly gives a positive result).

Another limitation is the lack of treatment strategies for many genetic disorders once they are diagnosed with genetic testing. One example is Huntington's disease, which affects 1 in every 10,000 people in midlife. This disease is caused by a mutation in one gene, which leads to a breakdown in the parts of the brain that control movement and cognitive function and, ultimately, death. Genetic tests are available to determine whether an individual whose parent has or had Huntington's disease carries the gene for the disorder and therefore will someday develop the disease. However, there is no effective intervention or preventive treatment for this disease. Some people who definitively learn, through genetic testing, that they will develop Huntington's disease will be anxious, whereas others will be relieved to know; some who learn they will not develop the disease will be relieved, but others may feel survivor's guilt if other members of their family have not been spared.

Concerns about Privacy and Sharing the Information

Privacy of health information is critical to the physician–patient relationship. Patients must be able to trust their physicians to respect the confidentiality of their intimate personal health information, which is essential to proper diagnosis and treatment of their conditions.

Genetic testing may raise several unique health information privacy concerns. Many people feel particularly strongly about keeping genetic test results private, because genetic information is linked to physical characteristics and even personality. Not only can it reveal information about your present condition, it also can predict aspects of your medical future. It divulges information not only about you but also about your siblings and children, and it has a history of being used to stigmatize individuals.

Several states have laws that explicitly protect the privacy of genetic testing information. Most of these laws prohibit obtaining, analyzing, retaining, or disclosing genetic test results without the informed consent or specific authorization of the tested individual, unless an exception applies. Typical exceptions include law enforcement purposes and paternity determinations, and some state laws make special provisions for research. Also, the federal 1996 Health Insurance Portability and Accountability Act (HIPAA) provides some privacy protection for genetic information.

The flip side of these genetic information privacy concerns is whether, in some circumstances, an individual who has undergone genetic testing should or must disclose the results. Consider, for instance, the case of a woman whose parent had Huntington's disease. She undergoes genetic testing, and the results are positive. Does she have an obligation to tell her fiancé before they get married and have children?

On the other hand, consider cases in which disclosure of a genetic test result can help family members prevent a disease. One example is individuals who have been diagnosed with MEN-2 (the disorder associated with tumors of the endocrine system, discussed earlier). In these circumstances, testing for the causative gene mutation in all first-degree relatives (e.g., siblings, children) is recommended so that a prophylactic thyroidectomy can be offered to those who inherited the mutation. Should carriers of known genetic risks be obligated to tell their relatives? Conversely, what should be done if a family member prefers not to be presented with such information? In these situations, in which privacy and confidentiality must be balanced with obligations to others, factors that should be explored thoroughly include the consequences of refusal to share the information and the reasons for refusal to share the information.

Concerns about Genetic Discrimination

Concerns about privacy protections for genetic information are linked to concerns that individuals may be treated differently by their employer or insurance company if the employer or insurer learns they have a gene mutation that causes or increases risk of an inherited disorder. The fear is that employers may have an economic incentive to use genetic information to avoid hiring individuals who would have higher medical insurance claims, higher absenteeism, and/or lower productivity, and that insurers may wish to use genetic information to avoid covering individuals who are more likely to receive costly care covered by insurance.

To lessen some of these fears, Congress recently passed the Genetic Information Nondiscrimination Act (GINA), which prohibits insurance companies and employers from discriminating on the basis of information derived from genetic tests. GINA forbids insurance companies from discriminating by reducing coverage or increasing premiums, and it prohibits employers from making adverse employment decisions based on a person's genetic information. In addition, insurers and employers are prohibited from requesting or demanding that an individual take a genetic test. Senator Edward Kennedy, who cosponsored GINA in the Senate, labeled the law "the first major new civil rights bill of the new century." Nonetheless, there are limitations in GINA's antidiscrimination protections. For instance, GINA addresses discrimination based on genetic information only with respect to employment and health insurance, not life, disability, or long-term care insurance.

Recommendations

You should consider the issues surrounding genetic testing, as described earlier, thoroughly in deciding whether to be tested. Because these issues are so complex and challenging, many people believe genetic counseling is important before and after the testing. Counseling from professional advisors who are experts in genetics can help you understand the nature, benefits, and limitations of genetic testing and think through, ahead of time, how a test might affect you. After the testing, counselors can help explain the significance of the results and what choices they present. Genetic counseling most often is "nondirective" in that the counselor provides enough information to allow you to determine the best course of action for you but does not make testing recommendations.

If genetic testing is offered without formal pretest counseling, the informed consent discussion between you and your doctor should be thorough and clear and should include the following (as applicable):

- The seriousness and variability of the genetic condition for which you are being tested
- Available therapeutic options

- The manner in which the disorder is transmitted, the significance of carrier status, and the probability of developing the genetic disorder if the test result is positive
- The reliability of the test and the test results
- Information about how the test results will be communicated to you and what will be done with the tissue samples on which the test is performed
- The possible social implications and emotional effects of a positive result
- The implications of a positive result for your children and other family members
- A warning that the test may reveal unexpected information (e.g., about paternity)

Conclusion

Genetic tests certainly will continue to play a significant role in modern medicine. As clinical practice standards, health policy, and laws related to genetic testing evolve, and we face complex and highly personal genetic testing choices, it is important that we neither overestimate nor underestimate their usefulness or their risks.

ELEVEN

To Be or Not to Be – A Research Subject

– Eric M. Meslin and Peter H. Schwartz

For most people, the terms *clinical trial, institutional review board, risk–benefit assessment*, and *informed consent* make as much sense as the instruction manual for a complicated piece of technology. Indeed, most people probably do not know that when medical research is conducted to test a new medicine, there are rules and procedures the scientists must follow to ensure that the research is both scientifically sound and ethically safe. Most people do not know there are different kinds of medical studies; some are conducted on people who already have a disease or medical condition, and others are performed on healthy volunteers who want to help science find answers. Yet both types of potential research subjects have many of the same questions, the answers to which can help them decide whether to participate in the study, what their rights are, and what decisions they may have to make. This chapter reviews the basics of being a research subject – including the potential benefits and risks of making this important decision.

The Basics

Once you become a patient, it won't be long before somebody asks you to be a research subject. For example, your doctor might want to enroll you in a clinical trial of a new medication, possibly for a condition for which other drugs are available – such as high blood pressure – or for one for which there are no approved treatments yet. Other research studies do not involve a medication or treatment at all; many just ask you to fill out a questionnaire or give a blood sample.

Of course, patients aren't the only people approached to participate in medical research. Many projects involve healthy people. In fact, the earliest stages of research on any new medication almost always involve testing in healthy people to determine side effects and correct dosages. Medical research is always going on all over the world, and there are so many different types of research, it may be hard to make any reliable generalizations. Even if you have never been a research subject, the effects of research certainly have an impact on your everyday life.

No matter what sort of research you are invited to participate in, or whether you are a patient when you are asked, it's entirely up to you whether or not to do it. This decision is important and may have many implications for your health and well-being, as well as those of other patients now and in the future. Making a good decision – the right one for you – requires you to become educated about topics you may not have thought about before, some of which may be quite complicated. This chapter explains the key issues to help you make a good decision.

What Is Research?

The first step in deciding whether to participate in a research study is to understand what research is and how it differs from medical treatment. According to some of the most important regulations, research is any "systematic investigation...designed to develop or contribute to generalizable knowledge" (common rule). For a project to count as *medical* research, the knowledge involved must be related to the effort to improve health and medical care. Of course, this endeavor encompasses a great variety of activities. Some discussions of research emphasize that it extends *from the bench to the bedside*, that is, from basic studies on molecules and animals in a laboratory all the way to clinical research conducted on humans to determine the effect of new medications and procedures. The sort of research you will be invited to participate in is called *human subjects research* because it involves human beings (you and others). Human subjects research is governed by special regulations and ethical principles and guidelines, which are discussed in this chapter.

Should I Be Concerned about Unethical Research?

Research involving human beings has a long and complex history. Although physicians and scientists have been studying the body for millennia, only in the past fifty years has research involving human beings been a major activity of universities, industry, and even nations. At the same time, an entire system for protecting human subjects from harm was developed in the United States and around the world, partly as a result of many cases of unethical research that came to light. These cases include the horrific concentration camp experiments conducted by the Nazis, some of which involved the torture and murder of many people. However, although those experiments were at the unethical extreme, many other cases of ethically problematic research occurred after World War II in prominent U.S. universities and were sponsored by the federal government. For example, the Tuskegee study that ran from 1932 until it was finally stopped in 1972 observed the progression of syphilis in poor black men in rural Alabama. In this study, researchers kept the men unaware of their infection and even took steps to make sure they did not receive medical treatment. Other studies, such as the Willowbrook State School experiments, in which children were intentionally exposed to hepatitis, and the Jewish Chronic Disease Hospital study, in which elderly patients were injected with cancer cells, resulted in public outrage and concerted action by the U.S. Congress to develop a comprehensive system of rules, regulations, and procedures to make sure all medical research is conducted ethically. Although the rules are quite complex, they involve three basic assumptions any person thinking about participating in a research study should know about.

1. All subjects must give "informed consent" before participating in a research study.
2. The risks to any humans participating will be minimized as much as reasonably possible, and a study should be performed only if the possible benefits outweigh the risks.
3. All studies conducted on human beings must have gone through an independent committee for review and ethical approval.

Research is a serious endeavor and is not an activity scientists undertake lightly. In many cases, researchers are funded to carry out studies with grants from federal research organizations such as the National Institutes of Health and the National Science Foundation – organizations supported by taxpayers. In fact, to receive these grants, researchers are legally bound to follow ethics regulations, including the requirement to obtain informed consent.

What Is Informed Consent?

Before you enroll in a research project as a research subject – before you undergo any tests or interventions – you must agree to it. Your agreement is called "informed consent" because you must be *informed* about the study so you can decide whether you want to join and you must give *consent* (approval) before anybody does anything to you. Some of the issues you must be informed about include the following three questions, which you should keep in mind:

1. *Why is this study being done in the first place?* Most researchers are committed to finding answers to health problems. So, it matters why a study is being done – is it just a frivolous wild goose chase or is it a serious search for the answer to a problem that might one day lead to a treatment or cure for a disease?

2. *What exactly will happen to me?* This is an obvious question, but the details are important. You should know whether your involvement consists of one visit or many visits, whether it involves an invasive procedure like a blood draw or something even more invasive, whether you will be answering surveys, and whether people will be contacting you for more information. The more you know about the actual study and what you will experience, the more comfortable you will be with your decision.

3. *What are the risks and potential benefits to me?* Knowing *what* will happen to you is not the same as knowing what the risks and potential benefits are to you from participating. Consider the idea of "benefits" first. It is common for patients to believe that if a doctor asks them to participate in research, they will receive medical care that will benefit them. This is not a good assumption for a couple of reasons. First, it makes sense to study a test or treatment for some condition only if there is uncertainty over whether there are real benefits from it. Second, although it is possible for a patient involved in a research study to get better treatment, research studies are not designed with this intention at all.

The goal of medical research is to obtain information that can improve health and medical care in the future, the sort of "generalizable knowledge" mentioned in the definition given earlier. For instance, many studies attempting to determine the effect of a medication include one group of subjects randomly assigned to receive no treatment at all (a placebo). (We'll say more about this later.) In considering whether to participate in a study, it is important to get a clear picture of what benefits you may receive, if any, as well as the benefits that may accrue to others.

Of course, the risks you will face are just as important as the benefits and depend on the type of research project in which you are asked to participate. If you are going to be given an experimental medication or undergo any procedures, the researchers must provide you with information about any possible side effects or complications. Even if the research project does not involve any medications or procedures – for instance, if you are just answering a questionnaire – the researchers must describe any negative effects there could be for you (e.g., a problem with confidentiality, i.e., someone getting information about you). The information the researcher gives you about risks may be very complex, and we'll also say more about how to handle that information later in the chapter.

Overall, there are many other things you might be told – and should be told – however, at the very least, the three key questions described earlier should be answered to your satisfaction. Moreover, these and other issues usually are detailed in a form (the informed consent document) that you will receive, read, and need to sign before proceeding. Remember, if you have learned about the study and you decide not to participate, that is your right too. *No one can (or should try to) force you to participate in research. It's your choice.*

Research on Those Who Can't Consent for Themselves

There are two situations in which you may be asked to give consent for research conducted on someone else. One situation involves children. Because children cannot give legal consent to participate in research, their parents or guardians must give consent before they can be enrolled. A child may be given some information, based on his or her ability to understand, and asked whether he or she would like to participate (the child's agreement is called *assent*); however, his or her parent or guardian must provide the informed consent. The other situation involves people who cannot consent for themselves because they have a mental illness, such as dementia. In this case, as with research involving children, the person's legal guardian must give consent before he or she can be enrolled in the study. The regulations concerning this type of research are particularly stringent and attempt to ensure that risks are minimized and the study truly is worth doing. If you are making a decision about research participation in one of these situations – for a child or another adult – you are expected to represent the best interests of that person, deciding for them as if you were deciding for yourself.

How Is Research Regulated and Reviewed?

Even before researchers start a project, and before inviting anybody to participate as a research subject, they must obtain the approval of a committee of experts who have reviewed the study in detail, including the informed consent document. In the United States, this committee is called an *institutional review board* (IRB). There are more than 3,500 IRBs in the United States located at medical centers, universities, and research institutions. In fact, the U.S. government requires any human subjects research study performed at an institution that receives federal grants or contracts to be reviewed and approved by an IRB. IRBs are made up of doctors, nurses, other researchers, community representatives, and other members who examine a range of documents the researchers must submit before they can go forward with their study. Again, the regulations the IRB applies are quite detailed, but they distill to the three general principles listed earlier: 1) informed consent, 2) minimizing risk to subjects, and 3) ensuring the benefits outweigh the risks. IRBs also review ongoing studies to make sure they are complying with regulations and with their previously stated plans.

Most IRBs are based at the institution, such as a university, where the research is being conducted; however, there are now some cases in which the IRB for a study is in a location other than the one where the study is being done. For instance, one IRB may oversee research being conducted at several universities or clinics. When you are approached to participate in a research project, it is perfectly reasonable to ask which IRB approved the study and how you can contact the board members if you have any questions. In rare cases, a research project may go forward without IRB review – for example, if it is being run by an organization that receives no federal grants or contracts. Therefore, you may want to make sure there was an IRB or other similar review of the study you are being invited to join. We think you should be somewhat skeptical of any study that was not approved by an IRB, especially if there is any risk to you from participating.

Besides IRBs, there are other bodies that review certain types of medical research. For example, if the project involves a new medication, the researchers must get permission from the Food and Drug

Administration (FDA) to perform the study. To get FDA approval, the researchers must show evidence that the drug to be studied has acceptable risks and real promise, based on data from laboratory and/or animal studies. Many universities have special bodies that review certain kinds of research – such as cancer or gene therapy studies – again, it is perfectly reasonable to ask which groups reviewed a project before you agree to participate.

What Type of Research Project Is This?

Although the issues we discuss in this chapter apply to all sorts of medical research, important differences exist among the various types of studies you might be invited to join. Therefore, you should know a little about each kind of research project so you understand the type of research involved, or at least the terminology being tossed around, in any study in which you might participate.

Clinical Drug Trials

In some ways, clinical drug trials are the prototypical research studies. Clinical drug trials are studies of new medications, or new uses for existing ones, to determine whether they can be used to treat specific diseases or other medical problems. If you are being invited to participate in a clinical drug trial, you should be aware of some specific issues and questions.

In what stage of testing is the drug? All drugs go through (at least) three stages of testing: phase I, phase II, and phase III. *Phase I* trials occur first and focus almost entirely on identifying the proper dosage for the medication as well as any side effects. These studies often are designed to begin with a very low dosage of the drug and then to increase it slowly until serious side effects are seen. *Phase II* trials focus on determining whether the treatment actually will help patients. These studies usually involve a smaller number of patients who receive the medication and have their responses to it measured carefully. *Phase III* trials are the large randomized, placebo-controlled studies that help clarify exactly how much benefit the drug has in treating the disease in question, whether it truly is safe, and whether it is an improvement over other medications used to treat that illness.

The take-home message is that if the study is phase I or phase II, there is relatively little evidence the treatment actually is beneficial and/or any better than other available treatments. In fact, the reason the researchers are doing the study is to look for that evidence. Therefore, you should be somewhat skeptical of any implication that a medication *probably* will help you; if the researcher knew that, they would not be doing the study. In fact, the IRB should refuse to let the study go on! The findings of a phase I study may be promising or give the study investigators hope, but, again, no one knows what future research will discover. By phase III, more evidence will evolve that the study investigators can use to explain the reasons for their hope, as well as any risks.

Will everybody get the treatment, or is there a control group?
In many clinical trials (especially phase III), not all subjects receive the study drug; some get no treatment (a placebo) or the currently accepted treatment. Therefore, if you are participating in a study to get a new treatment that has some promise, you should know whether there is a chance you won't get the study treatment. In many cases, neither the subjects nor the researchers know who is getting the experimental treatment and who is getting the placebo or standard treatment. This technique ensures that the subjects in the two study groups are not treated differently, which could bias the results.

Other Clinical Trials
Some clinical trials are designed to study a medical procedure or device, rather than a drug. For example, one study may compare two different ways of implanting a cardiac stent; another may compare two methods of repairing torn knee cartilage. As with clinical drug trials, clinical trials of procedures or devices raise several ethical issues, require a high level of regulatory scrutiny, must be reviewed and approved by IRBs, and cannot take place in humans without their informed consent. With regard to participation in this type of trial versus a clinical drug trial, many of the same questions arise: How much testing has been done so far on the benefits and risks of the test or procedure compared with the standard one? What benefits or risks have been seen so far? Is there a control group, or do all study participants get the experimental intervention?

Observational Research
Some studies are performed not to test a treatment or procedure, but to monitor people receiving a certain treatment. Investigators in these

studies record the participants' treatment and their response to it, talk to and/or examine the subjects, and may look at their medical records during and after treatment. If you participate in this sort of trial, called an *observational study*, the main discomfort or risk to you might be limited to blood tests or x-rays. Such studies also are important for improving medical care – by allowing researchers to figure out what is or is not working – and they involve much less risk than many clinical studies.

However, as with clinical trials – and all research studies, for that matter – you should think about the questions listed earlier regarding what exactly will happen to you and what the benefits and risks are to you. Don't accept vague answers: everything should be spelled out to your satisfaction. If someone refers to a particular medical test or x-ray you are unsure about, you have every right to ask for more information, including exactly how long the procedure takes and how uncomfortable it is.

Another risk of observational studies – and any study in which the researchers need to keep track of information about the participants – is the possibility someone will learn private information about you and inadvertently disclose it to someone else who is not authorized to have it. Privacy and confidentiality are important values in our society, so it is especially important for you to be aware of the plans in place to protect your privacy and confidentiality. The sort of information researchers collect is personal and may be related to your medical problems, your treatment, or any answers you provide on a survey. The researchers are obligated to keep this information private and to prevent anybody else from accessing it. Like banks, study investigators use various techniques – locked computers, passwords, and encrypted databases – to keep your information as safe as possible; however, sometimes there is a breach. The informed consent document must list this risk and describe how your information will be kept safe.

Of course some studies can be conducted without requiring researchers to collect personal information about you. Some research, such as public health surveillance studies or studies involving blood samples or other biological material, can be carried out without linking the research findings to a particular person. Studies involving anonymized data of this kind pose no specific risk to individuals.

Survey Research

In some studies, the researchers want nothing more than to speak to the participants and/or have them fill out questionnaires. If you participate in one of these surveys, basically your only important risk is any loss of confidentiality. In fact, this type of study carries so little risk, the researcher may approach you without asking you to read and sign an informed consent document and will ask for your verbal consent only when he or she is talking to you. Generally, an IRB still has to approve this type of study, but based on the fact that the risks are so low, there is no need to write everything down. However, you still are entitled to ask for as much information as you want. Again, it is up to you whether you want to take the time and effort to help, and there is no reason you should feel you have to do so. As always, participation in research is basically an altruistic action – for the good of people other than yourself – and you should feel good about volunteering if you decide to participate. There may or may not be some small token of gratitude (e.g., a gift card in a small denomination) to thank you for your time, and the researchers should act graciously toward you for helping them with their project and (hopefully) scientific advancement.

Biobanks

Finally, a special kind of observational research becoming more and more common is called *biobank* research. In biobank studies, researchers collect medical information from subjects and match it with biological data, such as blood or tissue samples or information from specific examinations (e.g., a physical exam or an x-ray result). Sometimes the tissue is left over from a medical procedure, such as a breast biopsy, and the researchers want the subject's permission to keep that extra tissue instead of throwing it out. Sometimes, the researchers want permission to call participants regularly to get updates on their medical history and even to look at their medical records at regular intervals. Such biobanks aim to collect and store information from hundreds to millions of people to find out more about how our genes and other facts about us affect our health and life.

As with all other research, if you are invited to join a biobank study, you should feel good about asking as many questions as you want to find out exactly what will be done and what the benefits and risks are to you. As in observational studies, the main risks to you are those associated with any procedure the researchers propose to do to collect the sample or conduct the exam, including a blood draw or other testing. In addition, because the biobank will be in place possibly for many years, the researchers must address what they will do to protect your information from unintended disclosure (i.e., to avoid loss of confidentiality). They also should explain a bit about who will use the biobank, how your information might be used in future studies, and how projects will be chosen in the future.

More Specifics and Complexities

The previous discussion is just an overview of research, the regulation of research, and the choices you will face if you are invited to participate in a research study. Hopefully, it will get you thinking about what to ask and what to consider if and when you are approached. However, for each of the topics described earlier, the issues get somewhat more complex when you look at them more closely. It is important for you to be aware of these complexities as you decide whether to participate in research.

When Medical Research Can Be Confused with Treatment

Sometimes participating in a research study may seem like receiving medical treatment, but, as we emphasized earlier, they are very different. They may seem similar because the procedures used in research (e.g., surveys, blood draws, administration of medicine) are typical health care procedures. Moreover, the interactions may feel the same – with a doctor and nurse talking to you about your medical history, symptoms, medications, and so forth – and may even occur in a doctor's office or hospital.

However, the two activities – medical treatment and medical research – are not the same. When you see your doctor, he or she has the primary goal and responsibility of protecting and/or restoring your health by treating any illness. In contrast, the primary goal and obligation of the researchers in a study (and any doctors and nurses who are involved) is to the research project. However, they also must watch out for your health and well-being, and there are many protections in place to watch over you while you are participating in the project. For example, in some clinical drug trials, there is a separate committee called a *data safety and monitoring board* that reviews the study on an ongoing basis. This committee has the authority to stop the study if it believes that patients might be harmed. However, the researchers' goals in doing the study, and their interactions with you as a research subject, are designed to increase scientific and medical knowledge and further (soon or someday) the ability to prevent or treat disease. The reason for doing the research is not to restore or improve your health.

So, let's go back to considering the benefits you might receive from participating in research. In some cases, the possible benefits to you might be very specific. For example, a drug not yet approved for use in medical treatment is being studied for a condition you have, and it already has shown some promising results. Your doctor may feel this treatment is the best one for you, even though it is unproven; thus, he or she may recommend that you enroll in a study of that medication. This sort of situation comes up often for patients with advanced cancer for whom all approved treatments were tried and failed to cure or control the cancer. At this point, with no other approved treatment available, doctors may recommend, or even encourage, these patients to enroll in a trial of some new medication.

In short, these patients are gambling that the new medication will be successful, whereas the drugs already studied and approved have failed; as such, their decision to enroll in the study seems more like a search for a new treatment than participation in research. However, it is important to understand that because the medication is being provided as part of research, the criteria for who gets the medication, the way it is given, and the sort of decisions the doctor or care team can make are driven by the study design, not by an effort to maximize patient care.

Many people looking at the ethics of research and informed consent have noticed that when patients in this type of situation are offered a research medication as part of a study, they may over-estimate the chance that the medication will actually help. It may be that the studies of the medication are in very early stages, and any possible benefit is completely unclear. In phase I studies, in which the goal is to determine the proper dose to use for future testing, there is little likelihood of benefit to any particular person. In other studies, such as phase III clinical trials, there is a group of subjects who get no treatment at all (the placebo group) so that the researchers can better determine the effects of the medication on people; in many cases, the research subjects, and even the researchers, do not know (until the end of the study) who got the research medication and who got the placebo.

In short, if you are thinking about participating in a research study because you think you will get a specific benefit – such as a medication you cannot get any other way – you should determine what the chances are that you will actually get the medication and that it will actually help you. In the end, whether to enter a study is a decision you should make mostly based on a desire to help advance science, as we discuss next.

Should I Participate in Research to Feel Good or Make Money (or Both)?

The differences in the nature of medical research versus that of medical treatment mean there are important differences in the motivation for participating in one or the other. When you agree to participate in a research project, you are doing it primarily for the benefit of others. The people who benefit from the knowledge gained from the study may have the same disease or condition you have or may belong to future generations. Or, your participation may be a contribution to increasing doctors' abilities to prevent or treat disease. These are important reasons for participating, but they are also very different from your reasons for getting medical treatment, in which the main goal should be to protect or recover your own health. Simply put, the difference may be one of altruism versus personal benefit.

Of course, not everyone has altruistic reasons for participating in research. Some people find it interesting to join a study; others may participate because there is a modest stipend. If you receive payment for participation, however, you should ask yourself whether the money is what convinced you to participate. No one is supposed to participate in research just for the money; the money is meant to defray participants' expenses or reimburse them for their time and is not meant to be payment like a paycheck. Although there are no set rates for remuneration, the general principle is that as the study risk or the subjects' involvement increases, so too will the amount of money provided. For example, a one-time blood draw to look for a certain enzyme or protein is far less risky than a study of the safety of a new medicine that involves multiple doses and tests over many weeks, so it will provide a smaller stipend.

There is evidence that some people participate in research only for the money. In particular, some research is carried out in healthy individuals, and a thriving community has developed made up of people who travel from place to place signing up for these studies. Although the payments are relatively small, these people – who call the practice "guinea pigging" – can make a modest living by doing this.

Informed Consent

To think more deeply about the process of informed consent, consider the last of the three key questions listed earlier in this chapter: *What are the risks and potential benefits for me?*

Consider a hypothetical study of some new medication for a condition you have. In this study, all the subjects will get the medication; make regular visits to the doctor's office, where blood will be drawn; and have an x-ray taken every 3 months for the next year. The main benefit to you in this case may be the chance that the medication can help: many cancer patients are in this situation when they are invited to join research projects studying new chemotherapy medications. Remember, however, that the whole idea of a research project is that doctors are still unsure whether the medication really works and what the possible side effects might be. Although it might be tempting to assume you will benefit, this is not certain.

Now consider the risks. Any trial of a new medication in human beings will occur only after there has been a significant amount of testing in animals and, in many cases, in at least some humans. Therefore, the researchers approaching you should be able to say something about the possible risks. Remember, though, that they will still be quite unsure of the side effects – which is the reason they are doing another study – and so they have to give you a list, which is usually long, of all the possible complications. Any of these complications might occur, they will tell you, but they can't tell you which ones. The previous research may or may not be able to give you a sense of the specific percentage of subjects who might get each side effect: Will it happen in two thirds of people taking the drug, or one third, or one in ten, or one in one hundred? Often researchers won't know, because determining these answers is one of the goals of research. Because current regulations require researchers to describe all the possible risks of an experimental medication or procedure, the informed consent document often looks like a laundry list of many, many bad things that could happen to you (but may or may not actually happen), and it is a good idea to ask how you are supposed to respond to such a form.

The first step in making sense of this form is to look at the words describing the possible complications and make sure you understand them. For example, the form may say that one possible side effect is *cerebral edema*, a term you may not understand. Even if it is described as "swelling of the brain," you likely would want to know more: Is it serious? Can it cause brain damage? Can any effects be reversed? A better description would be "swelling of the brain, which may cause confusion, or even coma and death." In the end, your understanding of the consent form depends on your asking the researcher to explain these terms, and you should never be embarrassed to insist on that. Because each person is different, there is no set of rules describing how much information must be given to explain a risk or its severity. For example, the term *cerebral edema* may be understandable for one person (he or she may be a physician or nurse), whereas others will need more information. In short, there is no shame in asking questions and expecting a conversation and answers.

Similar confusion may arise when the informed consent document tries to describe the likelihood of different complications occurring. Again, your understanding will depend on asking and getting answers to any questions you have. What about the description of edema as a possible side effect that "might" happen. What does *might* mean here? Is it a very remote possibility? A rare but real possibility? A 1 in 1,000 chance of it happening to you? A one in a million chance? Researchers and IRBs struggle to determine how much specificity is needed and whether that specificity will confuse people rather than educate them.

Try this experiment on yourself: Write a list of probability words, ranging from *never* to *always*; include as many words as you can think of, such as *might, usually, sometimes, rarely*, and so on. Then try to assign percentages to the words. For example, *never* should be 0% and *always* 100%. But what about the other words? You might put this list together and share it with a researcher who gives you an informed consent form containing words such as *might* and *possibly*. At the very least, this will be an opportunity to have an informed conversation because you may want to know more about a study than what is described in the consent form. You should expect to have questions about things written on the informed consent form (or about anything else the researcher describes), and you should feel free to ask them. Perhaps most importantly, don't bow to the subtle pressure people sometimes use to stop you from asking more questions. The doctor or researcher may look like he or she is in a hurry, but he or she is obligated to explain things to you in as much detail as you want. Don't be shy about asking for more information; remember, *they* are asking *you* to do them the favor of participating in their study.

What Happens If I Am Harmed or Injured In a Research Study?

Although all research involves some type of inconvenience (your time and effort), not all research is physically risky. The overwhelming majority of studies conducted in the United States do not result in any serious harm or injury. In fact, when serious harm does occur, it is a source of great concern. Several years ago, when a patient died in a gene therapy study, the entire system for reviewing and approving these types of studies was reviewed and revised to ensure it would not happen again. Still, research by its nature is an exploration of something new, and there is always the chance something bad might happen. A good informed consent document outlines the possible risks (both their severity and likelihood) clearly, letting you know what you can expect. However, another purpose of the consent form is legal – by informing you of the possibility of certain risks, your agreement to participate means you are prepared to accept the possibility that one or more of the harms might happen to you. Some of these may be minor, whereas others may be more significant. That's why it is such an important decision to participate and to be fully informed.

It is equally important for the researchers (and the consent form) to tell you what will happen if you do experience one of the identified risks. Will they treat you at the facility where you are participating in the study? Will they pay for it? Federal regulations for research in the United States require that consent forms tell you whether some form of compensation for injury will be available, but it is up to the researchers to tell you exactly what that involves. For many studies, the informed consent form will say that treatment of any injuries or harms must be covered by your own medical insurance. In this type of situation, it may be relevant whether you have health insurance or what your coverage is (e.g., your deductible).

What Are My Responsibilities?

Apart from the ethics of pay-for-participation, there are some other issues you should consider before agreeing to participate in such studies. For instance, if a person has undergone one study in January with one experimental medication, then undergoes a different study in April with a different experimental medication, it may be hard for researchers to tell whether a side effect that occurred in April was from the first or the second medication, or perhaps the interaction between them. This would mean that any research data from the second study could potentially be meaningless. Research is valuable only when it provides valid answers to important scientific questions. Research subjects play a very important role in this process, and they also have certain responsibilities. Giving accurate information about your health status to the researchers is one responsibility, so is making all efforts to comply with the study protocol, such as taking the drugs according to the schedule, coming in for scheduled visits, and cooperating with other aspects of the study.

Failure to carry out your responsibilities in these various ways can seriously hurt a study. If a participant has failed to follow the protocol, or has taken other experimental drugs without telling the researchers, then the study results may be based on tainted data. If too many patients fail to live up to their side of the bargain, the whole study might be in jeopardy. Researchers might draw incorrect conclusions, and reports in a medical journal or recommendations that doctors change their practice based on the study could have serious consequences for patient care.

Conclusion

We hope this overview of medical research, as well as its ethics and regulations, has given you a toolbox of ideas and questions to call upon when you are asked to participate in a research study. As we have emphasized in this chapter, you may feel unsure about what is being proposed and what the risks and benefits to you are, so it is most important that you have the ability to ask questions. This discussion comes back to the bedrock principles of research, which emphasize that informed consent is central and that participants must be free to decide, based on complete information, whether to participate. Only by gaining some understanding of the research process and the specific project in question can you make sure you are being treated appropriately. If this chapter empowers you to decide whether to participate in a research project and, if you do, if it has given you the knowledge you need to be involved with your eyes wide open, then it is a success.

TWELVE

Information That Will Help You Make Health Care Decisions for Adult Family Members

– Mark R. Wicclair

Unlike infants and young children, adults generally have the ability to make medical decisions for themselves. Because of genetic anomalies, illness, or accidents, some children will never acquire that ability as they grow into adults, and some adults lose the ability during their lifetime. This loss of what is called decision-making capacity or competency in an adult family member may be the result of an accident; an acute medical condition, such as a stroke or heart attack; a terminal illness, such as cancer; or a chronic progressive condition, such as Alzheimer's disease, multiple sclerosis (MS), or amyotrophic lateral sclerosis (ALS, or Lou Gehrig's disease). Generally, if an adult loses decision-making capacity, one or more family members will be asked to make decisions for him or her. That person is commonly called a surrogate (or an agent, representative, or proxy).

Medical decisions for family members literally may be about life or death. However, even when they are not, they can have very serious consequences and may be fraught with anxiety, stress, and uncertainty. Nothing can completely eliminate stress from hard decisions about loved ones. Therefore, the aim of this chapter is modest; it is to provide information that will help you if and when you are called upon to be a surrogate for an adult family member. Hopefully, this information will at least reduce the stress and uncertainty you will experience if you need to make health care decisions for a relative.

You already may be serving as a surrogate for someone in your family. Or, you may have family members in declining health and are expecting to be called upon to serve as a surrogate in the not-too-distant future. If you are in neither of these two categories, you nevertheless may be called upon to serve as a surrogate some day, perhaps for an aging parent, a spouse, or a sibling. The first section of this chapter is about preparing to become a surrogate and will be of particular interest to you if you are not currently serving as a surrogate. The remainder of the chapter should be of interest to you whether or not you currently are serving as a relative's surrogate.

Preparing to Become a Surrogate

As difficult as it may be to serve as a surrogate for a member of your family, there are a few steps you can take in advance that at least can help you avoid unnecessary doubt, discomfort, worry, and anxiety. First, it will help to understand what you will be expected to do if you are asked to become a surrogate. When a decision has to be made for a family member who no longer is able to decide, you likely will be asked to determine how that person would have decided in the circumstances. Hence, you can prepare to become a surrogate by learning as much as possible about the values, goals, and preferences of the family member(s) for whom you might be asked to make medical decisions.

If a relative has not already designated you as his or her surrogate, how do you know whether *you* will be asked to serve as a surrogate for a particular family member? Unless a patient has designated someone to serve as a surrogate, the law usually specifies a priority order of persons to serve as surrogates. A typical priority order is spouse, adult child, parent, adult sibling, adult grandchild, and close friend. Thus, if you are married, and your spouse is unable to make medical decisions, you likely will be asked to serve as his or her surrogate unless your spouse has designated someone else. If one of your parents is deceased or is not willing or able to serve as the other parent's surrogate, you and/or a sibling likely will be asked to do so unless your parent has selected someone else. However, surrogate decision making often is an informal process, and the legally specified priority order is not always observed. Understandably, several family members may want to participate in the decision-making process, and as long as there are no conflicts or disputes, they generally will have an opportunity to do so. Accordingly, you may choose to participate in decision making for a family member even if you aren't the primary legally specified surrogate.

Accidents and illnesses that result in a loss of decision-making capacity and a need for medical care may strike suddenly and unexpectedly and at any age. However, sometimes there are early warning signs that a family member sooner or later likely will require a surrogate. For example, a relative might have an incurable malignant brain tumor, early Alzheimer's disease, or ALS. Realizing that illness and loss of decision-making capacity may occur at any time, some of your relatives may engage in advance planning about their health care without waiting for early warning signs. Others may engage in such advance planning only after they are diagnosed with a condition likely to result in the loss of decision-making ability. In either case, advance planning might include initiating a discussion with you and other family members about health care–related goals and preferences. If a relative initiates such a conversation, you may feel like avoiding a frank discussion of illness, deteriorating health, and death. This is an understandable reaction. No one enjoys talking about such depressing and distressing topics. However, it would be a shame to pass up an opportunity to discover information that might enable you to be a more effective surrogate.

Sometimes people engage in advance planning about their health care by executing a living will. A living will is a document that provides general guidelines and/or specific instructions for health care decision making in the event the person is unable to decide. If a family member executes a living will, you have an excellent opportunity for a conversation about his or her health care goals and preferences. Even if a family member has a living will, it may be necessary for someone to help interpret it and apply it to the particular circumstances, and this may be a daunting task. A conversation with a relative may prove invaluable if you are called on some day to provide this kind of help. Accordingly, if a family member tells you he or she has a living will, or even if he or she gives you a copy, discussing it and your relative's wishes can help you achieve a clearer understanding of his or her intent and be a more effective surrogate.

Don't hesitate to initiate a discussion if a family member, especially one for whom you may be asked to serve as a surrogate, doesn't take the lead. Although you don't need to wait for early warning signs to begin to prepare for a potential role as a surrogate, their presence may make it easier for you to initiate the conversation. If you decide to execute an advance directive, you have an excellent opportunity to initiate a mutual discussion of health care goals and preferences with family members. As you explain your wishes, you can encourage your family members to reveal theirs. If a family member really does not want to engage in such a discussion, he or she can tell you. However, a family member's reluctance to initiate a conversation does not necessarily arise from his or her lack of interest, but perhaps because of a concern that such a discussion might upset you. By initiating the conversation yourself, you can break the ice and communicate your willingness to talk. It then is up to your family member to indicate whether he or she is like-minded.

Your goal when you engage in these conversations is not necessarily to get a detailed list of specific decisions. Even if a family member is known to have a specific diagnosis and prognosis, no one can foresee all the possible situations and all the possible decisions that will have to be made. Instead, the aim is to get a general sense of your relative's wishes. You might begin by discussing the big picture. Is there a line beyond which his or her quality of life would be so poor, unsatisfying, or devoid of meaning that he or she would not want to be kept alive? Would your relative consider life worthwhile if he or she were unconscious and never expected to regain consciousness or if he or she had permanently lost the ability to recognize and interact with you and other family members? Would your family member want to be given medication to prevent pain even if it might hasten death? Does your family member seek a "dignified death," and if so, what is his or her conception of death with dignity?

It may be helpful to consider specific cases, such as the experiences of relatives or friends and/or cases in the media. Are there relatives or friends whose end-of-life care is somewhat similar to what your family member would want? Are there friends or relatives who received medical care that your family member would not want in a similar situation? Are you and your family member familiar with any cases that were portrayed in the media, such as the case of Terri Schiavo, the Florida woman who was kept alive for thirteen years in a permanent vegetative state by means of medically supplied nutrition and hydration? If so, such cases can serve to focus a discussion of your family member's views. For example, the Terri Schiavo case presents an occasion to consider whether your family member would want to receive medically supplied nutrition and hydration if he or she were permanently unconscious.

One pitfall to avoid in these discussions is focusing on certain types of medical interventions without considering the medical context. For example, if a relative were to state categorically, "I never want to be on machines," he or she would not be the first to do so. This statement may be an understandable response to seeing an unconscious or semiconscious dying loved one or friend hooked up to various machines in a hospital intensive care unit (ICU). However, mechanical ventilation and dialysis also may be temporary measures to help people regain their ability to enjoy life. Accordingly, it would be appropriate for you to help your family member understand this point. Your role is not limited to that of being a passive listener. Your aim is to get an accurate understanding of your family member's actual goals and wishes. That aim would be thwarted if your family member's statements did not accurately reflect those goals and wishes because of a lack of information, misinformation, faulty reasoning, and so forth. Don't hesitate to ask questions to make sure you understand your family member's wishes accurately. Remember, if and when you become a surrogate, it will be too late to ask questions that might have helped clarify those wishes.

Finally, if and when you serve as a surrogate, you may have to weigh the expected benefits and risks associated with various treatment options. When talking to a family member, try to get a sense of the kinds of outcomes he or she would consider *benefits* and those he or she would count as *burdens* or *harms*. If possible, also attempt to get a sense of the relative value or disvalue he or she assigns to various benefits and burdens or harms. It is safe to assume that anyone would value physical and mental functioning and would dislike pain and discomfort. However, different people have different pain thresholds, and whereas some people would rather experience more pain than take medication that also causes diminished alertness, others would opt for pain reduction even it meant diminished alertness. Similarly, most, if not all, people value being alive and having both legs. However, some people are more willing than others to risk dying to save a limb. If you have to make medical decisions for a relative, the more you know about his or her specific preferences and priorities, the better.

Serving as a Surrogate for a Hospitalized Family Member

This section provides information intended to make it easier for you to be an effective surrogate. It also provides answers to some of the questions you might have if you serve as a surrogate for a family member. Because decision making for hospitalized relatives may be particularly challenging, that task is the focus of this section.

Decision-Making Guidelines

When you are asked to make medical decisions for a spouse, parent, sibling, or other family member, the choice may be obvious and may require little, if any, serious deliberation. You may not be married, but suppose you are and your middle-aged spouse suffers a heart attack. At the hospital, a cardiothoracic surgeon tells you that with coronary artery bypass surgery, your spouse likely will make a full recovery. You are told that if you do not approve the surgery, your spouse will die. If you had to make the decision, it is unlikely you would struggle over whether to authorize the surgery. Or, imagine you have a 78-year-old mother who lives in an assisted living facility. She is mentally alert – she is an avid reader and is better at remembering the names of other residents than you are – but she has arthritis and can no longer live independently. You receive a call from the assisted living facility informing you that your mother collapsed and was taken to the hospital emergency department. When you speak to the emergency department physician, she informs you that tests have revealed that your mother suffered a cerebral hemorrhage (bleeding in the brain). Later, you speak to a neurosurgeon who recommends surgery. He tells you that with surgery, there is a very good chance your mother will regain most, if not all, of her cognitive abilities. Without surgery, your mother will die. Again, it is unlikely that you would be uncertain about whether or not to approve the surgery. Finally, imagine you have an unmarried 22-year-old son. You receive a call from a hospital emergency department in the distant city where he lives. You are told he is in a coma due to a car accident. He is in the ICU receiving mechanical ventilation. The physician on the telephone recommends keeping your son on the mechanical ventilator (breathing machine) for at least a week because it is too soon to make any reliable prediction regarding whether he will regain consciousness. Surely, you would not think twice before accepting the physician's recommendation.

In each of these three cases, it is clear that the expected benefits of the recommended treatment far outweigh the risks, and, in each case, death is the expected outcome if the recommended treatment is refused. In such cases, surrogates generally can be confident they are making an appropriate decision when they accept a physician's recommendation. It is appropriate because the recommended treatment clearly is in the patient's best interests, and unless there is evidence to the contrary, it is safe to conclude that the patient would have wanted the treatment.

Unfortunately, however, decision making is not always so uncomplicated. It may be especially heart wrenching when relatives are terminally ill (i.e., they are expected to die within days, weeks, or months even if they receive all available medical treatments). Should a family member who is dying of cancer and has lost the ability to make medical decisions for herself be kept alive as long as possible in the ICU, or should life-extending measures cease and her care focus on the goal of keeping her as comfortable as possible while she dies? Decision making also may be heart wrenching when a family member has a devastating illness or condition that is not terminal but it nevertheless is questionable whether he or she would benefit from life-extending medical interventions. Should a severely demented relative who has advanced Alzheimer's disease and has lost the ability to eat and swallow be given medically supplied nutrition and hydration? Should an elderly relative who is neurologically devastated (her brain has suffered substantial damage) as the result of a stroke and who is not expected to regain significant cognitive function continue to receive mechanical ventilation?

If you are faced with making difficult choices for a family member, the generally accepted gold standard is called the *substituted judgment standard*. It asks you to put yourself in your relative's situation ("shoes") and attempt to make the judgment (decision) he or she would make. The primary limitation with this approach is that surrogates often lack sufficient information. As close as you might be to a spouse, parent, adult child, or sibling, do you think you know that person well enough to confidently say what he or she would decide in any of the situations in the preceding paragraph? Your answer may be yes, but if it is no, you are not alone. Studies tend to show that many people, when presented with a variety of scenarios, cannot accurately predict a close family member's health care choices.

Uncertainty about the decision a close family member would make is not necessarily the result of an inability to put oneself in another person's shoes. Suppose someone asked you right now what you would decide for yourself in each of the scenarios presented earlier. Are the answers obvious to you, or would you need some time to consider the options carefully and maybe talk to your loved ones? If the decisions you would make for yourself are not obvious to you, how can they be obvious to someone else, even a close family member?

As previously indicated, family members can lessen the burden on future surrogates by executing a living will. Sometimes a living will can provide unambiguous evidence of the decision a relative

who can longer decide would make. For example, living wills often
provide instructions to withhold or withdraw life-sustaining treatment
in the event of terminal illness or permanent unconsciousness. If the
terminally ill cancer patient in one of the previous examples had
a living will with these instructions, there would be no doubt the
substituted judgment standard would support a decision to withhold or
withdraw life-sustaining treatment. In fact, some people might claim
that because the living will's instructions are so clear and unambiguous
in the circumstances, there is no need for a surrogate decision maker.
However, a living will with these instructions would not provide
unambiguous guidance in the other two illustrative cases (the person
with advanced Alzheimer's disease and the stroke patient). In both
these cases, the instructions in the living will would be enhanced by
the surrogate's knowledge about the patient's values and preferences.
These cases illustrate how a surrogate's previous conversation with
his or her family member about the meaning and implications of
the living will would prove helpful. Recalling other conversations
also may provide helpful information. For example, the surrogate of
the Alzheimer's disease patient might remember that after she and
the patient visited a mutual friend who had the same condition and
was receiving medically supplied nutrition and hydration, the patient
exclaimed, "I don't want to be kept alive like that!"

In addition to living wills and personal statements, a relative's behavior, habits, and character traits also may provide useful information
when attempting to apply the substituted judgment standard. For
example, did he or she regularly visit physicians for routine examinations? Did he or she generally go to a doctor or emergency department
for actual or suspected medical problems? Did he or she usually agree
to have tests and procedures doctors claimed were urgently needed?
Answers to questions such as these might help you determine what
your relative would and would not want.

If you cannot make a reliable substituted judgment confidently,
how can you fulfill the responsibilities of a surrogate? A generally
accepted fallback standard is called the *best interests standard*. It asks the
surrogate to weigh the expected benefits and risks associated with each
option and select the one he or she thinks has the greatest net balance
of benefits for the patient. Ideally, when you apply this standard, you
should try to assess the benefits and risks in terms of your family
member's values, priorities, and preferences. For example, does your
family member value alertness more than the absence of pain, or vice
versa? Are independence and maintaining dignity important to your
family member; if so, how important are they?

Although it generally is thought that decision making should be *patient centered*, that is, focused on the *patient's* interests, patients aren't necessarily selfish or self-centered. When making health care decisions, some people consider the potential emotional and/or financial impact on loved ones, and it is perfectly appropriate to do so. For example, you might opt for a much less expensive and somewhat less effective medication to be able to pay for a child's college education. Accordingly, if you have good reason to believe a family member for whom you are making medical decisions would consider the impact on loved ones – including you – it is appropriate for you to take this into account when you apply the substituted judgment or best interests standard.

If you do not know enough about a relative's distinctive values and preferences, the usual advice is to weigh the expected benefits and risks from the perspective of a "reasonable person." What would a reasonable person want and not want? A few things in each category are fairly unmistakable: The former includes comfort and an ability to communicate, see, hear, walk, and eat; the latter includes pain, discomfort, and disabilities. What about life? Would a reasonable person always desire more life? Not necessarily. To be sure, some people may believe that life, no matter how poor its quality, is valuable and more life is always a benefit. However, people who are no less reasonable can believe that if their quality of life declines beyond a certain point (e.g., intractable pain or permanent loss of consciousness), life is no longer valuable and more of it is not a benefit. If you have not explicitly discussed your family member's views on this matter, you may have to rely on whatever you know about him or her and use your judgment. Take comfort in the fact that sometimes when we are faced with extremely difficult choices, there is no one right decision. Two or more options may be acceptable, and none may be unacceptable or wrong.

It also may be reassuring to know that a lot of people are faced with such life or death decisions, and many decide that the best decision for a family member is to withhold or withdraw treatment and specify patient comfort as the primary health care goal. Depending on the circumstances, such a decision can be both ethically appropriate and legal. Some physicians occasionally recommend withholding or withdrawing treatment, and many will present it as an option. However, some physicians are categorically opposed to withholding or withdrawing life-sustaining treatment because of their religious and/or ethical beliefs. Generally, if a physician has an objection to withholding or withdrawing life-sustaining treatment when it is legal and professionally acceptable to do so, he or she is required to help transfer the patient to another physician who is willing to follow these directives.

Shared Decision Making with Other Family Members

As previously stated, surrogate decision making may be a group process involving several family members. Hence, the responsibility for making difficult judgments is shared. Often, several family members each contribute relevant information, and some may have knowledge the others lack. Even if no one person has enough evidence about the patient's wishes and preferences to support a decisive judgment about what he or she would have wanted, putting together several different statements and stories may be sufficient to resolve the issue.

Some physicians may prefer to communicate with one spokesperson for the family. This arrangement may increase the efficiency of interactions with physicians and may be suitable for some families. However, you may find that the presence of several ears can increase the group's understanding of a physician's explanations. Some family members may hear or understand information that others don't, and some family members may think of important questions that don't occur to others. Choose the approach that is most suitable for you and other family members.

As valuable as group decision making may be, preexisting family discord can foster interpersonal dynamics that interfere with effective surrogate decision making. If the patient is seriously or critically ill, his or her family members likely are worried and under considerable stress, which may intensify interpersonal strains. If you do not trust a particular relative, are not on speaking terms, or harbor resentment due to a past episode, cooperation between the two of you may present a tremendous challenge. In such situations, it is helpful for everyone to try to put aside their feelings toward one another and focus on a common interest: the well-being of their ill family member. By focusing on the common goal of determining what their relative wants and what is best for him or her, everyone may be able to put aside feelings of resentment, anger, and hostility, at least temporarily. Hospital social workers and/or ethics committees often are called upon to help resolve interpersonal conflicts and may be able to help keep the focus on the ill family member. Hospitals generally provide brochures at admission that explain the various services available and how to request them. Nurses and hospital operators also can tell you how to request the assistance of a social worker or the hospital ethics committee.

Even if there is no preexisting discord, family members may disagree among themselves. A potential source of disagreement is a difference in how various family members understand key medical facts – the patient's condition and prognosis and the pluses (benefits) and minuses (risks) associated with the available treatment options. A helpful first step is to have a family meeting to determine whether everyone is on the same page. If there are disagreements about important medical information, request a family conference with a physician. The meeting will give everyone an opportunity to ask questions and come to a common understanding of the relevant medical facts.

Another potential source of disagreement is a difference in how various family members understand the patient's wishes. A family meeting at which each member presents his or her understanding of the patient's wishes and the evidence for it might help resolve the disagreement. Try to keep the focus on specifics. If everyone hears about a particular conversation a family member had with the patient, the group might be able to reach an agreement. If family members cannot resolve a disagreement by themselves, a social worker or the ethics committee might be able to help. Both are experienced at resolving conflicts in a manner that is both appropriate and acceptable to everyone.

Keeping Informed and Communicating with Physicians

As important as knowledge of your family member's wishes may be, it is no less essential to have an accurate understanding of his or her medical condition and prognosis as well as the expected outcomes for each treatment option. Therefore, if you are a surrogate, it is crucial to keep informed. Your relative's condition may change, and you cannot make an informed decision unless you have an accurate understanding of the *current* situation. Ask the physicians for regular updates, and let them know you want to be notified immediately if there are any significant changes.

Although keeping informed is essential, you might encounter obstacles. Physicians are busy, they have many patients, and some have other professional responsibilities, such as teaching and research. However, don't be timid. Insist on being kept up to date on your family member's situation. Although the Internet can be a source of general information about diseases and medical conditions, it is not a substitute for your family member's physicians. Only they know the specifics of your relative's current condition, prognosis, and feasible treatment options. You may find that nurses and social workers can be helpful in arranging for physicians to talk to you. If all else fails, consider asking for an ethics consultation. Ethics committees can help facilitate communication. There is more than a grain of truth to the expression "the squeaky wheel gets oiled."

Especially in larger medical centers and university-affiliated hospitals, there are regular changes in physicians. For example, ICU physicians, surgeons, and other specialists might change every week or two. Such changes may mean you will not be able to establish an ongoing relationship with one physician for the duration of your family member's hospital stay; however, you still can establish a relationship with each new physician. If your family member has a regular primary care physician (family physician or internist), that doctor may be able to provide some continuity despite all the medical staff rotations. Some hospitals have doctors called "hospitalists," whose functions include coordinating care and providing continuity. Nurses are another potential source of continuity.

As is true of people in general, physicians' attitudes and opinions may differ significantly. Some might see the glass as half (or 30%) full, and others might see the glass as half (or 70%) empty, and this difference in attitudes might be reflected in their respective recommendations. Such variations among physicians may be frustrating and confusing. One way to deal with these variations is to seek more specificity. For example, if a physician says there is a good chance a treatment will be successful, you might respond along the following lines: "Please explain what you mean by a 'good chance.' Can you give me a percentage or probability? What do you consider 'success'? Do you mean only that my husband will not die soon, or do you mean that he will make a full recovery and will be able to resume all his usual activities?" On the other hand, if a physician recommends a do-not-resuscitate (DNR) order because cardiopulmonary resuscitation (CPR) would be "futile," you might respond by asking for a clarification. Is the physician saying that if your family member's heart stops, even if it is restarted with CPR, it is next to impossible that he or she will regain consciousness or be able to leave the ICU? Or does the physician mean that if your family member's heart stops, it is next to impossible that it can be restarted with CPR?

Physicians also may disagree about medical judgments, such as the chances a patient on a mechanical ventilator will not need to stay on it indefinitely or the probability that a comatose patient will regain consciousness. If there is a difference between two physicians (e.g., between the current ICU attending physician and the previous one), you can request the opinion of a third physician. Similarly, if you want to confirm a diagnosis and prognosis before making a decision, you can request a second opinion. Don't worry that you will insult physicians; they should understand the importance of second (or third) opinions, and many are used to such requests.

Specialists may present another obstacle to understanding. When reporting on your family member's condition, a specialist might focus exclusively on the specific organ system or part of the body that is the subject of his or her specialty. A nephrologist might focus on your family member's kidneys, a pulmonologist on the lungs, a gastro-enterologist on the intestines, and so forth. For example, a nephrolo-gist (kidney specialist) might report, "Your father's kidneys are func-tioning better today." Or, she simply might tell you, "Your father has improved." What she may not be telling you is that your father's *overall condition* has not improved. If there still is only the slimmest chance he will ever regain consciousness, you may not think your father's condition has improved in any way that will affect your decision mak-ing. You can prevent misunderstanding if you question specialists to determine what they mean when they report an "improvement."

Nurses may be a valuable source of up-to-date information. How-ever, keep in mind they are not physicians, and they may highlight factors that are unrelated to your relative's overall condition and prog-nosis. For example, when a nurse tells you your relative's temperature has returned to normal or an electrolyte imbalance has been corrected, he or she may report it as "good news." As in the case of specialists' reports, however, these "improvements" may not indicate any overall improvement in your family member's condition. Nevertheless, it is understandable that nurses may prefer to communicate good rather than bad news. Listen carefully to nurses and physicians, but don't hes-itate to request clarification and ask questions whenever it will help you interpret and understand what they say.

If a relative is seriously or critically ill, physicians' statements for the first few days or weeks of hospitalization may seem encouraging. For example, they might say, "We are doing everything we can, and we will continue to do so," or "There still are other medications or procedures we can try." There is no reason to doubt the physicians are sincere and mean what they say. However, keep in mind they may fail to inform you that their best efforts might eventually prove unsuccessful. To be sure, some physicians may tell you from the outset that there are no guarantees and it may be necessary to reevaluate after a specified period to determine whether your relative's condition has improved, deteriorated, or remained unchanged. However, for a variety of reasons, others might not offer this information. They might not want to undermine your hope, or they simply might think there is no reason to provide such information. Whatever the explanation, if you are not made aware at the outset of a possible need for reassessment after a certain period, you may be taken aback when a physician who consistently seemed optimistic suddenly recommends that no effort be made to restart your family member's heart if it stops. As a consequence of such an unanticipated and seemingly dramatic shift, you may be reluctant to accept the physician's recommendation – even if it actually is reasonable in light of your family member's poor prognosis. To forestall such unpleasant and distressing situations, if physicians do not offer benchmarks for determining if and when it is time to reassess the goals of your family member's medical care, you can ask them to do so. Because providing you with such benchmarks can reduce the risk of future conflicts with you, it is in their interest to satisfy your request.

Physicians may present two or more options, or they might make a specific recommendation. However, even when a physician recommends only one test or treatment, there is always at least one other option: to forgo the recommended test or treatment. Although tests and treatments may have substantial benefits, they also may have unwanted and sometimes serious consequences. Accordingly, if the probability of any significant benefit is low whereas the probability of serious unwanted consequences is high, having the test or treatment may not be in your family member's best interest. This observation may hold true even when a patient is expected to die without a particular medical intervention. Because medical interventions can cause harm, such as disability, deterioration in health, pain, and discomfort, it is possible that even if it is assumed that continued life would be a benefit to the patient, the probability of any benefit is too low to incur a much higher probability of serious harm. Providing a potentially life-extending treatment can turn what might have been a "less bad" death into a "much worse" death. Bluntly stated, in some situations, death may be the *least worst* alternative, a point to keep in mind if you are faced with deciding whether to authorize last-ditch efforts to prevent a family member's death.

Disagreements with Physicians

Just as family members may disagree among themselves, there may be disagreements between one or more family members and physicians. The disagreement might be about medical issues – for example, whether the patient will ever regain consciousness. In such cases, an option is to request a second opinion. On the other hand, there may be agreement about the medical facts but disagreement about the appropriate treatment plan. For example, a physician and his patient's family members all agree the patient has irreversibly lost most of her cognitive function because of a stroke. The physician recommends ceasing all life-sustaining treatments, including medically supplied nutrition and hydration, and providing comfort measures only. The family members disagree. They insist on continuing nutrition and hydration. As a first step, it might be helpful to try to determine the source of the disagreement. Do the family members believe the patient will experience pain and discomfort if she does not receive nutrition and hydration? If so, the physician may be able to assure them that the patient can be kept comfortable without medically supplied nutrition and hydration. Did the patient explicitly tell her family members that in keeping with her religious beliefs, she did not want medically supplied nutrition and hydration to be withheld under any circumstances? If so, and the physician is made aware of the patient's beliefs and previously expressed wishes, he might be more inclined to honor the family's wishes. If an impasse is reached, a social worker or the ethics committee may help resolve the disagreement. Sometimes, however, the only feasible resolution is to find a physician who is willing to honor a decision the current physician refuses to implement.

Conclusion

Although you understandably may be reluctant to talk about illness, disease, and death with your family members, such conversations may prove invaluable if and when you are called upon to assist in decision making about a relative's health care. The knowledge you gain from these conversations will make it easier for you to serve as a surrogate for that family member, and your decisions are more likely to reflect his or her wishes. Hence, such discussions are in the interests of both of you.

If family members signal an interest in talking to you about their health care goals and preferences, encourage them to do so. Don't hesitate to ask questions that can help you better understand their wishes. You needn't wait for relatives to initiate a discussion of their health care preferences. Your own advance health care planning can provide an excellent opportunity for a mutual discussion with family members regarding goals and preferences.

If and when you are called upon to assist in decision making for a family member, start with the available evidence of his or her wishes, such as a living will and/or personal statements. The relative's behavior, habits, and character traits may be an additional source of relevant information. If there is insufficient evidence to reliably establish your relative's wishes, try to decide by weighing each option's expected benefits and risks and selecting the one with the best net balance of benefits.

Keep informed about your family member's condition and prognosis, and don't hesitate to request regular updates from physicians. If there are disagreements or conflicts between you and other family members or physicians, make use of all available resources, including social workers and ethics committees. Finally, keep in mind that sometimes there is no decision that is *the right one*. There can be situations in which two or more decisions are *acceptable* and none is *wrong*.

THIRTEEN

Caring for Individuals with Alzheimer's Disease

Ethical Issues along the Way

– Robyn S. Shapiro

A man does not consist of memory alone. He has feeling, will, sensibilities, moral being. . . . And it is here . . . that you may find ways to touch him.
– A. R. Luria (from a personal letter to Oliver Sacks)

What is the first and most important thing you as a caregiver can do for a patient diagnosed with Alzheimer's disease? Learn everything you can about the disease. This will help you not only in understanding what to expect but also in planning, managing, and making the most of available options.

Chapter Sixteen in this book, "Being and Thinking," describes the characteristics of dementia, which can have many causes. It is estimated that in industrialized nations around the world, approximately 60% of dementia is attributed to Alzheimer's disease. Every seventy seconds, someone develops Alzheimer's disease; as many as 5.3 million people in the United States are living with it now, and nine million cases are projected by 2040. This prevalent and devastating disease presents numerous challenges not only to patients, but also to caregivers. This chapter discusses a variety of issues that caregivers may confront in different stages of the disease and suggests further reading and useful resources.

Stages of the Disease

Although several scales have been developed to describe the progression of Alzheimer's disease, researchers and health professionals generally refer to three broad stages, characterized by the following usual symptoms:

Mild: The patient has difficulty concentrating and exhibits a diminished ability to plan and carry out household tasks, manage finances, or organize daily living. He or she cannot keep track of the passing of time or of his or her own age. The patient also may experience disorientation and the inability to find the right words to describe ordinary objects and their function.

Moderate: As symptoms progress, the patient may have difficulty recognizing people, although he or she usually can still recognize loved ones. He or she may need help with dressing and may show a lack of concern regarding his or her appearance and hygiene. Emotional problems and personality changes also may appear, including agitation, combativeness, paranoia, fear, anger, wandering, and depression. The patient may become withdrawn and antisocial. Close observation and care are necessary.

Advanced: At this last stage, it usually is no longer possible for the patient to respond to his or her surroundings. Communication is extremely limited. The patient cannot recognize loved ones. He or she suffers from incontinence, and basic functions, such as motor coordination and the ability to swallow, begin to shut down. Around-the-clock care is needed, and institutionalization most likely is required.

Truth Telling

Truth telling in the context of Alzheimer's disease should be handled as it is in other medical contexts. You should be as truthful and informative as you can while attending to the patient's need for emotional, relational, and practical support. This means that sensitive awareness on your part should take into consideration the patient's situation with regard to the differing issues that arise. A typical dilemma for caregivers occurs early on, as in the following scenario:

> *In the past year or two, your mom's memory has not seemed to be what it once was. She's never been good with names, but lately she*

has had trouble finding the right words and sometimes loses the thread of conversations altogether. She's anxious, even panicky more of the time, and often irritable. Many have suggested to you that your mom may have dementia, but you don't want to discuss this with your mom or have anyone else discuss it with her. You're afraid that if this is brought up with your mom, her emotional stability and cognitive capabilities will get even worse.

Your desire to protect your mom from this information is understandable. Yet, truthfully telling her about her condition and diagnosis allows her to plan several important aspects of her life, including how she wants to spend her remaining time with more mildly impaired mental functioning, and who she wants to make medical treatment decisions for her when she can no longer make those decisions herself. It also gives her a chance to seek help, such as counseling and support groups, which can help with the anger, fear, and depression that often occur. Some people actually are relieved when they know their diagnosis, because it lessens the embarrassment and annoyance they may have about their forgetfulness. Besides, your mom probably already suspects the diagnosis, anyway. If this is the case, withholding information can threaten the trust between her and the rest of the family.

Of course, it is important to be gentle and sensitive when informing loved ones about their diagnosis. Also, you may have to repeat the information several times on several different occasions, because affected individuals may not remember it at first.

In later stages of the disease, questions of truth telling may take on a different context. For example, should a patient who repeatedly insists her long-dead brother is coming for a visit be informed of the truth? Would it be kinder to say he phoned to postpone his trip? How much truth telling is required in the patient's interest? During the mild stage of Alzheimer's disease, there are good reasons for trying to orient the person to reality; however, in the later stages, imposing reality may become oppressive, resulting in the patient's agitation instead of enlightenment. The patient waiting for her brother would be best served by trying to refocus her attention elsewhere rather than forcing her to relive the pain of her bother's death or placating her with a lie.

Balancing Respect for Autonomy with Concerns about Safety

Lately, neighbors have noticed your Aunt Carol's erratic driving habits. You, yourself, saw her drive through a stop sign in a neighborhood with which she wasn't familiar a few weeks ago, and, on another occasion when you rode with her in the early evening, you noticed that she drove very slowly and crossed the center line a couple of times. She's also been more forgetful lately. Your aunt lives alone and has always enjoyed getting out of the house. When one of the neighbors asked your aunt about her driving, she denied there were any problems. What should you do?

Individuals with dementia may begin to have trouble managing independently in several aspects of their lives. Sometimes, others' questions or concerns, although well intentioned, are seen as an unwelcome interference by the affected individual. It may be difficult to know when and how an individual's independence needs to be limited – and limiting driving privileges is a particularly sensitive issue, because in many cases, driving restrictions severely threaten the person's freedom and lifestyle.

The situation involving your aunt presents a conflict between respect for autonomy, which directs us to respect others' life choices, and beneficence, which directs us to "do good" and protect others' well-being. Ideally, we can create a living environment for those affected by dementia that is both safe and respectful of their choices and independence. In your aunt's situation, it may be that partial limits are appropriate if, for example, she can drive safely in familiar surroundings, in good weather, and/or during the day. To encourage acceptance of such limits, she should be assured that adjustments will be made to fill the gaps posed by the limitations and to diminish the sense of loss (e.g., family members could offer to help with transportation). Responding to increased risks of danger posed by your aunt's dementia with this kind of gradual and negotiated approach to limitations would help keep her, as well as others, safe while maximizing her freedom and independence. It should be noted, however, that the time comes when Alzheimer's patients must give up driving completely; if this is postponed to the point at which a patient causes injury not only to him- or herself but to others, he or she may be held legally responsible.

Medical Care Planning

Your grandfather was diagnosed with Alzheimer's disease two years ago, and you have seen the progression of many symptoms. Your grandfather has become more forgetful, he's more unsteady on his feet, he's irritable, and sometimes he's combative. You worry about how

medical treatment decisions for your grandfather will be made as his
illness gets worse. How can you help?

People with decision-making capacity have an ethical right of
autonomy, or self-governance, and a legal right to direct their own
medical course. These rights mean that people can either accept or
refuse medical treatment, and these rights are not lost when individuals lose their decision-making capacity. When people clearly express
their treatment desires *before* they lose decision-making capacity, they
help assure these rights will be respected. As described by Professor
Ronald Dworkin, a noted philosopher of law, we must protect "prece-
dent autonomy" by honoring medical decisions individuals expressed
before their dementia set in.

Individuals' comprehension and judgment may still be relatively
intact in the early stages of a dementing illness; at this stage, they still
may be able to formulate and express preferences about their future
medical treatment. The capacity to make many medical treatment
decisions does not require that *all* aspects of cognitive functioning
are working optimally; people with a diagnosis of dementia are not
necessarily incapable of understanding medical treatment options and
making medical treatment choices. Also, some people with dementia
may have periods of mental clarity, during which they can better
understand the medical choices. Individuals diagnosed with dementia
who have decision-making capacity should be encouraged to execute
advance directives – documents that allow them to express their treatment
preferences with regard to the level of care they wish to receive when
they become more severely demented, in the later stages of their
disease.

The most common forms of advance directives are *living wills* and
health care powers of attorney. Although state laws on advance directives
vary, in general, a living will document directs an individual's health
care provider to withhold or withdraw life-sustaining procedures in
the event the patient is decisionally incapacitated and either terminally
ill or in a persistent vegetative state.

In a health care power of attorney document, individuals designate
a health care agent to make health care decisions on their behalf if
they become decisionally incapacitated. In general, the agent chosen
should be a person who has knowledge about and respect for the
affected individual's opinions and values and who is free from conflicts
of interest. The health care power of attorney document is activated
at the point of decisional incapacity. Unlike the living will, the health
care power of attorney document is not limited to directions about

withholding or withdrawing life-sustaining procedures in the event of a terminal illness or vegetative state. For example, if your grandfather had a health care power of attorney document and it was determined that he no longer had the ability to make health care decisions for himself, his designated health care agent could make all necessary treatment decisions for him, regardless of his diagnosis or prognosis. Under most state laws, the health care agent is directed to make health care decisions for the individual who signed the health care power of attorney document in accordance with that individual's treatment preferences or, if those preferences are not known, in accordance with the individual's best interests.

In addition to completing advance directives, it is important for people with Alzheimer's disease to discuss their values and preferences with their loved ones before their cognitive abilities become too impaired. Such discussions enable appropriate decision making in clinical situations that might arise later, and they are an invaluable supplement to the advance directive documents themselves.

Financial Planning

Your neighbor, John, has been living alone since his wife died two years ago, and he was diagnosed with early Alzheimer's dementia a few months ago. Last night, when John's son, Ben, came to visit, he took a look at his father's checkbook and realized it had not been balanced for some time. He also found a pile of unpaid bills on his dad's kitchen table. What should Ben do?

To prepare for eventual cognitive disability, the approach that is most respectful of autonomy with respect to financial matters – as is true for medical planning – is for individuals to make plans for themselves before reaching the stage where they cannot do so. For financial matters, such plans should include making a will and establishing a financial power of attorney.

Generally, to make and execute a will, individuals must be able to understand the extent of their property, their blood relations, and the general nature of their material and other assets, and they must have sufficient ability to make reasonable judgments based on this knowledge. If John is in the early stages of Alzheimer's disease, he may well satisfy these criteria.

A financial power of attorney document gives another person, such as a spouse or an adult child, the authority to manage one's property.

Authority granted in a power of attorney can be either general or specific (e.g., limited to selling a house, paying bills, or reviewing bank statements). Under most state laws, a general power of attorney becomes void if the person who granted it becomes cognitively incapacitated; therefore, it is important for those with early Alzheimer's disease to sign a *durable* power of attorney document. Durable power of attorney authorizes someone to act on behalf of an individual *after* he or she loses the ability to make his or her own decisions. If John had this kind of power of attorney, it would explicitly state that the rights that it grants to another can be exercised even if John becomes cognitively disabled.

Petitioning for Guardianship

Your Great Aunt Martha was diagnosed with Alzheimer's disease three years ago and has been in a community-based residential facility (CBRF) for the past two years. For the most part, Aunt Martha has managed well, but in recent months, she has been wandering at night and her forgetfulness has become worse. Administrators from the CBRF recently suggested to Aunt Martha's daughter that she initiate guardianship proceedings for her mother. Aunt Martha's daughter wonders if that's a good idea.

It is not uncommon for organizations providing services to cognitively impaired individuals to worry about their responsibility for the well-being of those individuals. In most respects, care providers' concerns about the affected individual's abilities to safely manage independently are beneficial and appreciated. Sometimes, however, care providers' concerns about their own responsibilities conflict with the recognition of and respect for, to the maximum extent feasible, affected individuals' choices and abilities.

Guardianship proceedings formally clarify an affected individual's legal status as an incompetent individual and transfer decision making about that individual to someone else. In some situations, this is necessary to assure protection of the individual's safety and well-being. However, this step must be taken thoughtfully, because a judicial declaration of incompetence and the imposition of guardianship limit the affected individual's legal rights. To make sure autonomy is not restricted unnecessarily, if guardianship occurs, it should be at an appropriate time, and the timing should be determined on the basis of the affected individual's interests, not the care provider's risk management concerns.

Considering Chemical Restraints

Peter's wife, Mary, was diagnosed with Alzheimer's disease several years ago. He has been caring for Mary at home since then. Presently, Mary has had frequent periods of agitation, and she wanders around the house most nights. Peter wonders whether there are some medications that can help.

Behaviors such as those exhibited by Mary may be frightening and difficult. Although some medications may be able to control these behaviors quickly, sometimes the best course is to seek more-limited approaches that are less likely to damage whatever cognitive abilities the affected individual still has. Many experts believe that chemical restraints should be used only as a last resort, after less-invasive measures have been exhausted. Richard Martin and Peter Whitehouse argue that "behavioral interventions (i.e., making modifications in the environment) are generally preferable to medications for the treatment of most behavioral problems" exhibited by those with dementia. These authors point out that although medications may be important to address depression, psychosis, anxiety, and sleep disturbances, psychoactive drugs should be used only when the target symptom is well defined, and such drugs should be started at low doses, with slow increases and careful monitoring for side effects.[1]

Another reason to avoid chemical restraints is they may have harmful side effects, which should be thoroughly discussed with the treating physician.

Institutional Placement

There comes a time in the course of caregiving when the question of institutional placement arises. The *Alzheimer's Caregivers Guide* suggests two factors to be considered: your physical and mental state as a caregiver and the physical and mental state of the patient. As a caregiver, you must determine how much you can do and when you have reached your limit. Some caregivers reach their limit early on, some reach their limit in later stages, and some are able to cope throughout.

There are a variety of options for institutional care. Several nursing homes have special units for Alzheimer's patients, and there are smaller kinds of supervised living situations, such as board and care and personal care facilities, that care for Alzheimer's patients. In assessing what type of care is best suited for your patient, as well as what each facility offers, it is important to be vigilant, because quality of care is not uniform. The hunt may be long, but the more thorough you are in your search, the more you can be assured of the best match for the patient.

The Aging Parents and Elder Care website (www.aging-parents-and-elder-care.com/Pages/Checklists/Alzheimers_Chklst.html) is especially helpful in choosing an Alzheimer's care facility. The site provides checklists for both nursing homes and assisted living facilities to help you determine what to look for in each. You can take these checklists with you when you tour the various institutions.

Stopping Artificial Nutrition and Hydration

Betty was diagnosed with Alzheimer's disease ten years ago and now is in an advanced stage of dementia. When she first experienced trouble swallowing almost three years ago, Betty had a gastrostomy tube placed. At that time, although Betty was often confused, she enjoyed activities at her nursing home and was able to interact with others. Now Betty is bedridden, in a fetal position, unable to do anything for herself, and unaware of her environment. Betty's sister does not believe Betty would want continued artificial nutritional support under these circumstances and wonders what to do.

Decisions about withholding or withdrawing artificial nutrition and hydration are among the most difficult ones faced by caregivers of cognitively impaired individuals. In most states, the law protects a caregiver's determination to stop tube feeding for a loved one if that decision is clearly in accord with the affected individual's likely treatment preferences under the circumstances. If, in the early stages of Alzheimer's disease, an individual decides he or she would not want to be artificially fed during later, more advanced stages, those preferences should be documented clearly in an advance directive. If such wishes are not expressed clearly before the loss of decision-making capacity, the laws in some states may not allow artificial nutrition and hydration to be withheld or withdrawn.

Even if a caregiver is certain about an affected individual's feelings about artificial feeding, the decision to withdraw tube feeding that has been administered over a period of time often is more difficult than deciding to withhold it at the outset. Many ethicists, however, contend that there is no moral difference between withholding and withdrawing treatment, including artificial nutrition and hydration, if information about the benefits and burdens of the treatment and the patient's likely preferences under the circumstances are clear.

Caring for Caregivers

A crucial ingredient in caring for the patient is caring for yourself. As caregiver, depending on your relationship with the patient, you have your own sense of grief and loss. The demands of caring for an adult whose functions are reduced in so many ways are unceasing and draining. Under these circumstances, it would not be unusual for you to begin to feel worn out, frustrated, and resentful, particularly knowing your efforts will not result in a cure for your loved one and that more of the same will follow. Guilt and even depression often result. However, there are a variety of resources to help you. In addition to talking with your physician, there are support groups, personal counseling, respite care, and adult day care. Start exploring these options early, before you reach a desperate state. Particularly useful websites include:

> www.nia.nih.gov/Alzheimers/Publications/caregiverguide.htm
>
> http://alzheimers.about.com/od/caregivers/a/Rules_Response .htm
>
> http://helpguide.org/elder/alzheimers_disease_dementia_support_ caregiver.htm

Enhancing Quality of Life

How caregivers view the patient through the stages of the disease is a determining factor in shaping the patient's own experience. If the person with Alzheimer's is perceived primarily as a dysfunctional burden, then he or she likely will not be afforded the respect that would otherwise be unquestioned. However, as Kitwood points out, well-being is possible to varying degrees as the disease progresses, and the patient's quality of life can be much enhanced by recognizing and exploring ways to reach the emotional, relational, and aesthetic aspects of the person.

Regarding the capacity of patients to respond to emotional stimuli, in his *Musicophilia*, Oliver Sacks explores the comforting power of music and observes that he has witnessed deeply demented patients respond to music, even pieces with which they were not familiar. This phenomena suggests to Sacks that such patients are capable, at least at such times, to experience the entire range of human feelings and these responses demonstrate, according to Sacks, that there is still a self that can be summoned, even if only by music.

These emotional connections for patients may come from very simple additions to their daily lives. The family of one patient found that placing a birdcage with a canary in the patient's room provided a focus of affectionate interest and attention. Another patient, a man for whom dancing had been an important pleasure, was soothed and comforted by his favorite music. A former university professor, for whom reading no longer was possible, took great pleasure in accompanied neighborhood walks. Attentive caregivers look for ways to work with the patient's remaining capacities for the patient's benefit.

Conclusion

Caring for a loved one with Alzheimer's disease is a challenging experience that poses new dilemmas with each changing level of ability. As Ronald Reagan noted in his November 11, 1994, letter to the American people, "Unfortunately, as Alzheimer's disease progresses, the family often bears a heavy burden." It should be noted, however, that the burden also comes with the opportunity of providing the patient with a final gift. As Alzheimer's patients become increasingly unable to decide for themselves or act to implement their values, those tasks, to the degree necessary, can be assumed by others. With the assistance of caregivers, patients can continue to experience a measure of self-governance and thus be assured as the disease progresses of ongoing respect for their safety and human dignity.

REFERENCES

[1] Martin RJ, and Whitehouse PJ: The clinical care of patients with dementia. In *Dementia Care: Patient, Family, and Community*, edited by N. L. Mace (Baltimore: Johns Hopkins University Press, 1990): 25.
[2] Sacks O: *Musicophilia: Tales of Music and the Brain* (New York: Knopf, 2007): 201–231.

SUGGESTIONS FOR FURTHER READING

Bell V, Troxel D: *The Best Friends Approach to Alzheimer's Care* (Baltimore: Health Professions Press, 1997).
Binstock BH et al. (ed.): *Dementia and Aging: Ethics, Values and Policy Choices* (Baltimore: Johns Hopkins University Press, 1992).

Center for the Study of Bioethics at the Medical College of Wisconsin: *Making Day-to-Day Decisions Wisely: A Practical Handbook on Ethical and Legal Issues for Caregivers of Individuals with Alzheimer's Disease*. (Milwaukee: Medical College of Wisconsin, n.d.).

Kitwood T: *Dementia Reconsidered: The Person Comes First* (Buckingham: Open University Press, 1997).

Mace NL (ed.): *Dementia Care: Patient, Family and Community* (Baltimore: Johns Hopkins University Press, 1990).

Mace NL, Rubins PV: *The 36-Hour Day* (Baltimore: Johns Hopkins University Press, 1991).

Morris JC (ed.): *Handbook of Dementing Illness* (New York: Marcel Dekker, 1994).

Post SG: *The Moral Challenges of Alzheimer's Disease* (Baltimore: Johns Hopkins University Press, 1996).

Sabat SR: *The Experience of Alzheimer's Disease: Life Through a Tangled Veil* (Oxford: Blackwell, 2001).

To learn about services, research centers, research studies, and publications about Alzheimer's, contact the following resources:

Alzheimer's Disease Education and Referral (ADEAR) Center
800-438-4380 (toll-free)
www.nia.nih.gov/Alzheimers

Alzheimer's Association
800-272-3900 (toll-free)
www.alz.org

Alzheimer's Foundation of America
866-232-8484 (toll-free)
www.alzfdn.org

National Institute on Aging
Alzheimer's Disease: A Caregiver and Patient Resource List
http://www.nia.nih.gov/Alzheimers/Publications/resourcelist.htm

FOURTEEN

When the Patient Is a Child

– Timothy S. Yeh

As we train to become pediatricians, one of the first things we learn is that children are not small adults. Those who care for young patients should heed this lesson each day. If you are a parent, this concept may seem obvious, but it nonetheless is helpful to remember how important it is, because when your child is ill, you are your child's best advocate. The illness that brings your child to the hospital may be unique to children, or it may be something that can afflict people of any age. One difference is that most adults are capable of understanding their illness, making decisions about their own care, and understanding what is happening to them. Newborn babies and young children are entirely dependent on others for their care and well-being. As they grow older, they begin to acquire a sense of the world around them; they develop an ego or self-awareness and can gradually understand more complex ideas (e.g., what causes illness and how the illness affects them personally).

Decision Making for Children

A patient's competence is one of the most important factors in making informed decisions. It represents his or her ability to understand the situation and possible outcomes and to consider the consequences of each choice he or she makes. In addition, a patient must be able to take this information, put it in the context of his or her values and goals, and then make a voluntary decision. Regardless of age, a person's competence may be limited by several things. To be able to consent to treatment, a person must be conscious. For example, an unconscious automobile accident victim cannot consent to treatment by the hospital team. Similarly, a person who is severely limited in intelligence may be unable to consent to treatment, even though he or she is conscious. An individual who cannot make rational decisions also is limited in the decision-making process. For instance, a three-year-old child is no more able to consent to surgery than is a delusional adult. Children are limited by their ability to reason because they have not reached the developmental (cognitive) stage of being able to think abstractly. Patients also may be limited by knowledge or perception with regard to their health care issue. This is especially true for children, who, as they mature, gradually acquire the ability to process complex concepts, such as the fact that unseen viruses can cause an illness. Young children usually cannot differentiate between symptoms and the causes of illness and may believe illnesses are transmitted "magically." Also, children have limited experiences, significantly affecting their ability to make decisions for themselves. For example, diabetic adolescents may refuse to take their insulin because they do not like the injections. At this age, their experience with diabetes may be limited, and they may be unable to understand the potential life-threatening complications of untreated diabetes. Finally, all states have legally determined age limits defining what a minor is. Among other things, these statutes regulate health care decisions, financial transactions, and the ability to vote and obtain a driver's license. Adults can make decisions for themselves, whereas a child (minor) legally cannot.[1]

Emancipated Minor

Although there are laws defining the age or situation in which a person transitions from being a minor to an adult, the definitions are somewhat arbitrary and may not coincide with an individual's "developmental" age. Patients who are legally deemed to be minors cannot independently make decisions about their health care, with certain exceptions. For example, most states allow minors aged thirteen through eighteen to provide consent for some medical care, which may include contraception and care for sexually transmitted diseases, pregnancy, alcohol and drug abuse, and psychiatric problems. In the United States, a minor (i.e., someone less than eighteen years of age) can become "emancipated" by obtaining a court order after demonstrating he or she is financially independent from his or her parents or guardians, is legally married, or is a member of the armed forces.

Surrogate Decision Making

Apart from the exceptions noted previously, health care decisions for minors are made by their parents or guardians. This is known as surrogate or proxy decision making. *Surrogate decision making* also applies to adults who lack the ability to give informed consent to their own treatment. Except in cases in which abuse or neglect is a concern, it is assumed that a parent or guardian will act in a child's best interest. One essential difference between surrogate decision making for children and surrogate decision making for adults is that, in many cases, adults have previously expressed their wishes either verbally or through a written advanced directive, whereas children (especially infants and young children) have not. Thus, the surrogate for a child must decide not only what is in the best interests of the child, but also what that child would want if he or she were capable of giving informed consent. This choice is made in the context of the child's family's values and beliefs, as well as the values and tenets of the society in which the child lives.

Some health care decisions for children are relatively straightforward and noncontroversial. For example, a father may bring his ten-year-old daughter to the hospital because she has developed abdominal pain, vomiting, and fever. After examining her and performing a series of blood tests and imaging studies, the doctor diagnoses probable appendicitis. The doctor recommends that the patient be taken to surgery to remove her inflamed appendix. The patient's father weighs the benefits and risks of consenting to the surgery or not, and then makes the decision for her. These choices are as follows:

Proceed with surgery

Risks   Complications from the anesthesia
           Bleeding
           Problems with healing
           Postoperative infection
Benefits   If the appendix is infected, it can be removed before it causes
           further problems

Do not proceed with surgery

Risks   Further complications of the appendicitis, including perfora-
            tion and spread of infection throughout the entire abdomen and
            bloodstream
Benefits   Avoid anesthesia exposure
            Avoid an unnecessary operation if the diagnosis is incorrect

In this case, the likelihood that this is appendicitis (high) far out-
weighs the potential complications from the surgery itself (low). Most
parents, as the child's surrogate decision maker, would consent to the
surgery.

Best Interests of the Child

A child cannot make health care decisions independently, so how
does his or her surrogate decision maker decide what choice is in that
child's best interests? There are several ways to approach this. As a
parent or guardian, you know your child better than anyone else and
are best able to articulate his or her wishes. You also understand that
your child is part of an entire family and that each decision can have
an impact on your family. At the same time, you must decide what
the best medical choice is based on an objective view determined by
factual information presented to you by the health care team. Your
child's best interests are served when you incorporate all these factors
into your decision making.

Disagreement between the Health Care Team and Surrogate Decision Makers Regarding Care

Unfortunately, sometimes the decisions we make are not simple, either
for the child's parents or for the health care team. For example, a ten-
year-old girl has a highly malignant blood cancer (leukemia). In most
cases, this type of leukemia has been incurable with the available
treatments. She has undergone chemotherapy, radiation therapy, and
bone marrow transplantation, yet despite all these efforts, her cancer
has returned. These treatments have taken their toll on her as well,
causing her great discomfort during the course of their administration.
She now is in constant pain and requires medication to provide some
relief.

The patient's doctors tell her parents there is a new, experimental
treatment available for patients in their daughter's situation. This treatment is associated with significant side effects, and the likelihood it

will lead to a remission or cure is small. The next step in the decision-making process is extremely important and can take one of several paths. The parents and the health care team may agree that because the chances of a beneficial outcome from the new treatment are so small and the side effects superimposed on their daughter's current medical problems are so great, the best choice for her would be to forgo the new treatment and do everything possible to make her comfortable at the end of her life. On the other hand, both the parents and the health care team may agree that despite the side effects and the slight chance of success, they do not want to deny the patient of any possible treatment.

Suppose the parents and the health care team are in disagreement. This might be the case if the health care team insists on giving the patient every possible treatment, whereas her parents believe their daughter has gone through enough. Or, the parents may wish to proceed despite the small probability of benefit, whereas the health care team may feel it would only prolong the patient's discomfort to no avail.

How does one make the "right" decision when there is agreement or disagreement between the parents and the health care team? In the previous scenarios, there is no absolute "right" choice. Rather than focusing on what is "right," it is more important to ensure that the decision serves the child's best interests. In these situations, good communication and frank discussions between the health care providers and the parents or guardian are essential. The health care team must be very clear about the goals of treatment and realistic about what it can offer. You, as a parent or guardian, must be equally clear about your own concerns and the reasons for your decision. When the decision is difficult, it often is helpful to consult with others outside the immediate care providers, including seeking the help of extended family and clergy, obtaining a second medical opinion, or consulting with a medical ethics group. In most cases, even those complicated by the uncertainty of outcome, a plan can be reached that will serve the child's best interests.

Cognitive Development and Decision Making

As noted earlier, a person's ability to consent to medical treatment depends on his or her being deemed competent. Rationality (or reasoning), knowledge and perception, and experience are all factors in determining decision-making competence that children acquire as they develop and mature. It has been observed that some children with chronic diseases such as cystic fibrosis or cancer seem "mature beyond their years." Although chronologically they are not older than children their age, their experiences (especially with medical treatments and hospitalizations) allow them to acquire the knowledge, perception, and experience necessary to understand and participate in their care. Children who have a terminal illness may know others with the same disease who have died, thus they understand the implications of their illness, whereas their healthy peers are only beginning to understand their own mortality.

When should you involve your child in his or her health care? The American Academy of Pediatrics stated that "as children develop, they should gradually become the primary guardians of personal health and the primary partners in medical decision-making, assuming responsibility from their parents."[2] Clearly, there is no specific age that is appropriate for all children. Your child, as well as the circumstances relating to his or her medical issues, will help provide you with a guide on how to approach this question. If you believe your child can understand his or her medical problem, the treatment indicated, and the expected outcome, then it would be appropriate to encourage his or her participation. Members of the health care team (e.g., physicians, nurses, social workers, child life specialists, nutritionists, and others) with expertise in child development can provide you with a professional assessment of what your child is capable of understanding.

Other than the special circumstances mentioned earlier, minors cannot legally consent to medical treatment. However, whenever possible, if you and the health care team feel it is appropriate, your child should be involved in decision making and be allowed to provide assent for treatment. Assent for treatment is beneficial in that it provides children with a sense of control over their own life and a feeling that their opinion matters, and it is helpful in their compliance with treatment. Informed consent can be given only by minors with legal entitlement and decisional capacity (e.g., emancipated minors); otherwise you, as a parent or guardian, must provide permission.

Whether or not your child is an active participant in health care decision making, providing him or her with developmentally age-appropriate information is extremely important. Also, be careful not to talk as though your child "is not there" and cannot understand the conversations occurring in his or her presence. It is appropriate for you to remind members of the health care team, physicians included, that when speaking in the presence of a pediatric patient, they should be inclusive rather than exclusive and address the child as well as the parents. Children usually are much more observant than adults give them credit for. Even if they do not understand the exact meaning of words, children become experts at reading body language at a very young age. Children as young as six years of age often take an active interest in understanding their illness.

One issue when incorporating children in the decision-making process is whether they can make a voluntary decision. A truly voluntary decision is made independently, without undue influence from others. In the case of an adolescent or older child who assents to a specific treatment, one must always be sensitive to the fact that the decision may partly be in response to what the child views as the response desired by authority figures (parents, guardians, physicians, and other health care providers). The child's assent may be based solely on a desire to comply with their wishes. Older children and pre-teens tend to conform to social norms and expectations. On the other hand, later in adolescence, there is a risk that the child is disagreeing with the proposed treatment specifically to defy the wishes of those in a position of authority. Listening very carefully to the perceptions of the patient often will assist in determining the meaning of a child's assent.

The Adolescent Patient

How can we tie all this together for adolescent patients? Typically, by late adolescence, cognitive development has progressed to the point at which complex concepts are readily understood. In addition, an understanding of mortality, including one's own, is usually acquired during these years. However, the limits of life experience may hamper the medical decision-making process. Similarly, adolescents may be conflicted by the need to conform versus the desire to become more independent. Most importantly, continual open discussions are necessary. It is known that knowledge of the illness and treatment options increases a child's feeling of control and ability to cope with the illness.

Potential problems arise when an adolescent and his or her parents or health care team disagree on how to proceed with treatment. It is difficult, if not impossible, to force adolescents to accept treatment they do not want. Patience, consistent communication, and an acknowledgement of the adolescent's needs and wishes are essential to work through the problems.

In certain circumstances, there are exceptions in which minors can consent to treatment and have a privileged and confidential relationship with the health care team. These situations involve emancipated minors and minors (thirteen through eighteen years) seeking treatment for certain problem-related conditions, including contraception, sexually transmitted diseases, pregnancy, alcohol and drug abuse, and psychiatric problems.

Support for Children and Their Families

As the parent or guardian of an ill infant, child, or adolescent, you are not alone. Every physician who cares for children should know what resources are available to children and their families within their community. Every hospital should provide the support families in crisis need. Medical centers specializing in the care of pediatric patients have social workers, child life specialists, and patient care advocates. These individuals can address the needs of their pediatric patients as well as their families and are integral members of the health care team. Social workers help patients and families (including siblings) cope with the stress of hospitalization and identify resources that are invaluable when the routine of life is disrupted by illness. Child life specialists use their knowledge of child development to help patients adapt to hospitalization and prepare them for what lies ahead. Patient care advocates, the ombudsmen of the hospital, are the official representatives of patients and their families. They are your allies and are available for your benefit.

Family-Centered Care in the Pediatric Setting

The importance of family-centered care in pediatrics is well recognized. Your child is wholly dependent on you, his or her guardian, for physical, economic, and emotional support. This does not change if he or she is admitted to the hospital, although parents often feel they have lost control over what happens when their child is hospitalized. It is true that medical therapies, the daily routine, and minute-to-minute decisions often are predetermined. Hospitals operate twenty-four hours a day, seven days a week, and 365 days a year. The health care team functions together and separately at the same time. Important information is communicated in written form (the patient chart or medical record) with notes and orders as well as verbally among staff members. The nursing staff may work eight- or twelve-hour shifts. Physicians and other members of the health care team make "rounds" to visit patients at least once a day to discuss the patients for whom they are responsible. Medications, meals, and therapies are given at prescribed times throughout the day. Diagnostic procedures such as x-rays, scans, and blood tests are routinely scheduled. It is vitally important to your child that you remain the constant in this continuous whirlwind of activity.

A hospital that provides family-centered care incorporates the entire family of each child they care for. Parents can feed their child and accompany him or her during procedures. Child life specialists can assist parents in preparing their children for procedures and testing. As the parent or guardian of a patient, you should feel comfortable asking questions and participating in discussions that take place with your child's health care team. For prolonged hospitalizations, periodic family–patient care conferences should be held to review the plan of care, answer questions, and make appropriate changes based on input that includes the parents or guardian. In addition, in-hospital school programs enable children to keep up with their schoolwork during their absence. Pet therapy programs allow specially trained and certified animals to visit patients when appropriate and can provide benefits in the healing process.

Many hospitals have visiting policies for pediatric patients that may include extended hours and special circumstances. In fact, most pediatric medical centers provide accommodations for parents or guardians to "room in" with their child. Most hospitals also recognize the need for siblings to understand what has happened and to visit the patient in the hospital. This not only is beneficial to the patient but can also alleviate some of the anxiety and even guilt that siblings associate with an illness in a family member. Additionally, other accommodations allow the pediatric patient to have some sense of control. These include allowing the child's friends to visit, allowing special comfort items to be brought in (blankets, stuffed toys, music), and having children choose their own meals (or even having food brought in from home).

Other issues may arise from the hospitalization of a child with siblings. Parental absence may lead the child who remains at home to express anger at the parents or the sick child by acting out and by attention-seeking behavior. It is perfectly normal for parents to feel guilty for not being able to spend more time with their other children. The hospitalization invariably leads to disruption of family routines such as meals and school activities. For all these reasons, it is important for the parents or guardian to consider the entire family during this stressful period. In addition to bringing the other children to visit the child who is sick, parents can take turns staying at the hospital while the other parent maintains the usual daily routine at home. It also is extremely important for parents to make sure they themselves are as well rested and nourished as possible so that they can be there for all their children. Your hospital social worker can be of great assistance in helping you with these issues.

Finally, take advantage of any resources the hospital may have to keep those who are unable to visit informed. Family resource centers often have access to computers and the Internet, allowing you to post progress reports on Web logs created for your child and to link to parent support groups. One such service, the Caring Bridge (www.caringbridge.org), is used by more than twenty million families each year.

The Well-Informed Ethics Committee

There are occasions when disagreements arise during the course of providing care to children in the hospital. Very frequently, these disputes can be resolved through continued dialogue with all of those involved in caring for the patient, including parents or guardians. The conflict may be the result of poor communication and misunderstanding and thus easily resolved. Social workers and patient care advocates can work on the family's behalf to try to reach an agreement that will serve the child's best interests. When these measures are unsuccessful, it may be useful to request the involvement of the hospital's institutional ethics committee (IEC).

The Joint Commission on Accreditation of Healthcare Organizations (JCAHO) accredits and certifies more than 15,000 health care organizations in the United States. It stipulates that every accredited hospital have an established mechanism to address conflicts. In most hospitals, this requirement is met by the IEC (or bioethics committee).

The IEC is composed of individuals from both the hospital and the general community. Participants from the hospital community usually include physicians, nurses, social workers, and representatives from administration. The general community may be represented by community leaders, clergy, and members of advocacy groups (e.g., groups representing disabled people). Many committees have as permanent members or consultants individuals with special training in bioethics.

The IEC is responsible for providing ethics consultations as well as developing policies and educational programs for staff about ethical issues. When an IEC is asked to do a consultation, it must adhere to the same principles as any other medical consultation, including maintaining confidentiality, gathering information, and formulating a recommendation. In addition, the IEC may serve as a mediator in ongoing discussions between the patient or family and the health care team.

A typical IEC may receive a request for consultation from a physician, nurse, social worker, or any member of the health care team. An IEC consultation request also may come from a patient or family member. The case is presented to the committee by the health care team, and the patient or family member may ask to present his or her perspective. After the information-gathering portion of the consultation, the committee discusses the issues identified and makes a recommendation to the health care team. The committee also may be asked to share its recommendations with the family. The committee's recommendations are advisory; ultimately, it is up to the family and the health care team to reach an agreement that best serves the patient.

When the consultation involves patients who are children, it is important for the IEC to have representatives with specific expertise in pediatric issues when patients cannot represent themselves or when they are legally unable to make medical decisions for themselves. Knowledge and experience in the areas of surrogate decision making and cognitive development should be available to the committee, either through its members or by consultation with appropriate individuals.

In rare instances, a disagreement cannot be resolved. Although it is always preferable to continue trying to work through the dispute, occasionally the matter may be brought before a court. However, this should be the avenue of last resort, after all other attempts at resolution have been exhausted. Few judges or juries have the degree of medical knowledge needed to deliver an educated judgment in these cases.

Family Presence during Medical Procedures or CPR

Naturally, parents want to protect their child. However, when the child requires medical treatment, the entire process may run counter to their instincts. Children with serious illnesses often are subjected to multiple uncomfortable or painful procedures and treatments. Although parents may not be able to change the procedure itself, they may be able to decrease the amount of emotional and physical discomfort by supporting their child. Child life specialists can teach a child and his or her parents techniques such as visualization and relaxation that can make a procedure less traumatic for the child. When appropriate, the parent's presence during a procedure can decrease the child's anxiety. Some hospitals allow a parent to remain with his or her child during difficult procedures or while the anesthesiologist administers the medications that will put the child to sleep before the procedure. This usually makes the procedure itself much less traumatic for the patient.

In the tragic situation in which a child requires cardiopulmonary resuscitation (CPR), his or her parents may want to remain with the child. Although the child may not be conscious during CPR, the parents may be comforted by the fact that they are with their child during what may be the last moments of life. Whatever the outcome, they may feel that their child is aware on some level of their presence and that they can help or provide comfort to the child.

Numerous studies have found that given the option, more parents choose to stay with their child during complex medical procedures and CPR. In one study, nearly all those who chose to remain with their child during procedures and CPR said they would make the same decision again. Many family members who were present during CPR said that it reassured them that everything possible was done for their loved one.[3]

However, although it seems there is a trend toward parents wanting to remain with their child during complex procedures or CPR, the practice remains controversial among clinicians (physicians, nurses, respiratory therapists, and others), and it is not standard practice at all hospitals caring for children. There is still a concern that the family member may disrupt the treatment being administered or that, if the family member cannot emotionally handle the situation, he or she may require medical attention as well. However, the experience reported in the medical literature does not appear to support these concerns. Still, you should be aware that in some hospitals, and with some physicians, you might meet resistance to such requests. In any case, if you find yourself in such a situation, you can make the request. If the health care team agrees, it will designate one of its members to stay with you and support you. On the other hand, if you do not feel comfortable being present during a crisis situation, you should not feel pressured to do so. You should make the decision that is best for you as well as your child.

Family Members as Potential Organ Donors

Unfortunately, some children develop a disease that leads to the need for organ transplantation. In the case of kidney, liver, or lung failure, a living donor may be an option for the child. A healthy donor may donate one of his or her kidneys or a portion of his or her liver or lung to save the life of the child who receives it. Because it is important to have the closest tissue match possible to minimize the chances of the child's body rejecting the transplanted organ, living related donors are sometimes the best potential donors. For many reasons – medical, ethical, and legal – living related donors usually are adults. An adult can legally consent to the donation and make an informed decision. The risks and discomfort from removing the donor organ may be significant. Moreover, even adults may be unduly influenced (pressured) by others if they prove to be a suitable match for a child who needs an organ. The instances of minors donating kidneys are rare. It is important for the entire health care team to be involved and supportive of both the potential donor and the recipient. The medical social worker's role is critical in identifying issues that may arise regarding the decision to donate, and he or she can mediate and intervene in the best interests of all those involved. Input and insight from the other members of the health care team are essential.

In 2000, the Live Organ Donor Consensus Group issued guidelines for minors as organ donors.[4] They stated that 1) the donor and recipient must be highly likely to benefit (e.g., donation to an immediate family member); 2) the surgical risk for the donor should be extremely low (kidney); 3) a child should be the donor of last resort and should not undergo donor evaluation until all other options are exhausted, including the potential for a deceased donor; and 4) the child should agree freely to donate, without coercion and with a full understanding of the process. The American Academy of Pediatrics added that the emotional and psychological risks to child donors must be minimized.[5]

On the other hand, several blood diseases (e.g., blood cancer, or leukemia) and metabolic disorders can be treated with stem cell transplantation. As is the case with organ donation, a living related donor might be the best potential donor. Stem cell donation generally is considered less traumatic and carries fewer risks than other forms of organ transplantation. However, there are still serious ethical issues that arise when minors are considered as a potential source of stem cells. The use of siblings who are minors for stem cell donation is both an ethical and a medical dilemma. First, one must consider whether the circumstances satisfy the five criteria presented by the Live Organ Donor Consensus Group and the American Academy of Pediatrics. Next, one must consider the medical aspects of being a stem cell donor. There are two methods for obtaining stem cells from a living donor. The first is by inserting a needle into the center of a bone (marrow) and drawing the stem cells out. The second is by taking blood from a vein and then separating the stem cells in the blood for the donation. The first procedure is more invasive and painful and requires an anesthetic, whereas the second requires the donor to take a medication that boosts the number of stem cells in the circulating blood. The problems with using the second method in children are that no one knows the long-term effects of giving the stem cell–stimulating medication, special catheters must be placed to withdraw the blood, and the amount of blood removed from a smaller child may require a blood transfusion afterward.

The question of whether minors should be considered for organ donation has not been answered. Although it not a common situation, it serves as a reminder of all the considerations that must be addressed when a child is involved in a health care decision – surrogate decision making, assent, and what serves the best interests of the patient (in this case, there are two patients, the recipient and the donor). Medical advances are made every day, and although it is difficult to anticipate the types of challenges we will face in the future, the principles for providing care for children will remain the same.

Medical Research and Your Child

When children are patients, their parents may be approached by the health care team to ask their permission for their children to participate in a research study. Research studies may take many forms. Some studies involve minimum risk to your child, possibly using information already obtained during the course of routine treatment (e.g., lab test results, demographic information). Others may require interventions with potential but uncommon side effects, such as a separate needlestick to obtain blood for a specific test needed for the study. In this case, the brief discomfort, possible bleeding, or infection at the puncture site might be considered acceptable if the research itself would be of significant benefit to others (and possibly to the child as well). Other studies may involve the use of treatments that have not been previously tested and approved. These most often involve new drugs or devices to treat specific medical problems that may not be adequately controlled with current therapies.

The Children's Oncology Group (COG), a national collaboration of hospitals caring for children with cancer, creates treatment protocols, or procedures, directed at all forms of childhood cancer. By enrolling patients in its studies, the COG builds on the experience and results from treating thousands of children with cancer using carefully designed protocols.

Whatever the nature of the research, you should carefully weigh the risks and benefits of the study in which you are asked to enroll your child. Just as a study should not be dismissed because it will be of no direct benefit to your child (but will potentially help others), you should not automatically agree to have your child participate in a study that might be helpful to him or her. In fact, many studies randomly assign patients to two groups: one group receives the new treatment and the other receives the standard (current) treatment.

Before consenting to your child's participation in a research study, you should be mindful of the same things that are important in any medical decision involving your child, such as including your child in the discussion and obtaining his or her assent if developmentally appropriate. In fact, the Office of Human Research Protection of the Department of Health and Human Services states that any approved research study involving children must include an assent process with the child (if developmentally appropriate) as well as an informed consent process (permission) with the parent or guardian.[6]

Summary

Our children depend on their parents and guardians to provide for and protect them. They are most vulnerable when they become ill. Their "family" of caregivers becomes larger as the health care team joins their parents to help them recover. This requires an understanding of surrogate decision making, cognitive development, and age-appropriate involvement of the child in the decision-making process. It is everyone's responsibility to keep the child's best interests at the fore and to be the child's advocate.

REFERENCES

[1] Gaylin W, Macklin R (eds.): *Who Speaks for the Child? The Problems of Proxy Consent* (New York: Plenum, 1982).
[2] Committee on Bioethics: Informed consent, parental permission, and assent in pediatric practice. *Pediatrics* 1995, 95:314–317.
[3] Markovitz Barry P: *AAP News* 2005, 26:11.
[4] Office of Human Research Protection, Department of Health and Human Services: *Protecting Human Research Subjects: Institutional Review Board Guidebook*, 1993.
[5] Live Organ Donor Consensus Group: Consensus statement on the live organ donor. *JAMA* 2000, 284:2919–2926.
[6] Friedman Ross L, Thistlethwaite JR: the Committee on Bioethics: Minors as living solid-organ donors. *Pediatrics* 2008, 122:454–461.

FIFTEEN

Care of Elders

– Claudia Landau and Guy Micco

This chapter discusses what you need to understand about the care of people who are "of a certain age." What exactly that "certain age" is, we aren't saying (because we don't know). However, we will call someone who has reached such an age an *elder*, because we believe this is a more respectful term than *old*. We begin by saying a bit about what happens as we age and what's different about being an elder. We then discuss what we can do about the deleterious effects of aging on our bodies and how to maintain our health and vitality for as long as possible. Along the way, we address how to effectively interact with our doctors and the medical system.

In general, changes associated with aging are caused by repeated exposure to the stresses of life, which, in turn, lead to a progressive decrease in function of organs and the body as a whole. We take *stress* to mean the inability to cope with a perceived threat, real or imagined, to one's mental, physical, emotional, or spiritual self. One of the fundamental features of the body is its attempt to maintain a constant internal environment. This requires continual adjustments and interactions in and among the body's regulatory and repair mechanisms. Physiologists refer to this as the maintenance of *homeostasis*. As we age, for a variety of reasons, our ability to do this becomes impaired.

This in turn leads to the burdens of dysfunction, disability, and disease that accumulate with aging. *Allostasis* is a term used to describe this accumulation. One view of this process was suggested by the biologist Thomas Kirkwood: On a cellular level, we can imagine an interplay between the negative impact of a stressful life and the positive effect of a healthy lifestyle. Both individual and environmental stress may result in an accumulation of cellular defects or damage. Over time, these defects multiply and result in the changes and diseases we associate with aging. However, the body also has a system for repair, and a healthy lifestyle may be able to slow or even decrease the accumulation of cellular damage.[1]

There are two important points to make: 1) As our body ages, our adaptive and repair abilities decrease and 2) we can affect these abilities in both positive and negative ways through how we live.

What Changes with Aging?

All systems of our body are affected by aging. For example, as we age we all will have a decrease in hearing, vision, muscle mass and strength, memory, heart and lung function, and so forth. However, the degree of functional loss differs from person to person, based on genetics, disease, and lifestyle factors. Again, it is important to note that we can affect our body's ability to function both positively and negatively; we are not completely at the whim of our genes.

What is different about being an elder? How the changes that aging effects in our bodies interact to produce disease differ from one person to the next; in addition, how these age-related diseases present in elders may be quite different from what happens in a younger body. For example, in elders, symptoms of serious disease may seem vague or trivial. Therefore, if you have persistent, vague symptoms – for example, just feeling poorly or a significant decrease in your ability to function and perform your usual activities – you should call your doctor. In addition, some symptoms require investigation sooner than they did when you were younger; therefore, you should not delay when you have a new bothersome problem (see Table 15.1).

Here is a classic example. Mrs. P. is eighty-eight years old and lives with her husband of sixty years in their own home. Mr. P. is hard of hearing, somewhat depressed, and not involved in the care of their home, but he does take pleasure in shopping and preparing most of their meals. One day, Mrs. P. falls. She doesn't think she hurt herself but does notice that she is very tired. She takes to sleeping all day long. Her husband notes that she is not eating well. Her daughter,

Table 15.1. Classic problems of elders that present
differently than in younger people

Infection without fever
Depression without sadness
Heart attack without chest pain
Heart failure without shortness of breath
Serious abdominal organ pathology without significant pain
Cancer without specific symptoms
Thyroid disease without specific symptoms

visiting soon after – and, coincidentally, having just read this chapter –
insists that her mother go to her doctor. Mrs. P. resists, saying, "It's
really nothing; I'm just a little tired out. I am eighty-eight, you know."
However, she accedes to her daughter's wish. Her doctor, Dr. L., takes
a good history and does a physical examination. She notes that Mrs. P.
has a cough and a temperature of 99°F, her blood pressure is 110/62
mm Hg, and her pulse is 88 bpm (beats per minute). Her heart, lung,
and abdominal exams are unremarkable. Being a fine geriatrician,
Dr L. knows that Mrs. P.'s usual temperature is 97°F and that a serious
infection can occur in an elder without a high fever. She also knows
that an elder may have pneumonia but have a normal lung exam or
even a normal chest x-ray. In this case, Mrs. P.'s chest x-ray shows
a small pneumonia. Because she was seen early in the course of this
illness, Dr. L. believes Mrs. P. can be treated at home; by coming
in early, she avoided hospitalization. The doctor asks her patient to
increase her fluid intake and prescribes an antibiotic. She also sets up
a home visit by the visiting nurse for the next day.

   Here's another example of the importance of paying attention to
new symptoms, especially in elders: depression without sadness. At
ninety years of age, Mr. D. was very active in his community and an
avid exerciser despite his arthritis. He was always upbeat. One day
he went to his physician because he was concerned about decreasing
energy. He ascribed this to his arthritis, but this problem really hadn't
changed significantly. His doctor asked him about his mood – was
he feeling sad or depressed? "No," was Mr. D.'s reply. However, on
further questioning, it became clear that he was staying at home more,
exercising less, worrying about his health, and being less socially active.
Because of these signs, his doctor thought Mr. D. was depressed. He
searched for other causes of fatigue, such as anemia, heart disease, and
low thyroid, but also prescribed an antidepressant medication. Over
the next two months, Mr. D. began to notice his energy level returning

to normal – he was back to his daily exercise routine, and his social calendar was full.

Geriatric Syndromes

The term *geriatric syndrome* refers to a problem or set of problems that is more common in elders. Such a syndrome may be complex, having more than one cause and affecting more than one body system. In addition, it may lead to other medical problems. Take, for example, insomnia. This common problem may be caused by pain, anxiety, depression, medications, heart or lung disease, heartburn, sleep apnea, or a neurological condition (to name only a few causes). Insomnia, in turn, may lead to its own psychological problems and to fatigue, less ability to exercise, weakness, falls, memory loss, and more.

Another example is urinary incontinence. It is important not to ignore this problem – common in both men and women – because it may be an early sign of a serious disease, such as urinary tract infection, bladder cancer, diabetes, or neurological problems. Also, urinary incontinence itself may lead to other geriatric syndromes, most notably depression, skin breakdown, and falls.

Mr. G. is an elder who had a runny nose and sneezing for a few days. He finally went to his pharmacy and bought a cold remedy. (Cold remedies have medications in them that can affect bladder and prostate function.) He began having trouble urinating, with associated dribbling of his urine. He went to his physician about this and was given yet another medication for his prostate. This new medication (commonly used for prostate problems) caused his blood pressure to drop significantly when he stood up. Two nights later, on getting up to go to the bathroom, he got dizzy, fell, and broke his hip. He was taken to the hospital, underwent hip surgery, and died a week later from a blood clot to his lungs. Stopping the original cold medicine would have "cured" his urinary problem and prevented his death. This is an extreme, but not all that uncommon, example of how one problem can lead to another, in this case needlessly.

Sometimes the treatment of a geriatric syndrome may be quite simple and can significantly enhance the quality of a patient's life. Mrs. H. is eighty-four years old and has been having increasing trouble hearing for the past few years. Her husband complains that "she can't hear a thing." She resists this claim, which leads to numerous heated arguments. Mr. H. and their children keep asking Mrs. H. to see her doctor and get a hearing evaluation. Finally, she relents. She is found

Table 15.2. Geriatric syndromes (symptoms
common in older adults that may be
caused by many factors)

Insomnia
Weight loss
Urinary incontinence
Balance problems/falls
Frailty/weakness
Pressure sores/skin breakdown
Osteoporosis (thinning bones)
Dizziness
Memory problems
Delirium (temporary confusion)
Special sense loss (hearing, seeing, taste, smell)

to have severe hearing loss in both ears and is referred to an audiologist for hearing aids. After a few months of adjustment to the aids, Mrs. H., Mr. H., and their children all agree that the household is much more peaceful now.

We want to emphasize that many physicians fail to ask about geriatric syndromes, out of either ignorance or a perceived lack of time. Thus, considering the previous examples, your doctor may not ask you how well you are sleeping at night, what over-the-counter medications you are taking, or whether you have had a problem with leakage of urine or getting to the bathroom on time. You must be your own advocate and tell your doctor if you have any of the geriatric syndromes. Table 15.2 offers a comprehensive listing of these.

What Is Different – but Not as Different as You Might Think – about Being an Elder

Yes, our bodies change as we age – we sag, wrinkle, slow down physically and mentally, and become more susceptible to chronic disease. And, yes, we have less ability to cope with acute stressors. However, the good news is that often we can do something about the most serious of these problems. For instance, decreased flexibility and muscle mass do occur with aging but are as much a function of use (or disuse) as of age per se. Your muscles can become stronger and your flexibility and balance can improve, even at age ninety. Your endurance – for example, your ability to walk – likewise can be enhanced. It will, of course, take time and commitment; there is no quick way to effect positive change. This is so important that we strongly suggest that

Table 15.3. What's different about medication use in elders compared with younger patients

---

Medications have more ill effects
Multiple medications interact with each other (polypharmacy)
Some medications should be used cautiously or not at all
There is a need to start low and go slow (see text)

---

all elders – even those with disabilities – be engaged in a regular exercise program. Before you begin a new program (or add to an existing one), you should consult your physician and a physical therapist or certified trainer, who will monitor you so you do not injure yourself.

Age rarely is an absolute reason *not* to be treated for any particular medical problem. This is true even for most surgeries. In other words, you still can be treated for cancer, heart disease, and many other illnesses, regardless of your age. Much more important than age are your state of health and your functional ability.

Medications

Elders take more medications than any other age group in our society. These drugs may be life improving, even lifesaving; however, they also account for 10% to 20% of hospital admissions. In one study, adverse drug events were the fourth leading cause of hospital deaths. As you age, any medication is more likely to produce ill effects (see Table 15.3). In fact, the likelihood of having an ill effect increases as the number of medications you take increases. In addition, some medications should be used very cautiously in elders, and some should not be used at all (see Table 15.4). However, some doctors still prescribe these drugs inappropriately.

Table 15.4. Drugs that usually should be avoided in elders

Meperidine (Demerol) – we *always* avoid this drug; there are good
    alternatives
Diphenhydramine for sleep (Benadryl and others)
Certain antidepressant medications; always avoid amitriptyline (Elavil),
    doxepin (Sinequan), and imipramine (Tofranil)
Long-acting benzodiazepines, e.g., diazepam (Valium)
Long-term nonsteroidal anti-inflammatory medication use, e.g., ibuprofen
    (Motrin, Advil), naproxen (Naprosyn), aspirin
Iron sulfate tablets (325 mg) more than once a day

What can you do to ensure that you are on the correct medications and that you minimize the chance of having a bad reaction? First, bring all your drugs (including over-the-counter medications, supplements, and herbal preparations) in a bag to every visit, and review them with your doctor. Second, make sure you know why you are taking each medication, and periodically ask your physician if you can stop taking any of them. Third, if your doctor suggests you start a new drug, ask if there is any nonpharmacologic (nondrug) treatment that might be effective. The idea, again, is to take the fewest medications possible, and to take each of them only for a good reason. Last, and perhaps most important, is the admonition to "start low and go slow." This means, compared with a younger person, an elder usually should begin with a significantly lower dosage and should increase the dosage slowly until the desired effect is attained.

In some ways, the preceding information concerns the overtreatment of elders with medications. However, there also is a problem with undertreatment, even nontreatment, of certain medical problems. For instance, a physician may heed the admonition to start low and go slow with a certain medication, then fail to increase it to its effective dosage despite the absence of ill effects. This frequently occurs with the treatment of depression and pain.

When to Call a Doctor

Many elders are reticent to call their doctors. However, as we have emphasized, as we age it is essential for our well-being to intervene early when we become ill. Please remember, serious illness may present with vague symptoms. In other words, if you are at all worried, *call your physician*; do not wait. Be your own advocate. It may be lifesaving or at least minimize trips to the hospital.

There are some symptoms that you should never ignore and for which you should seek immediate medical attention (see Table 15.5). In addition, you must learn the symptoms of any disease you have and, in consultation with your physician, know when to call for help. If you miss an appointment, make another one. If you miss an appointment because you feel too sick, make sure you talk to your doctor the same day.

How to Communicate with Your Doctor – and What to Communicate

Your relationship with your doctor, including how well you talk to each other, affects your care. A good relationship – one in which you

Table 15.5. *Never* ignore the following symptoms – call your doctor!

Decreased energy, fatigue
Fever
Change in your ability to function, e.g., you can't manage making the bed
    anymore
Nausea and vomiting
Diarrhea
Dizziness

Call 911! Then call your doctor for the following:
Chest pain or chest pressure
Shortness of breath or other breathing problems
Weakness or numbness on one side of the face or body
Trouble talking or swallowing
Sudden loss of vision or sudden onset of double vision

and your doctor share information and work together to make the best decisions about your health – will result in the best care. If you feel uncomfortable asking questions, or leave the office unsatisfied with the encounter, bring an advocate with you to your next visit. When in doubt, it is always advisable to bring someone with you to your doctor.

Be prepared. Doctors are very busy. Keep and bring with you a list of the most important questions you want to discuss as well as an up-to-date list of your medications, including all over-the-counter pills you take, as a part of your portable medical record (see later). In the optimal situation, your doctor would write down all pertinent new information for you at the end of your visit, such as any medication changes, tests he or she wants you to have, or symptoms that should prompt a call. At the very least, *you* should write these things down, so be sure to bring paper and pencil with you to your visit.

One final point: don't assume your doctor understands your beliefs about your body, aging, or health care in general. If there are important aspects of your background and culture you feel your doctor should know, tell him or her directly.

Hospitalization

Hospitalization usually is a time of physical danger and high stress. Although this would be an opportune time to benefit from the care of a personal primary care doctor whom you know and trust, you may not be able to count on him or her being available to you; you may have a hospitalist caring for you. Hospitalists are a benefit in that they are physicians well trained in acute care medicine who are quite efficient at working up and treating the problems that bring patients to the hospital. The downside is you don't know who will be your admitting doctor, and even that person may not be the one who sees you on subsequent days. The days of primary care doctors following their patients both in and out of the hospital are quickly leaving us; we must make do.

If your primary doctor is unavailable in the hospital, there are several points for you to keep in mind to minimize problems. First and foremost, you and/or your family and friends must be your vigilant advocates throughout the hospitalization, including discharge planning and follow-up care. By *vigilant advocates* we do not mean harassing the doctors and nurses. They virtually are always on your side, trying their best to help. We simply mean helping them prevent, and keeping an eye out for, problems that may occur even with the best of intentions.

One simple first step to prevent problems from arising is to bring your portable medical record to the hospital with you (see the following text for details). If you have an advance directive (and you should) – which tells physicians what you would want given possible end-of-life scenarios – bring this as well. This document, which should be kept up to date, will give your hospitalist much of what he or she needs to know how to care for you. This is especially important if you are so sick you cannot concentrate sufficiently to give the doctor the details of your medical history.

Another simple, often forgotten, step is to call your primary care doctor to tell him or her you are in the hospital. This will give your doctor the opportunity to call the hospitalist to discuss your problems and care.

Here are a few of our comments and suggestions for making your life easier in the hospital:

1. Pain relief is your right. In the hospital, your pain level is considered the fifth vital sign; it should be tracked along with your other vital signs, such as your blood pressure, pulse, breathing rate, and temperature. There is virtually no reason you shouldn't be given adequate pain medication to afford you the relief you desire. If there is a reason, you have the right to be told and understand what it is.
2. Bowel movements are important! Be sure you are given the opportunity to "evacuate your bowels." If you are having trouble doing so, or have not done so in three days, tell your doctor or nurse. And, speaking of bowel movements, having a commode available at your bedside, especially for nighttime use, may be a real benefit.

3. Bring your hearing aids and glasses to the hospital. If you forget, ask a relative or friend to bring them. Being unable to hear or see well can add to the confusion of being sick in a strange environment.

4. Vital signs often are taken around the clock, including once or twice in the middle of the night. This necessitates awakening you from what little precious sleep you may be getting. If this occurs, don't hesitate to ask your doctor or nurse if you can forgo blood pressure, pulse, and temperature checks during sleeping hours. Often it is possible to do so.

5. When you are well enough to be considered for discharge, it is very important that plans be carefully made for home and follow-up care. How will you be cared for at home and by whom? What equipment or expertise will your caregiver need? Will a visiting nurse or home health aid be available to you? When and with whom will you have follow-up doctor visits?

6. Finally, be sure to ask your hospitalist to write out your new medical problem list (or add to your old one). This should include a careful listing of all the medications – new and old – that you should be taking. Please remember that, just as you may be given one or more new drugs to take at home, you may also be asked to stop one or more of the medications you were taking before you entered the hospital.

What Is Geriatrics?

Geriatrics is the branch of medicine concerned with the diagnosis, treatment, and prevention of disease in elders and the problems specific to aging. (It comes from the Greek *geron*, meaning "old man," plus *iatreia*, meaning "the treatment of disease.")

Geriatricians receive specialty training in medicine and have the special concerns of elders in mind. Geriatricians help their patients to preserve functional capacity, to live as well as possible with chronic diseases, to prevent and treat geriatric syndromes, and to use medications judiciously.

In addition to physicians, there are other trained health professionals who specialize in caring for elders (see Table 15.6). Sometimes they work independently, sometimes as a team working together toward a more comprehensive and effective evaluation and treatment plan. A good geriatrics team works holistically, considering an elder's medical history and present medical condition, as well as his or her social and psychological well-being. Team members focus on a person's functional capacities and consider his or her ability to perform activities of daily living (ADLs) – such as bathing, dressing, and eating – and their instrumental activities of daily living (IADLs) – such as the ability to prepare and shop for meals, take medications properly, and manage

Table 15.6. Geriatrics team members (not an
all-inclusive listing)

Gerontologic nurse specialist or nurse practitioner
Social worker
Physician
Nutritionist
Physical therapist
Occupational therapist
Pharmacist
Gero-psychiatrist or psychologist

finances. Although the geriatrician may serve as a point person, he or she often is not the team leader. Each member of the geriatrics team is a skilled health professional. All play an important role in the proper assessment and care of an elder.

When Should You See a Geriatrician?

You should see a geriatrician when:

• You have symptoms or difficulties that your present doctor minimizes
• Your doctor does not know what to do
• You have problems functioning independently or you want to improve
• You have problems with thinking or memory
• You have multiple chronic medical problems and multiple physicians
• You are on too many medications
• Family members and friends feel stressed as caregivers
• Your pain is not controlled
• You have fallen or are worried about falling
• You feel you are too weak or frail
• You have a geriatric syndrome, and your physician says it's "just old age"

Finding a Geriatrician, or Not

Suppose you or one of your parents or friends decide there is a need for a geriatrician. Where do you find one? First, you should know there are not a lot of them. Geriatricians generally are associated with university medical centers and Veterans Administration (VA) hospitals. If you are a veteran, call the nearest veterans center; if not, call your local hospital or university medical center and ask if it has, or can refer you to, a geriatric clinic or a geriatric evaluation unit. The American Geriatrics Society referral service can also help. You can call them at (800) 563-4916 or submit your request via their website: http://www.healthinaging.org. Also, some communities have geriatric care managers for private hire. They may be nurses or social workers and may be able to direct you to a physician sensitive to, and experienced with, the needs of elders.

What if you can't find a geriatrician, or the one you find just isn't for you? What should you look for in a geriatrician, or any physician? In general, the following qualities are necessary to be a "good" doctor: *Competence* – it is easy to name this but more difficult to discern. How can you tell if your physician is competent? You should probably look for board certification; however, although this may be helpful, it is no guarantee. Similarly, a good reputation is a useful – but not infallible – sign. In this regard, we have found that nurses who are actively engaged in health care may provide a more reliable assessment of competence and other positive physician qualities than others in the community.

Kindness – under this rubric, we include characteristics such as empathy and compassion and skills such as being able, and taking the time, to *listen* to you. Yet, as we've mentioned and you know, physicians these days are very busy; however, a certain amount of time is required to understand an elder and his or her often complex and multifarious problems. You have a right to expect that your physician will take the time necessary to understand you. But, please help them use this time wisely. Prepare for your visits; bring your medical history. Write down all your questions. (See "Designing Your Own Portable Medical Record" for specific suggestions.)

Other important qualities include a doctor's *availability* and *responsiveness*. A good doctor responds to your phone calls within a reasonable time, and he or she is available to you, especially in emergencies, or has made provisions for another physician to cover the practice while he or she is unavailable. If you are not feeling well or have a new symptom of concern, you should at least speak to your doctor, his or her on-call person, or a nurse *the same day*. A good doctor recognizes that a percentage of these calls may not be urgent. You and your doctor, over time, will be able to clarify what things can wait. So, don't be shy when you are concerned about your health. Symptoms of serious illness in elders often may be subtle. Call, and expect a response.

What You Need to Know about Your Own Health

You should know:

1. Your blood pressure. If you have high blood pressure, are not eating or drinking well, and/or have lost weight, ask your doctor if you should take

a lower dose of blood pressure medication. If you are dehydrated or have lost weight, blood pressure medications can make your blood pressure drop when you stand and cause you to be dizzy and possibly fall. It is optimal to have, and know how to use, a blood pressure kit so that you can check your own pressure at home.

2. Your medications. Know more than the color of the pill. Also know what each one is for and what drugs it interacts with. When you are sick, understand how your medications might need adjustment, and ask your doctors if any medications should be changed.

3. Your baseline temperature. If your temperature is normally 97°, a temperature of 99.8° may be more significant than if your baseline is 98.6°.

4. Something about any chronic disease you may have. Some insight into the nature of your condition and treatment will facilitate communication with your doctor and help you to better participate in your health care.

Prevention

Prevention is becoming a buzzword in today's health economic climate. Of course, if you prevent a disease, that will be cost-effective for the system, but more importantly, you also will save yourself the burden of that disease! Given this insight, what kind of preventive health care should you pursue? We offer a list in Table 15.7. Note that exercise is number one *and* two. Physical activity is reported to help prevent numerous diseases, from heart attacks to diabetes to Alzheimer's disease. The exercise you do doesn't have to be strenuous. People are surprised to learn how healthful walking is – regular walking reportedly not only decreases heart disease, but also decreases death from all causes.

Social Engagement

To *socially engage* means to connect with others and do things that please you. An activity with others that includes exercise is a way to include exercise with engagement. Hike, play tennis, golf, bowl, or just walk with others. There are many ways to find this sense of connection and community, from spiritual and religious groups to a bridge or reading club. What seems to be important is the engaging.

To some, *prevention* has a more medical ring to it than exercise and social engagement. They think of blood tests like the PSA (prostate-specific antigen), or colonoscopy, or a treadmill. Some of these approaches may be very useful; however, not all screening tests are worth the cost and inconvenience, and some may actually be

Table 15.7. Preventive health care

---

1. Exercise
2. Exercise!
3. Engage socially
4. Have preventative screening
   a. Blood pressure – yearly
   b. Vision, hearing, and balance – yearly
   c. Blood tests
      i. Glucose (sugar) – yearly
      ii. Thyroid function – yearly for women, every 5 years for men
      iii. Blood count – how often is controversial
      iv. Vitamin D level – at least once
   d. Osteoporosis screening – unless there are risk factors, begin at age 65 in women, age 75 in men
   e. Cancer screening – discuss with your primary care doctor
      i. Mammogram – every 1–2 years beginning at age 50, continue up to age 78, then discuss with your doctor
      ii. Pap test – every 1–2 years to 75, if 3 have been consecutively normal
      iii. Colonoscopy – every 10 years beginning at age 50 (earlier if there is a family history of colon cancer); stop at age 75
      iv. PSA test?
5. Keep up with vaccinations – pneumonia, influenza, diphtheria/pertussis/tetanus, herpes zoster (shingles)
6. Prevent accidents – check at home for proper/safe lighting, throw rugs (slip → fall!), rails, smoke alarms

---

dangerous to your health. How can this be? Take the PSA test for prostate cancer. Men who have prostate cancer generally have a high PSA level in their blood. Many physicians believe a yearly PSA test can detect early prostate cancer, which then can be cured by surgery or radiation therapy. The problem is that no study to date has shown that men who have the test done routinely are any less likely to die from prostate cancer. Some prostate cancers may be so aggressive that it doesn't matter if they are found early. Furthermore, it is possible that some prostate cancers are relatively benign (not harmful) and would not progress much before a man died from an unrelated cause. A man with either of these types of cancer would not benefit from a PSA test and, in fact, might actually be harmed by needless surgery or radiation. Until the ongoing studies show, one way or another, whether the PSA test is worthwhile, it will remain controversial. We (along with the American Geriatrics Society and other organizations) recommend that men do not automatically get a PSA test but that they speak with their doctors about the potential risks and benefits of the test and decide whether it's worthwhile. In fact, this is good advice regarding any screening test. Be sure you understand how such a test might benefit you and what the downside is to having it done.

Designing Your Own Portable Medical Record

To ensure you receive the best possible medical care, it is essential that your medical history be available whenever you see a doctor. However, in reality this is not always the case. The way our system is presently organized, your medical chart is not always available when it is needed. Therefore, we suggest that you create a portable medical record that you can carry with you. Your portable medical record should contain all the information mentioned in the following list. You should take this with you to each and every medical encounter, including visits to your doctor, the emergency room, specialists, and hospitals.

1. Keep track of all the names, addresses, and phone numbers (and fax numbers, if possible) of all the physicians you have seen. Include all doctors you have seen, even if only for a referral. Include the date you first saw them.
2. Create a list with all your medical problems, both current and past, including:
   a. Your surgeries
   b. Any other hospitalizations and serious illnesses
   c. Emergency room visits
3. List *all* your medications (include herbal and over-the-counter medications)
4. List your allergies and medication you did not tolerate
5. List the major tests you have had, including:
   a. Radiologic tests: x-ray, CT scan, MRI, nuclear medicine
   b. Heart tests: echocardiogram, stress tests, electrocardiogram (ECG)
   c. Laboratory (blood) tests
6. State your goals of care
7. Include your advance directives (your wishes if you cannot speak for yourself)

Conclusion

The care of elders is complex. To optimize your own care, you should know and keep a record of your medical history, have the best possible communication with your doctors, and take an active part in your treatment. You must be knowledgeable, proactive, and assertive if need be to get the best care possible. We hope this chapter gives you some of the tools you need to be successful. Now, we suggest you go out and exercise (exercise!), learn, play, dance, laugh, and connect with others.

REFERENCE

[1] Kirkwood TBL: Understanding the odd science of aging. *Cell* 2005, 120:437–447.

SIXTEEN

Being and Thinking

– Ilina Singh, Claudia Jacova, Paul Ford, and Judy Illes

This book is about survival strategies for challenges related to our health and well-being. This chapter is specifically about surviving challenges to our brain health – disorders that render young children overactive and unable to learn or attend well to their tasks, disorders of aging that affect memory and personality, and disorders of cognition and consciousness that arise when a person suffers an injury to the head. The contributing authors of this chapter each tackle one of these topics. Professor Ilina Singh of the BIOS Centre for the Study of Bioscience, Biomedicine, Biotechnology and Society describes how proper diagnosis and treatment of childhood attention difficulties can provide relief from the associated upheaval that occurs in the home or at school. Professor Claudia Jacova of the University of British Columbia describes dementia as a journey that implicates the full range of a person's network and, ideally, involves a caring team of family members, friends, and health professionals. Professor Paul Ford of the Cleveland Clinic describes the significant uncertainties that can accompany patients in intensive care units specializing in brain injury and disease.

This chapter is a multinational effort involving scholars and clinicians from Canada, the United Kingdom, and the United States.

The geographic borders are irrelevant, however, as each section contributes to a common theme that we address in our own voices: the life-changing nature of unexpected abnormalities of brain function. This combined effort is reminiscent of an Indian story from the Jataka tales in which the collective strength of the trees in the forest withstands the power of the storm:

> *United, forest-like, should kinsfolk stand;*
> *The storm o'erthrows the solitary tree.*

Although there is no doubt that some children grow out of their developmental disorders and thrive while others do not, there is equally little doubt that most people who are affected by a degenerating brain succumb to its ravages and that recovery from brain injury is as unpredictable as it is heterogeneous, with "back to normal" (and the inherent complexities of what "normal" really is) as the best possible outcome. Our goal here is not to suggest otherwise, or to capture all possible circumstances – that would be impossible. Rather, we seek to provide information that is clear and forthright and that conveys survival tips intended to be empowering. In undertaking this task, we join with you as a community – as a forest – so you do not have to stand as a tree alone in the storm of the disordered brain.

Part I
ADHD Diagnosis and Treatment in Children:
Fact and Fiction

Ilina Singh

Someone thinks your child may have attention-deficit hyperactivity disorder (ADHD). That someone may be you, your child's teacher, your aunt, or a neighbour. If you are like most parents, you will have mixed reactions. ADHD is one of those childhood conditions that many people like to judge and comment upon, as though they have considerable personal knowledge. This continuous social commentary can make it difficult for parents or carers to sort out fact from fiction. It also means that most people find the process of having a child evaluated and then treated for ADHD particularly stressful and emotionally confusing. Even if you agree that your child has some of the classic symptoms of ADHD – hyperactivity, inattention, and impulsiveness – part of you will wonder whether the symptoms are severe enough to warrant a journey to the doctor. Part of you will worry about the consequences of that journey to the doctor – the pressure on your child, the potential stigma of a medical label, the embarrassment of having to take medication. You will hear about the horrors of overdiagnosis of ADHD and medication side effects, especially if you go on the Internet. This section should help you sort through some of these social and ethical issues.

What Is ADHD?

You are sure to get many different answers to this question, depending on whom you ask and where you look. From the point of view of medical research, ADHD is a behavioural disorder caused by a mixture of genetic and environmental factors. The core symptoms of ADHD are inattention, hyperactivity, and impulsiveness. There are two kinds of ADHD – inattentive type and hyperactive/impulsive type. The first kind describes kids who are usually quiet but lack focus; they tend to be disorganised and daydream a lot. The second kind describes kids who also can't focus or organise themselves, but they are hyperactive and act impulsively. It's not unusual for these children to be aggressive. The first kind of child often is overlooked, especially in crowded classrooms, because he or she doesn't cause much trouble. The second kind of child is often a red flag and a thorn in the side of teachers and peers, is likely to be identified as "problematic" more quickly, and is more likely to be recognized as having ADHD.

At this point, it often becomes clear to parents and carers of a child that the question "What is ADHD?" does not have a straightforward scientific answer. Children's "problematic" behaviour will always be defined and evaluated in accordance with social and educational expectations. These expectations vary depending on a variety of factors, including the type of family, the school, the socioeconomic background, and the national setting of the child. Therefore, a child with hyperactive behaviours who is in a well-resourced classroom with a small number of students and an experienced teacher may not be identified as possibly ADHD, whereas the same child in a different type of school and classroom setting might be.

Acknowledging that there are social and cultural factors that influence how quickly a child is referred for an ADHD diagnosis is not the same as saying that ADHD does not exist. This is an important distinction because there are those who will tell you that ADHD is a myth perpetuated by lazy parents and teachers, intolerant school systems, and overworked physicians. If you are fighting to get your child evaluated or his or her condition recognised, this critical point of view may feel hurtful. In media reports, parents especially are subjected to ethical scrutiny and moral reprobation. Children's problem behaviour frequently is attributed to rejection or neglectful parenting, or parents are seen as seeking an ADHD diagnosis because treatment would provide them with a "quick fix" for their problems. If your child has been diagnosed properly (more on good diagnoses later), you should feel confident that he or she has a real disorder that requires medical treatment and an appropriate educational response.

On the other hand, if you feel you are being pressured into an evaluation for ADHD, it is in the best interests of your child for you to consider whether you and your child might be falling victim to coercive social influences. These influences may come in many forms. For example, parents often feel pressure to "fix" children who aren't performing or behaving well. Pressure may be exerted by teachers, family, spouses, friends, or internally – many feel it's part of their job to ensure the success of their children. If you are feeling this sort of pressure, it's worth discussing it with the doctor when you take your child in for an evaluation for ADHD.

How Is ADHD Diagnosed?

Many of the accusations hurled against parents and physicians as part of the debate over ADHD are unfair and untrue. However, it is the case that ADHD diagnoses and stimulant drug use to treat this condition have risen sharply over the past decade throughout the world. In some areas, ADHD is underdiagnosed, but in other areas, it is clearly overdiagnosed. It is the physician's obligation to perform substantive diagnoses that follow good practice guidelines, such as those set by the American Academy of Pediatrics. Sometimes, however, primary care providers don't know enough about how to diagnose ADHD properly; other times, they simply don't have enough time to do a good job amidst a busy day. That's where parents and carers come in; if they are armed with knowledge and understanding of what makes a good diagnosis of ADHD – such as the approved child behaviour checklists and the need to obtain information on the child from multiple informants – they can help gather the relevant information or, where necessary, insist that the medical evaluation follow good practice guidelines. Taking the time to ensure a rigorous diagnosis of ADHD means that parents and carers contribute to a rise in properly diagnosed children with ADHD, and a decline in misdiagnosed children. If your child does end up with a diagnosis of ADHD, such action also will help your family defend against accusations that the diagnosis is not "real" and will increase your confidence in the treatment strategy chosen.

Stimulant Drug Treatment for ADHD

This section focuses on social and ethical issues related to stimulant drug treatments. This is not to be taken as an indication that behavioural therapies and/or parent training programmes are not helpful and effective in managing children with ADHD. Indeed, many children benefit from learning how to self-manage their problem behaviours in conjunction with medication. Parents also tend to benefit from courses tailored to the particular challenges presented by a child with ADHD. In the United Kingdom, such parent training courses are now considered the first line of treatment for ADHD; medication is used only in severe cases or when other approaches don't work. Your doctor may be able to recommend courses for parents and carers, as well as for children, to attend. Or, you can ask for a referral to a practitioner who will provide behavioural therapy or family counselling. There also are active patient and family support groups, such as Children and Adults with Attention Deficit/Hyperactivity Disorder (CHADD), that provide a wide range of services for families of children with ADHD.

What Stimulants Are and What They Do

Stimulant drugs (e.g., Ritalin, Concerta, Adderall) are the most common form of treatment for ADHD. In the largest study of ADHD treatments to date, stimulants were found to be more effective than behavioural therapy, and more effective than behavioural therapy combined with stimulant drugs.[1] That sounds straightforward, but unfortunately, it isn't. This study also suggests that over several years, the initial advantage of stimulant drugs over these other interventions wears off.[2] No one is quite sure why this is, but it may be that over time, and particularly as they get older, children take their medication less consistently.

What Stimulants Do Specifically for a Child

In most children, stimulants help improve focus and attention – which means you will find your child is more able to listen to you, absorb what you are saying, and respond appropriately. Children often say they suddenly can "hear a little voice inside my head that tells me not to do something." If your child is hyperactive, stimulants probably can help calm him or her down. Because of their positive effects on focus and concentration, stimulants also can help improve children's performance on academic work in the short term.

Side Effects of Stimulants

Stimulants also have side effects, although these usually are mild. However, they may interfere with sleep and appetite, and they may suppress a child's growth very slightly. Usually, you can improve problems with sleep and appetite by changing the timing or the amount of the medication dose. More severe side effects are rare. In the vast majority of cases, stimulants will not turn your child into a zombie. Children who are taking the correct dose of medicine usually tolerate it well. In fact, the most common report from parents is that things do get better with medicine, but the child is not a dramatically different person.

You may hear people worry about the impact of stimulant drug treatment on a child's growing brain. There is no firm evidence (meaning evidence that turns up repeatedly in scientific studies) that stimulant drugs interfere with brain growth, alter brain growth, or cause areas of the brain to die.

More and more children in the United States start on one drug for a psychiatric condition and end up on several drugs – a drug cocktail. For example, children with ADHD quite often are prescribed a sleeping medication in addition to a stimulant. Avoid drug cocktails for your children if possible. We have reasonably good safety data on stimulant drugs when they are taken on their own. However, we have a poor understanding of the impact of these drugs on a child's system when they are taken in combination with other medications.

Psychological Impact

Do children become psychologically dependent on stimulant drugs over time? Stimulant drugs are short-acting drugs, meaning that they move in and out of the body within four to eight hours, depending on the type of drug prescribed and the physiologic makeup of the child. This means children normally spend a fair amount of time having to manage various social and cognitive tasks without the benefit of medication. When asked to talk about their capacities to perform these tasks with and without medication, most children respond with a balanced understanding of the relationship between their own efforts, and the boost they get from the medication. Many children admit to using their diagnosis of ADHD and/or the medication to treat it as an excuse for poor performance or behaviour – but their admission that this is an excuse points to a degree of independent thinking that is not characteristic of psychological dependence.[3]

Does Being on Stimulant Drugs Encourage Children to Experiment with Other Drugs, Such as Marijuana or Alcohol?

There is evidence that children taking stimulants for ADHD are more likely to abuse illegal substances in adolescence.[4] However, it also is important to note that no one knows whether taking stimulant drugs *causes* this behaviour. Indeed, many children with ADHD have temperament and personality styles that make them more likely to engage in risky behaviours.

Will Taking Stimulant Drugs Stigmatize My Child?

The answer depends on the kind of school and community of which your child is a part. In certain areas, research suggests that the stigma of ADHD behaviours is *worse* than the stigma of an ADHD diagnosis or stimulant drug treatment. However, it also is the case that children with ADHD are sometimes called names, such as "druggie," and accused of "taking drugs." This kind of bullying seems to be less frequent in the United States than in the United Kingdom, and less frequent to nonexistent for children who have the inattentive type of ADHD. It is worst for boys with ADHD who are also aggressive.

Children also may indulge in a kind of self-stigmatizing, whereby they think of themselves as "different" in a negative way. Because medication is a concrete sign of their difference, they may react against it. Most children don't like taking the medication, for no other reason than it seems annoying. A child's desire not to be different sometimes interacts with the annoyance, resulting in his or her refusal to continue taking medication.

The key to supporting your child against stigma is to have well-informed adults and peers in the community. You can inform teachers and the families of your child's close friends (if your child agrees) by sharing educational resources with them. To adequately support your child, teachers certainly ought to be informed. Children with ADHD who have support within their peer group tend to have fewer problems with social stigma and bullying.

Ethical Concerns

If I Give My Child Stimulant Medication, Will He or She Stop Taking Personal Responsibility for Problematic Behaviour?

No, not unless your child is encouraged in this direction. As noted previously, children tend to be realistic about what this medication does for them. Adults are the ones who sometimes attribute greater powers to these drugs. Moreover, many parents say that drug treatment actually helps improve their child's behaviour when he or she is off drugs as well, because when children are taking medication, they are more capable of learning how to manage their behaviours. This learning appears to translate to improved behaviour management, even when the child has not taken medication.

Will Stimulant Drugs Squash My Child's "Real" or "Authentic" Self?

We do not have a lot of research evidence on this important issue. The available research suggests that in middle childhood (ages eight to twelve), children do not appear to experience taking medication for ADHD in terms of a loss or diminishing of their real selves. However, it does seem that they believe medication helps change them – for the better. Some children with ADHD have low self-esteem and tend to believe their real selves aren't so great. Taking medication can help these children feel better about who they are.

As children near adolescence, they are more likely to get upset at any perceived or actual threats to their identity. Adolescents with ADHD do begin to question whether medication oppresses their real selves. The best way to handle this is to try to talk to your adolescent about this conflict and to encourage him or her to think about the benefits and disadvantages of medication. You also can engage trusted friends, family members, and teachers in this effort. Remember that the task is not to talk your adolescent into taking medication; it's to get him or her to be thoughtful rather than reactive. Interim solutions sometimes help here, such as agreeing on medication holidays – times on weekends or during school holidays when medication is not taken.

Is It True that Some People Use Stimulants to Enhance Their Children's Academic Performance Even When They're Not Diagnosed with ADHD?

Stimulants do improve focus and attention in "normal" people – that is, adults and children without a psychiatric disorder. Sometimes this results in improved performance in testing situations. It probably is the case that some parents give their children stimulants to give them a competitive edge, but because few parents would admit to this practice, we don't know how common it is. We know that students will procure stimulants independently of their parents as study aids or to enhance performance on tests. At universities in the United States and the United Kingdom, the practise of taking stimulants to study and to take tests is increasingly common.

Because of these enhancement practices, there is a small danger that your child's medication could be stolen, or that he or she might be convinced to sell it to peers. Anecdotal reports suggest that adolescents are more likely to give their medication to friends if asked to share, rather than sell it to them.

Some parents worry that stimulant drugs may be abused for their amphetamine properties of increasing wakefulness and transiently improving attention. The slow-release forms of methylphenidate – the active ingredient in Ritalin – cannot be abused; however, short-acting medications such as Ritalin may be ground up and snorted for a high.

A Last Word

In research with children who have ADHD, they tell us they wish there were more people they could talk to about what it's like to have ADHD and to take medication (if they do). Doctors often are too busy to have a conversation with a child patient, and teachers may be intimidating to talk to, especially for younger children. Parents and carers often are the best people to talk to children about their experiences and concerns. Just taking the time to listen to your child and to ask questions on a regular basis can make a big difference.

Part II
Dementia: A Long Journey

Claudia Jacova

Background

None of us needs to be reminded that memory impairment and dementia are leading public health concerns worldwide. In 2001, there were an estimated 24 million dementia sufferers, with the number growing at a rate of approximately 4.6 million new cases every year. In North America, among people aged sixty-five or older, 6% to 10% have dementia. As populations age, the number of people affected is expected to proportionately increase. These numbers trouble each of us, not only because of their societal impact but also because of the distressing question of whether we ourselves will fall victims to a dementia disorder.

Who is at risk for dementia? – probably everyone, in one form or another. After age sixty-five, the likelihood of developing dementia doubles every five years and approaches 50% by age eighty-five.

Therefore, the older you are, the more likely it is that your neurological symptoms may be the early signs of a neurodegenerative disease. However, approximately 10% of all dementia sufferers are younger than age sixty-five, with some still raising a family, at the peak of their working lives, or both. Women carry a greater risk of developing dementia, particularly Alzheimer's disease (AD), with advancing age: there is a very sharp increase in dementia incidence for women, from 2.9 in 1,000 persons per year at ages sixty-five to sixty-nine to 100.9 in 1,000 persons per year at age ninety or above, compared with 2.0 in 1,000 and 53.8 in 1,000 for men in the same age groups. Having a first-degree relative, such as a parent, with AD increases your risk for this disease approximately two to three times.

What Exactly Is Dementia?

The term *dementia* describes a clinical syndrome of memory, attention, perception, and personality impairment sufficiently severe to cause problems with tasks of everyday life. Dementia may be caused by several neurodegenerative diseases, with AD being the most common and accounting for 50% to 70% of reported cases.

All neurodegenerative diseases affect the brain in a progressive manner, with the specific pathology spreading from localized regions to most areas of the cortex and subcortex. The progression of brain pathology is paralleled by increasing symptom severity.

Indeed, dementia has been described as a journey. This journey may last many years, with the estimated life expectancy after diagnosis ranging from two to sixteen years. As there currently is no treatment to halt or reverse any of these diseases, it is very important to obtain an early and accurate diagnosis. This section focuses on the beginning of the dementia journey, but one must be aware that the challenges do not end here. Although living with the middle and late stages of dementia is beyond the scope of this section, there are many excellent readings on that topic.

What Symptoms Should Concern You?

The Case of Douglas

Douglas, a lively and pleasant seventy-two-year-old man still operating his own insurance business, comes to the clinic with his wife, Maureen. He complains of increasing forgetfulness. He often misplaces belongings, forgets business and social conversations, and has difficulty with days and dates. Maureen feels Douglas's problems are just a natural part of getting older and that all their friends face similar difficulties. Maureen raises a crucial question: Is memory loss part of normal aging?

It is widely recognized that normal aging may entail mild performance declines on memory tasks that require recall of recent events. These declines occur over decades rather than months, improve with cueing (hints that trigger recollection of the "lost" memory trace), and have little or no impact on everyday living skills. There is no clear-cut separation between these normal changes and early dementia symptoms, but any impairment beyond this benign profile or that is out of step with previous levels of ability should prompt you to consult a doctor. AD and related disorders can manifest initially with symptoms not related to memory, including difficulties producing or understanding language, disorientation in familiar surroundings, and changes in mood, social behaviour, and personality. The first person to suggest a doctor's visit may not be you but rather a family member or close friend. What if you feel nothing is wrong? It would still be in your best interest not to ignore your relative's or friend's concern, especially when subtle changes in social behaviour and personality are brought to your attention – these are the changes that are most difficult to detect on your own.

Is It Dementia?

An assessment of a cognitive complaint will require a full history of current and past illnesses, a review of your current medications, and a physical and neurological examination. The clinician will take an in-depth history of your cognitive symptoms. Be prepared to discuss the nature of the symptoms you have noticed, when and how they started, and whether you think they have become worse since you first noticed them. This history will be far more detailed and valid if the clinician can interview both you and another person who knows you well and can offer an objective perspective on the type and extent of cognitive changes you may be experiencing. Although you may not feel ready to share your problems, you need to weigh your desire for privacy against the accuracy of the symptom description and, ultimately, of the diagnosis. The assessment also may include a history of dementia in your family to determine the extent of your genetic risk. The clinician will want to know who has been affected, how the diagnosis was obtained, and at what age each affected family member developed the disease. For this reason, you may wish to collect as much family history as you can track down in advance of your visit.

The Case of Harold

It has been an exhausting morning for Harold, an eighty-one-year-old retired lawyer; he had an interview with the clinician, cognitive testing, a session with a genetic counsellor, and an MRI scan. He is now waiting to see the clinician again. Harold's son, who has accompanied him to his appointments, understands what his father most needs now: certainty regarding the significance of his symptoms, so he can make appropriate decisions and move on with his life.

In addition to his medical history, Harold's diagnosis will be made on the basis of well-validated checklists, including the Diagnostic and Statistical Manual of Mental Disorders (DSM-IV-R) and the International Classification of Diseases (ICD-10). These checklists require the presence of several clinical features that cannot be accounted for by other medical disorders. They accurately identify dementia in 60% to 95% of cases, as confirmed by examination of the brain after death. Once the presence of dementia is established, a differential diagnosis must be made to identify the type of degenerative dementia causing the symptoms. This step is very important for the prognosis and management of the disorder.

Objective cognitive testing is an essential step in evaluating a cognitive complaint because it allows the determination of the presence and overall severity of impairments in relation to the average abilities of one's peers. At a minimum, every patient should receive a brief cognitive test such as the Mini Mental Status Examination (MMSE). This type of test includes questions to probe memory, orientation, naming and comprehension, and spatial abilities.

The Case of Eva

Eva is a fifty-four-year-old mathematics professor at the peak of her career. In the past year, she has noticed increasing difficulty preparing for and keeping track of her lectures. As part of her assessment, she has been given the MMSE. It has been a distressing experience: "I did not expect I would ever be asked as a test of my mental faculties which city we are in. I felt I was being unnecessarily humiliated. At the same time, it dawned on me that if I have early dementia, in a few years I might not be able to answer correctly. That terrified me."

Like Eva, many people experience this type of test as more intrusive than a physical examination. One potential workaround that researchers are exploring is a computerized approach in which people can self-administer the test, either in the doctor's office or perhaps at home. This promising approach is not yet widely established.

In some situations, brief cognitive tests are not sufficient. Impairments may be too subtle for the somewhat blunt probes of these tests and may not be centred on memory per se. In these cases, the clinician may request more in-depth cognitive testing – neuropsychological testing – of a broad range of memory and non-memory functions. Neuropsychological testing not only contributes to the diagnostic workup, it also is important for the longer-term management of cognitive symptoms. It can assist with vocational decision making for people still in the workforce and enable cognitive rehabilitation interventions where possible and appropriate.

Supportive Clinical Investigations

Brain imaging with magnetic resonance (MRI) or computed tomography (CT) is done to rule out non-dementia disorders and to assess for the presence of cerebrovascular disease. In some instances, specialists will order a positron emission tomography (PET) scan or a cerebrospinal fluid analysis when the clinical symptoms do not allow differentiation between AD and, for example, a more rare, related disorder such as frontotemporal dementia.

There currently is no established disease biomarker for AD or other dementias, although the search for biomarkers is intensive. Promising techniques include the tracing of specific brain regions on MRI, the determination of Alzheimer's pathology–related metabolites in cerebrospinal fluid or cerebrovascular disease, and the measurement of in vivo brain metabolism with PET. Recently, a chemical has been developed that, when injected into the bloodstream, binds to beta-amyloid, the toxic protein that aggregates into plaques in the brain of people with AD. These and other techniques may change the face of dementia workup dramatically in the years to come.

Is Early Diagnosis Important?

The Case of Josephine

Josephine is a seventy-eight-year-old retired teacher. She has been diagnosed with mild cognitive impairment (MCI), a state of cognitive functioning below normal but short of dementia in severity. MCI puts her at higher risk than someone with normal cognition of developing dementia in the future. When invited to join a program to monitor her functioning over time, she refuses. She wants to be able to enjoy life without knowing about the disease until forced to address this reality.

Do you share Josephine's reluctance to obtain an early diagnosis? There still is no sure cure, so this may be a very reasonable choice. However, there are advantages to early diagnosis that you also should consider. These advantages pertain especially to proper diagnosis of the brain disorder, treatment that can slow down the progression of the disease, and the opportunity to plan for the future.

Evaluation is essential to proper diagnosis and to assigning treatment that can cure treatable brain disorders and control the disease process in untreatable forms, including those that cause dementia. Current treatment approaches for all dementias are aimed at alleviating symptoms. The most commonly prescribed medications for mild to moderate AD are cholinesterase inhibitors (ChEI). Clinical trials of these drugs have shown small but reliable benefits for six to twelve months and even longer on measures of cognition, everyday functioning, and behaviour.

However, these studies offer few answers to the questions that matter most to patients and their treating physicians: Who will derive benefits? How long should treatment continue? And most importantly, Will symptom progression be slowed for the long term? If the benefits are uncertain, continuation on the medication needs to be weighed against possible side effects and against the cost of the medication. Not all private health insurance carriers provide coverage. You should address all these questions with your doctor when you are being treated with a ChEI medication. Some people choose to participate in experimental drug trials directed at testing next-generation treatments, including anti-amyloid, anti-inflammatory, and neurotropic interventions. If you and your family feel there is potential benefit in participating in experimental drug research, you should find out about ongoing trials through your doctor or clinic.

Early evaluation and diagnosis also can identify medical risk factors, such as vascular disease, that may accelerate the onset of dementia and its rate of progression. Studies have shown that treatment for high blood pressure and stroke prevention can reduce the risk of dementia and cognitive decline. These are now recommended medical practices in the management of dementia risk. Treatment of high blood cholesterol and heart disease also may have a preventive effect, although studies have not been consistent in this regard. Even in the face of varying results, all patients should revisit their lifestyle habits and adopt positive strategies for good health through diet, exercise, and minimal stress.

No doubt, a diagnosis of dementia would have a devastating impact on you and your family and extended network, but learning about it early also gives you the advantage of reflecting on your future, reevaluating your priorities and preferences, and making your wishes known. You will want time to review your legal and financial affairs, and it is important to authorize someone you trust to look after your finances when you can no longer do so yourself. Similarly, you will want to reflect on who should make health care decisions for you when your own competency to do so is compromised. It is best to think about living arrangements while you can still care for yourself: Who can assist you when you will need help? Should you move in with a family member? What options will be available when you require a safe environment in which you will receive assistance with daily living? What care facilities would you find acceptable? These decisions require the time that you may not have later in the disease.

Who Is the Right Doctor?

Who is the right doctor? Someone you trust. In most countries, the first step is to consult your family physician. If your doctor has known you for several years and has some expertise in dementia, he or she can diagnose and manage your problem. However, if your symptoms are very mild or atypical, your family physician may refer you to a specialist or dementia clinic for further evaluation. Depending on your symptoms and your age, you may be seen by a neurologist, a geriatrician, or a psychiatrist. In the dementia clinic setting, these specialists will work within a multidisciplinary model of care along with other health professionals, including neuropsychologists, social workers, and genetic counsellors. Genetic counselling plays a prominent role in dementia care because of the recognized role of genetic factors in neurodegenerative disorders and, in consultation with your physician and the team, can provide information about your own risk and that of your family members.

How Do We Manoeuvre through the Maze of Uncertainty in Dementia?

Unless there are concerns about your safety and security, seeking a consultation that might yield the life-changing diagnosis of dementia is a very personal choice. There are good reasons to act early, but every person has to weigh these against personal life circumstances, goals, and values. When the time is right, get as much information as you can about the assessment, management, and follow-up of MCI and dementia. More progress has been made in understanding the pathophysiology, causes, and treatment of dementia in the past fifteen years than in all the decades since Dr. Alzheimer first reported on the disease named after him in 1906. There was no hope before, and although there is no cure now, hope resides upon the shoulders of scientists who are vigorously hunting for an answer and the matrix of medical management strategies and social support systems our society has created. Every step of the dementia journey involves many people. Establish that trustworthy network for yourself.

Part III
The NICU: Navigating Complexity and Uncertainty
Paul Ford

If your loved one has a severe brain injury, has undergone brain surgery, or is in the terminal stages of a brain disease, he or she may spend time in a neurological intensive care unit – the NICU. The NICU is a place for patients who are currently critically ill or need to be watched carefully. The NICU is full of high-tech machines, unfamiliar language, and constant commotion. Decisions made in the NICU often have long-lasting implications and may need to be made very quickly. These decisions involve complicated and detailed medical facts with high levels of uncertainty. The uncertainty stems from the variability in recovery of injured brains and the incomplete knowledge we still have of brain processes. Many choices involve risky procedures that may impair cognitive function even while improving survival. The NICU is a place where your observations of a patient may lead you away from the truth about the likelihood of recovery or from what is actually occurring in the patient. For instance, a patient may appear awake when he or she actually is not, or a patient's lack of movement on one side of the body may be a sign of damage on the opposite side of the brain. When you are asked to make decisions about the treatment of a loved one in the NICU, it is essential that you understand the goals of treatment and likely outcomes. This involves listening carefully and asking for clarification when information does not appear to match what you are seeing at the bedside. The discussion that follows is intended to help you navigate the world of the NICU experience and the usually heart-wrenching reason your loved one is there. I start with common bits of information that can help you find the right questions to ask.

Damage Is Unrecoverable, but Some Function May Return

Very commonly, NICU patients have suffered some type of damage to the brain. Damage to the brain generally is irreversible and may result from one or more causes. A lack of oxygen is one. Part of the brain may be without oxygen either because of too little blood circulating to it (ischemic damage) or because the blood that gets to the brain has either too little oxygen in it (hypoxia) or no oxygen in it (anoxia). Other ways brain tissue may be damaged include infections (virus, bacteria, or prion), an immune system attack on the brain (e.g., multiple sclerosis or lymphoma), traumatic injuries (e.g., from a gunshot or car accident), or tumours. Although the damaged area may not regenerate, other healthy parts of the brain may take over and help a person recover partially. This process, referred to as *brain plasticity*, may take a very long time and require difficult and strenuous therapy. Usually, function is never fully recovered. To make fully informed decisions, it is very important to understand the cause of the injury and the chance another part of the brain can take over the function of the lost portion.

Brain damage often is seen in pictures of the brain taken by machines such as an x-ray, CT (computed tomography), MRI (magnetic resonance imaging), PET (positron emission tomography), or SPECT (single photon emission CT) scanner. However, damage may be present even if it cannot be seen on an image. There is no good way to see all brain damage. Clinical symptoms, medical causes, and speed of recovery serve as the best predictors of the most likely outcome. Simply put, irreversible damage may be present even if the doctor cannot show you a picture of it. Although it is a good thing to ask if there are pictures to confirm the story you are being presented, it is even more important to ask for the specific types of evidence the doctor has for his or her medical opinion.

Location, Location, Location

The degree of impact an injury to the brain or spinal column has on a person depends on exactly where the damage occurs. For instance, a very small stroke in the pontine region of the brain may cause a patient to be "locked in": fully conscious but with limited ability to move or communicate. This is nicely demonstrated in the autobiography of Jean-Dominique Bauby – *The Diving Bell and the Butterfly* (produced as a movie in 2007) – wherein Mr. Bauby is locked in but communicates by blinking one eye to dictate his memoirs. The opposite of a small injury with a large effect is a large injury with smaller or subtle effects. The most famous case is that of Phineas Gage, who in 1848 survived an iron rod penetrating through his head (frontal lobes) from a dynamite accident. Although he seemed to recover fully, it became clear later that his personality was dramatically changed. Given the striking volume of damage compared with that experienced by the locked-in patient, it was surprising that Mr. Gage survived to walk and talk, yet a small blood clot left Mr. Bauby unable to move or talk. Similarly, the precise location of spinal damage dictates the level of pain, sensation, and residual movement experienced by a patient.

In considering the location of a brain injury, you should first remember that the brain is divided into two hemispheres that appear to be mirror images of each other. Although both sides look similar, there are differences. Many functions in the brain are crossed. For example, the right hemisphere controls the left side of the body, and vice versa. Language is a particularly important feature of human interaction. Unlike the creation of new memories, a task believed to be shared by both hemispheres, language often develops primarily in one hemisphere or the other. In approximately 95% of right-handed individuals, language resides in the left hemisphere. Language also is interesting in that it has two important components, each controlled primarily by different portions of the brain. *Receptive language* broadly refers to the ability to understand language. *Expressive language* refers to the ability to create language. When a patient loses one (or both) of these language abilities, the doctor may refer to him or her as *aphasic*. It is important to ask for clarification on what the doctors mean if they use the term *aphasic*. It might mean loss of expressive language, receptive language, or both. Language is such an important part of human function that physicians often are very protective of it in surgery. Further, physicians may raise concerns about a patient's quality of life if he or she loses the ability to communicate and understand other people. There are many interesting stories of those with brain injury that demonstrate unexpected and unusual results, depending on precisely which areas of the brain are damaged.[5] When thinking about brain or nerve injury, the important issue is not always how much is damaged but often the location of the damage.

Not Waking Up: Coma and the Persistent
Vegetative State

Understanding why your loved one is not waking up or does not respond to you may be very confusing. The description of a patient as being "in a coma" is not a diagnosis but rather just a description of being in a deep unconscious state. The unconsciousness may be the result of a brain issue, another medical condition, or medication. For instance, when a patient has continuous seizures (*status epilepticus*), a physician may use a medication (e.g., pentobarbital) to purposely suppress consciousness to allow the brain to "reboot." Even when all medications are removed, the patient may remain unconscious as a result of failure of some other organ, such as the heart, liver, or kidneys. Or, it may be that the brain is damaged in ways that will prevent the patient from ever regaining awareness (e.g., persistent vegetative state) or have intermittent minor awareness (e.g., minimally conscious states). Always ask! The many different causes of unconsciousness may serve as indicators of whether a patient is ever going to wake up and, if he or she does, how much he or she will be able to do.

Notions of consciousness after brain injury also are complicated by body movements that may be deceptive and even counterintuitive. A patient's failure to suppress some basic reflexes may be a sign of a lack of consciousness rather than a sign of consciousness. This fools many people because we normally think of movements as conscious actions. The most deceptive of these are the startle reflex, hand grasping, and spine-mediated movements. Just as a newborn baby cries reflexively every time a noise occurs, a person's body may move reflexively in relation to a loud noise. Patients with no cognitive awareness may still close their hands reflexively when an object or a loved one's hand is placed into their palm. In reality, the appearance of squeezing is nothing more than an automatic reflex of the nervous system. If you see movements in your loved one and the doctor tells you the patient is not moving intentionally, ask him or her to come to the bedside to give you an explanation of the movement. Generally, the movements are reflexive; however, occasionally doctors miss something, or your loved one may be responding meaningfully to familiar voices. It is important to recognize that for the doctors to provide you with answers to these questions, they may need to perform clinical examinations that test various reflexes. Although some of these tests, such as pinching the patient very hard or shooting ice-cold water into his or her ear, look torturous, they usually are necessary to understand the patient's ability to respond consciously. One of the most important tools doctors have for predicting a patient's ability to regain consciousness is related to how much change occurs in these clinical exams during the first few days after a brain injury. In general, be open-minded to the fact that some of what you are observing may be misleading you, and use reliable information resources, such as your doctors.

Pressure Buildup

A pressure buildup within the skull may be very dangerous for patients. It may be caused by swelling, bleeding, tumour growth, or an increase in the volume of cerebrospinal fluid. The doctors may describe the brain as having "herniated," meaning the pressure has reached such a dire level that part of the brain has been pushed into places it should not be. If the pressure becomes too high, it may cause severe irreversible brain damage and death.

To control pressure, patients may receive medications, have a tube inserted to drain the fluid (ventriculostomy), or have part of their skull removed (craniectomy). With all these interventions, patients may live, but with devastated cognitive function. Quick decision making is vital because delays can allow the damage to render the treatment attempt futile. The decision whether to attempt such a lifesaving intervention is not only a medical one, but also one of quality of life.

Decision Making in the NICU

When trying to make significant decisions in any intensive care unit (ICU), the first and most difficult task is to establish what quality of life the patient would accept in the long term and how much treatment burden he or she would accept to reach that goal. ICUs generally are complex places to navigate. The Society of Critical Care Medicine maintains a helpful website – http://www.myicucare.org – to guide families on general ICU issues. These decisions are particularly challenging in the NICU because many of the outcomes relate to cognitive impairments ranging from loss of some function to a permanently vegetative state. Once you achieve some clarity about your loved one's acceptable goals and acceptable treatment burden, it is important to get the treating doctors' best estimate of what is reasonably possible and likely in your loved one's case. These decisions must be made with a full view of the outcomes in the near future as well as in the long term.

Sometimes, people have to make decisions about their loved one even though no one really knows how to treat his or her illness. In these instances, some physicians conduct research whereas others simply offer an untested therapy (innovation). The differences among receiving standard therapy, receiving innovative therapy, or being part of research study may be extremely confusing. Standard and innovative therapies are given for the primary benefit of the patient. A research study is designed to gain information to help future patients, although it may help the patient taking part in the study. Some families ask whether their loved one is going to be a "guinea pig" or if the procedure is "experimental." This language will not get you a straight answer, because people use these terms to mean different things. NICU patients and, more generally, neurosurgical patients often are vulnerable, so it is important to be clear what is being done for research or as innovation.[6] Rather than asking the "guinea pig" question, it would be better to ask the following questions:

1. Is this the usual therapy for the disease?
2. If there is no proven therapy, why do you think this therapy will work?
3. Is this medical plan solely for my loved one's benefit?
4. Are you asking him or her to be part of a research protocol?
5. If this is innovation or research, has a doctor unconnected with the research or innovation provided a second opinion?

This series of questions should illicit important responses, including whether steps have been taken to independently confirm whether the proposed plan is medically reasonable. Although standard therapy is provided in most NICU cases, knowing when it is not being offered will improve your ability to make decisions.

Most serious cases in the NICU involve a cast of many physicians and nurses from a variety of medical and surgical specialties. If there is considerable uncertainty or a particularly big decision must be made, you should ask for the relevant specialties to meet with you to establish a care plan toward the patient's goals. Although this is not practical for small decisions, if you are feeling very uncertain about an aspect of your loved one's care or you seem to be getting different messages from different doctors (who often rotate weekly in big institutions), you are justified in asking for a team meeting. There are at least three reasons you might be hearing different messages from different doctors:

1. There is a genuine professional difference of opinion about outcome or diagnosis.
2. The doctors mean the same thing but are using different words.
3. Each doctor is speaking only in terms of his or her specialty (e.g., a kidney specialist may say a patient is much improved but may simply mean the patient's kidneys are working better even though his or her overall condition is far worse).

In each case, meeting the doctors can help clarify the issues and restore a trusting relationship. This type of meeting also can provide an opportunity to remind the doctors of the acceptable outcomes for the patient and to revisit what goals are reasonable at that time. Many hospitals have mechanisms for resolving conflicts related to values and ethics.[7] These resources are often valuable when meetings with the medical team have left unanswered questions or when distrust continues. Once the plan of care has been set and is being followed, the next major choices involve the end of the NICU stay.

The End of the NICU Stay Approaches

The NICU stay is complete when a patient's condition has improved, there are no further therapies available in the ICU to help, or death occurs. Intensive care doctors and nurses strive for the first of these types of discharges. Even among patients who improve, rehabilitation at home or at a skilled nursing facility normally is required for those who have spent significant time in an NICU. Before discharge, the health care team should explain the range of rehabilitation options available, articulate plans for follow-up by an outpatient doctor, define any long-term restrictions on activities, and delineate expectations for functional and cognitive recovery. You should have a frank discussion with the team regarding what actions are to be taken in the future if the patient's condition deteriorates or there is a relapse. This type of planning is essential for patients with progressive disease who are nearing the terminal phase. Some patients make the choice not to be readmitted to the NICU if their long-term prognosis is poor.

Patients who have exhausted all therapeutic options in the NICU and are not improving may be transferred to a more appropriate care setting. For some, that setting may be a hospice, where they will be made comfortable and allowed to live out the remainder of their days in a non-hospital setting. For patients who need long-term ventilation with artificial nutrition and hydration, a long-term acute care facility may be the only appropriate setting. Again, a clear discussion regarding the patient's long-term care goals and prospects for readmission to the NICU is a fundamental part of good communication and realistic expectations.

Ultimately, some patients die while in the NICU. In some cases, despite aggressive medical attempts to save a patient, cardiac arrest, a large bleed in the brain, or an overwhelming infection may result in his or her death. In other cases, patients or their surrogates request that unwanted therapies, such as ventilators or dialysis, be withdrawn.

In still other, rarer cases, patients die while on life support, but their hearts continue to beat. These patients are determined to be dead based on neurological criteria (formerly called "brain death"). These are derived from a set of tests to determine whether a patient is dead despite being attached to machines that continue to circulate blood and air. When the criteria are applied correctly, there is certainty that the patient is dead. Each of the aforementioned forms of death has sadness attached to it. Many medical centres have bereavement or support services, which often are valuable in helping people cope with the imminent death of a loved one.

Navigating the NICU while your loved one is there will be easier if you educate yourself on basic information about the brain and nervous system and if you ask members of the care team to help you understand anything you find perplexing.

Concluding Perspectives

Our health care systems may not be perfect, but physicians and nurses, psychologists and social workers, ethicists and clergy, and bereavement specialists and other professionals are available to provide survivors with the support they need. It is a two-way street. Be informed. Ask good questions, and, above all, be honest with yourself and others about the values of the person for whom you are caring. As two of the seven Ojibway grandfather teachings say:

To cherish knowledge is to know wisdom
Honesty in facing a situation is to be brave[8]

Good luck.

Acknowledgments

This work is supported in part by NIH/NIMH 9R01MH84282–04A1 (J. Illes), CIHR/CNE #85177 (J. Illes), and the Ralph Fisher and Alzheimer Society of British Columbia Professorship in Alzheimer's Research to Howard Feldman (C. Jacova). The authors gratefully acknowledge the assistance of Neil Chahal and Carole Federico at the National Core for Neuroethics (UBC).

REFERENCES

[1] Jensen PS, Hinshaw SP, Swanson JM, Greenhill LL, Conners CK, Arnold LE, Abikoff HB, Elliott G, Hechtman L, Hoza B, March JS, Newcorn

JH, Severe JB, Vitiello B, Wells K, Wigal T: Findings from the NIMH Multimodal Treatment Study of ADHD (MTA): implications and applications for primary care providers. *Developmental and Behavioral Pediatrics* 2001, 22(1):60–73.

[2] Jensen PS, Arnold LE, Swanson JM, Vitiello B, Abikoff HB, Greenhill LL, Hechtman L, Hinshaw SP, Pelham WE, Wells KC, Conners CK, Elliott GR, Epstein JN, Hoza B, March JS, Molina BS, Newcorn JH, Severe JB, Wigal T, Gibbons RD, Hur K: 3-year follow-up of the NIMH MTA study. *Journal of the American Academy of Child and Adolescent Psychiatry* 2007, 46(8):989–1002.

[3] Singh I, Keenan S, Mears A: The experience of treatment and care for ADHD. In: *National Collaborating Centre for Mental Health. Attention Deficit Hyperactivity Disorder: Diagnosis and Management of ADHD in Children, Young People and Adults.* National Clinical Practice Guideline Number X. 29 April 2009. Available at http://www.nice.org.uk/nicemedia/pdf/ADHDConsFullGuideline.pdf. 2008.

[4] Molina BS, Flory K, Hinshaw SP, Greiner AR, Arnold LE, Swanson JM, Hechtman L, Jensen PS, Vitiello B, Hoza B, Pelham WE, Elliott GR, Wells KC, Abikoff HB, Gibbons RD, Marcus S, Conners CK, Epstein JN, Greenhill LL, March JS, Newcorn JH, Severe JB, Wigal T: Delinquent behavior and emerging substance use in the MTA at 36 months: prevalence, course, and treatment effects. *Journal of the American Academy of Child and Adolescent Psychiatry* 2007, 46(8):1028–1040.

[5] Sacks O: *The Man Who Mistook His Wife for a Hat and Other Clinical Tales* (New York: Summit Books, 1985).

[6] Ford PJ: Vulnerable brains: research ethics and neurosurgical patients. *Journal of Law, Medicine, and Ethics* 2009, 3(7):73–82.

[7] Boissy AR, Ford PJ, Edgell RC, Furlan A: Ethics consultations in patients admitted to neurological centered hospital units: a seven year retrospective review. *Neurocritical Care* 2008, 9(3):394–399.

[8] Banai-Benton E: *The Mishomis Book: The Voice of the Ojibway* (St. Paul, MN: Indian Country Press, 1979).

SEVENTEEN

A Patient's Guide to Pain Management

– Ben A. Rich

Some (hopefully not all!) of what you are about to read in this chapter may strike you as quite strange and perplexing. The reason is that since the rise of more scientifically and technologically oriented medicine in the middle of the last century, physicians and laypersons have had very different (and sometimes even conflicting) views about the relationship between pain and suffering and the responsibilities of the medical profession to effectively relieve them. Surprisingly, before the rise of the modern era, physicians took their responsibility to relieve pain much more seriously than they do now. It is as though the less physicians could do to treat or cure disease, the more assiduously they strived to ensure their patients were at least comfortable and certainly not suffering from pain or other distressing symptoms of illness when the means of relief were available somewhere in the physician's toolkit.

With the rise of modern medicine and the many remarkable advances in medical science and technology, many previously incurable diseases became curable or at least manageable for increasingly longer periods of time. As the focus shifted to making a prompt and accurate diagnosis and then selecting and effectively implementing the most appropriate treatment, what appeared to fade into the background was the patient's experience of illness, including pain and other symptom distress.

Pain – and more importantly, the perceived duty to promptly and effectively treat it – receded so far into the background that by the late twentieth century, there arose what only quite recently (at least when considered in the broad scope of the history of medicine) has come to be recognized as an epidemic of undertreated pain. Indeed, so great is the epidemic in both significance and scope that it belatedly has been recognized as a major public health problem. That such an epidemic could develop and be tolerated for decades is fraught with implications for all of us who are, or who sometime in the future may become, the victims of serious pain.

An epidemic of undertreated pain could not, of course, be considered a major public health problem if pain itself did not constitute a health problem in the individual patient, as opposed to simply an uncomfortable situation for the person experiencing it. It is important to understand that the epidemic of undertreated pain is not the result of callous or sadistic physicians. Rather, it followed from a risk–benefit calculation physicians made between the relative burdens of undertreated pain and risks they believed to be associated with the use of pain relievers, particularly those known as opioid analgesics (sometimes colloquially referred to as "narcotic painkillers"). The problem with this risk–benefit assessment process, however, is that in undertaking it, too many physicians had flawed or inaccurate information about the risks of pain management with opioids and the health benefits of pain relief. In many instances, the former were greatly exaggerated and the latter were significantly underestimated.

Why Pain Is a Problem

Pain, in a positive sense, is a defense mechanism and a survival strategy. There are certain individuals with maladies that prevent them from feeling pain, even when they sustain a severe injury. These people are not "blessed" by this condition, for it places them at grave risk of serious injury or even death. Pain is an alarm system we desperately need to protect ourselves. However, once we have been made aware of the harm or injury and have responded to it appropriately, including seeking medical care, the persistence of that pain becomes a problem that itself must be addressed.

Previously, many physicians were very reluctant to provide patients with pain relief because they looked at pain as an important piece of medical information they would need to monitor, either to diagnose the underlying condition that caused the pain (diagnosis) or to determine the effectiveness of treatment. If a patient reported new or persisting pain after surgery or some other form of treatment, it might indicate a complication from the procedure or a progression of the condition despite the treatment. Providing the patient with effective pain and symptom management was considered counterproductive, because the patient would then not be able to report distress and alert the physician to the new or continuing problem.

Today, this point of view largely has been discredited. There are many ways to follow how patients are doing with regard to their underlying medical condition, such as monitoring vital signs (pulse, respiration, blood pressure, body temperature), which does not require patients to endure pain that can be effectively managed. Furthermore, we are much more aware today of the many harmful consequences of unrelieved pain. These adverse effects are physiological in nature and are not related only to the subjective unpleasantness of the painful stimulus. Unrelieved pain has been found to delay recuperation from surgery, hinder rehabilitation, and limit the effectiveness of chemotherapy in cancer patients, among other problems. It also is one of the most common reasons patients must be readmitted to hospitals only days or weeks after their discharge.

Another reason pain – or more particularly, securing prompt and effective management of pain – is a significant and long-standing problem is that pain essentially is a subjective experience. There are no purely scientific, objective, or reliable means of determining whether someone's reports and descriptions of pain are accurate. Unfortunately, some physicians (and nurses) have developed a mindset that certain medical conditions are consistently associated with particular types and levels of pain. Thus, when a patient reports a type or severity of pain that exceeds the clinician's preconceived notions, the report is met with skepticism. In such circumstances, the patient is at risk of being labeled as one who likes to complain, is prone to exaggerate, is seeking attention or sympathy beyond what his or her medical condition warrants, or, worst of all, is a "drug-seeking" patient. In a later section of this chapter, we return to this issue and discuss how to pursue effective pain advocacy for yourself or a loved one.

Such skepticism on the part of clinicians often is unwarranted and unfair and fails to acknowledge the fundamental fact that whereas a discrete disease entity may constitute an objective, scientifically based determination, the patient's experience of the illness linked to a particular diagnosis, including pain and symptom distress, is unique to that individual. Indeed, it is in recognition of this fundamental fact that the health professions have been compelled to move from the former biomedical model to the biopsychosocial model, and some thought leaders are now urging yet another transition – to a biocultural model of patient care. The evolution in thinking reflected in these models is that high-quality, compassionate patient care must be directed to the uniqueness of the individual and not merely the disease entity that constitutes the diagnosis.

Although all patients with pain are vulnerable to undertreatment because of the knowledge deficits and regulatory concerns of health care professionals, recent studies reveal that certain types of patients are at a significantly increased risk. Among them are racial minorities (especially blacks), those of low socioeconomic status, and the elderly. Inadequate pain treatment has been found in acute care settings such as emergency departments, chronic care facilities such as nursing homes, and even among cancer patients.

Knowledge, Skills, and Attitudes of Physicians Concerning Pain

There are two essential components to addressing pain in patient care: assessment and management. Unfortunately, many physicians are well behind the learning curve, because, as remarkable as it may seem, medical schools and residency programs (postgraduate training of physicians required for national board certification in any specialty) provide very little education and training in pain assessment and management, despite the fact that this is the most common reason people seek medical care. As disconcerting as it may be to patients, in the case of pain, it is not reasonable to assume your physician's knowledge, skills, and attitudes about pain and its assessment and management are up to date and adequate to the task.

A great deal of enlightenment on the nature of pain, its importance for quality patient care, and currently available approaches to relieving it has been achieved during the past fifteen to twenty years by the thought leaders in pain medicine. However, despite recent and quite significant efforts to disseminate this information to primary care professionals and specialists alike, we have a long way to go before the custom and practice of physicians are consistent with the state-of-the-science and quality standards that could be achieved by consistently following nationally recognized clinical practice guidelines. When you are in the process of choosing a primary care physician, or are about to undergo a surgical procedure or course of treatment in which pain or unpleasant symptoms might reasonably be anticipated, consider politely but straightforwardly asking the physician who will primarily be responsible for your care some or all of the following questions:

- What is your philosophy on pain management?
- What training (including continuing medical education) have you had in the past ten years in assessing and managing pain?
- Are you familiar with the Agency for Health Care Policy and Research's clinical practice guidelines on pain management or those of another national professional organization, such as the American Pain Society or the American Academy of Pain Medicine?
  - If so, do you consistently follow such guidelines in the care of your patients?
  - If not, would you be prepared to consult such guidelines in my care or request a consultation with a pain medicine specialist?
- How important do you consider pain management to be in patient care?
- Do you believe the medical board of this state expects and encourages physicians to assess and treat pain promptly and effectively? If not, how will that affect your willingness to ensure that my pain is effectively managed, including the prescribing of opioid analgesics if necessary?

The same suggestion applies if you likely will be involved in the care and treatment of a loved one. The more serious the diagnosis or complex the procedure(s) or treatment, the greater the patient's need for an advocate. As patients, we should strive to be our own advocates, but we also should never hesitate to enlist the support of relatives and close friends as advocates as well. If any physician to whom you pose the preceding questions (on behalf of yourself or a loved one) reacts in a negative, dismissive, or evasive manner that suggests he or she is uncomfortable with or disturbed about being asked, you should seriously consider seeking another physician who shares – which a conscientious and compassionate physician should – your beliefs about the important role of pain relief in quality patient care.

Types of Pain

Pain often is divided into three broad categories: acute, chronic, and terminal/end-of-life. The third category formerly was characterized as cancer pain, but with the many recent advances in cancer treatment, pain associated with cancer or the consequences of its treatment may pose a challenge for patients and physicians for years. Acute pain is pain associated with a traumatic injury, surgical procedure, or other medical condition that is not expected to persist for more than several days or, at most, a few weeks if the patient receives appropriate care and responds as reasonably anticipated. Depending on the nature and severity of the pain, a wide variety of prescription medications are available and usually effective in achieving pain relief. In some instances, non-medication approaches such as relaxation techniques, meditation, biofeedback, or massage therapy may be used instead of or in addition to pain-relieving medications.

Chronic pain is a pain condition that persists for months (six months is a common benchmark). Some medical conditions may cause pain that may not become chronic if proper treatment is provided in a timely way, but other conditions may produce chronic pain despite good-faith efforts to treat it. Chronic pain can be very challenging to physicians, patients who suffer from it, and the patients' families. In some instances, in which the original condition precipitating the pain has resolved or reached maximum medical improvement, chronic pain becomes an independent diagnosis and the primary focus of treatment.

With regard to both acute and chronic pain, the complete obliteration of pain is neither achievable nor necessarily desirable. The common term *pain management* is used to describe the process by which health care professionals seek to reduce a patient's pain to a tolerable level with a minimum of adverse side effects from any medication that may be prescribed. Often, a balance must be struck between pain relief and alertness, including the ability to maintain a level of function necessary for activities of daily living, family responsibilities, or work-related duties. It is very important for the patient and the person or persons providing care to agree on how that balance should be achieved.

There are several very important terms (and the phenomena they denote) both patients with pain and the professionals caring for them must understand. You should not assume that just because someone is a physician or nurse, even a highly experienced one, he or she fully comprehends these distinctions. The clinical surveys suggest otherwise. Two key terms that must be distinguished very carefully are *physical dependence* and *addiction*. Physical dependence is a natural response of the body to medications such as opioids. After as little as a week or two, the body adjusts to the medication in a way that makes any abrupt discontinuation of it problematic, because the discontinuation may cause symptoms of withdrawal. The appropriate means of discontinuation is to gradually reduce (taper) the dosage over time. It is extremely important to remember that physical dependence is not an indication of addiction or that the patient is at risk for addiction; on the other hand, it is a complex disorder with biological, psychological, and social aspects and implications. Unlike physical dependence, addiction is highly problematic. It is characterized by compulsive use of the drug, a craving for the drug, and continued use of the drug despite harm. The risk that a patient may become addicted to a pain medication is roughly the same as that for developing any other form of addiction. A personal or family history of any form of addiction does increase the risk, but never to the point at which it becomes more likely than not. It also is important to remember that even patients who are currently addicted may have serious pain that should be treated. However, such patients need treatment for their addiction disorder as well, and the complexity of their condition probably warrants consultation with a pain medicine specialist.

It is important to distinguish between genuine addiction to a pain medication and *pseudo-addiction*, a phenomenon in which a patient with serious unmanaged pain demonstrates drug-seeking behaviors in a legitimate pursuit of pain relief. Pseudo-addiction is an iatrogenic condition, meaning it is caused by physician behavior in the failure or refusal to manage the patient's pain adequately. To label a patient who manifests pseudo-addiction as a drug-seeking or drug-addicted patient is to add insult to injury.

Another important term both patients and professionals need to understand is *tolerance*. This phenomenon occurs when a patient requires an increased dose of an opioid medication to maintain the level of pain relief he or she originally achieved. Tolerance usually is not an issue in acute pain management. In chronic pain care, the need for higher doses of the same medication also may indicate a worsening of the underlying condition (disease progression in the case of cancer). Most patients with stable underlying conditions can be managed on relatively uniform doses of medication. However, there also is the phenomenon of breakthrough pain, especially in patients with advanced and terminal conditions, for whom another medication may be needed to address temporary situations in which the primary pain reliever is inadequate.

Relief of pain, as well as other distressing symptoms associated with terminal illness, often is provided within the context of an ever-increasing number of palliative care services or units in acute care hospitals, or through enrollment in hospice. Hospice services can be provided in a range of settings, including inpatient hospice units, skilled or assisted living facilities, or the home of the patient or a family member. Incredible advances have been made in identifying the essential features of quality end-of-life care, which, like chronic pain care, involves a wide range of medications as well as non-medication strategies to help the patient and those close to him or her cope with the challenges of the dying process and the natural grieving that goes along with it. We discuss these concerns further later in this chapter.

Social, Political, and Legal Issues Related to Pain Management

To help you understand why pain management has been characterized by confusing discontinuities, paradoxes, and deficiencies in professional performance, we need to spend a little time describing the social, political, and legal environment that has exerted so much (often negative) influence on the attitudes and practices of health care professionals. In 1971, President Nixon was the first to informally declare a "War on Drugs" (there was no official legal proclamation), borrowing, some have suggested, from other military-style calls to arms, such as the "War on Cancer," which also began during the first Nixon administration, and President Lyndon Johnson's 1964 declaration of a "War on Poverty." The original target of the War on Drugs was the notorious and illegal street drugs of abuse, such as cocaine, heroin, methamphetamines, and marijuana. More recently, however, legitimately prescribed pain medications increasingly have been diverted to non-medical uses, raising concerns about whether prescribing professionals are adequately screening their pain patients for addiction disorders or a propensity for diverting drugs to such illegitimate uses.

Most prescription pain medications are deemed "controlled substances" in the sense that their manufacture, distribution, prescribing, and dispensing are regulated by the federal Controlled Substances Act. The act sets out five "schedules" of drugs based on two factors: 1) the extent to which the drug meets a legitimate medical need and 2) the risk of addition that it poses. Schedule I drugs, which include cocaine and heroin, are deemed to have no legitimate medical use and to be highly addictive. Many of the strongest pain medications that are effective in treating moderate to severe pain, such as morphine and hydrocodone, fall into schedule II.

The Drug Enforcement Agency (DEA), a branch of the U.S. Department of Justice, is charged with enforcing the Controlled Substances Act. To prescribe controlled substances in compliance with this law, health care professionals must be registered with the DEA and issue prescriptions only to patients, for a legitimate medical purpose, and only in the course of sound professional practice. Many states

have also implemented what are called prescription-monitoring programs, which allow the tracking of prescription drugs. Professionals
who are deemed to be engaging in inappropriate or otherwise illegal prescribing practices are vulnerable to criminal prosecution under
the Controlled Substances Act or disciplinary action by their state
licensing board.

There has been a widespread perception among physicians that the
DEA and state medical boards have a special concern regarding the
prescribing of schedule II drugs, particularly over significant periods of
time for conditions characterized by chronic pain. Consequently, there
is a well-documented disinclination on the part of many physicians
to prescribe stronger (schedule II) pain medications, even when pain
relievers in the lower schedules have proven ineffective in achieving
an acceptable level of pain relief. Indeed, studies have shown that even
cancer patients do not consistently receive the type of prescription
pain relief they need to be comfortable.

The War on Pain

Although there has been no official declaration of a "War on Pain" as
there was with the War on Drugs, in the past ten to fifteen years, there
have been major public policy initiatives to promote improved pain
relief. As a patient in pain or a person who may need to become an
advocate for a loved one who is in pain, you should be aware of these
initiatives, because they can make you a more persuasive and effective
advocate.

In 1998, the Federation of State Medical Boards issued model
guidelines on prescribing pain medications to patients and urged each
individual state board to adopt and promote the use of similar guidelines by physicians. One important goal in promoting these guidelines
was to persuade physicians that state medical boards strongly support effective pain relief for patients, including the use of the strongest
(schedule II) available medications when appropriate to ensure patients
do not suffer unnecessarily. Effective pain relief now is widely recognized as essential to quality medical care. The model guidelines were
expanded and updated in 2004 and are now referred to as a "model
policy." The federation also recently published *Responsible Opioid Prescribing: A Physician's Guide*, written by the noted pain medicine specialist Dr. Scott Fishman. The purpose of the book is to translate the
federation's model policy into practical office-based pain management
guidelines.

The entity with the most influence over the quality of care patients receive in the hospital is the Joint Commission, known until recently as the Joint Commission on the Accreditation of Healthcare Organizations (JCAHO). To be eligible to receive Medicare and Medicaid reimbursement, hospitals must be reviewed, or "surveyed," periodically by the Joint Commission and be granted "accreditation." In 2001, the voluminous Joint Commission accreditation standards were modified to specifically include pain management. The new bottom line according to the Joint Commission pain standards is that "every patient has a right to have his or her pain assessed and treated." What is important for patients and their advocates to understand, however, is that the existence of these standards does not eliminate the need to be attentive and assertive about securing effective pain management. Awareness that the Joint Commission and the Federation of State Medical Boards view this as essential to good patient care can strengthen one's conviction in pursuing it and serve as an effective reminder to health care institutions and professionals that this is part of the standard of care they must provide their patients.

Finally, Congress has declared the decade beginning January 1, 2001, to be the "Decade of Pain Control and Research." The declaration constitutes an official recognition by the federal government that improving pain relief for patients and expanding research in this field are a national priority. It is yet another reminder that undertreated pain is bad for patients, their families, and our society.

An Overview of Good Pain Care

The purpose of this section is not to be a mini-medical school course in pain management. Rather, it is to help patients and their families recognize the essential features of competent, compassionate, and thorough pain care, as well as some of the red flags or warning signs of deficiencies. Remember, professionals may err on the side of being too aggressive or cavalier in their approach to pain relief as well as too passive or indifferent. Either approach is inconsistent with the standard of care and poses a risk of significant harm to the patient. The following are important elements of a sound pain assessment and management approach:

1. A thorough "pain history" including items such as how long pain has been present and whether it is continuous or intermittent, its location, its character (e.g., sharp, dull, tingling), what makes it feel better or worse,

its effect on physical function, and measures to relieve the pain that have been tried thus far. One recommended strategy for assessing pain is the acronym PQRST, with the letters standing for **P**rovocation (what triggers the pain), **Q**uality (characteristics), **R**egion (location), **S**everity (using a numeric scale with 0 being no pain and 10 being the worst pain one can imagine), and **T**emporal (onset, progression, changes).

2. At a minimum, a focused physical exam associated with the pain description is another important component of a good pain assessment and is particularly important if there is little or no prior relationship between the physician and patient. Physicians who are prepared to prescribe strong pain medications without a thorough history, pain assessment, and physical exam are placing their patients and their practice at risk. Whether any diagnostic tests, such as x-rays or blood work, are necessary depends on too many variables to be answered in this context. Results of recent diagnostic tests should be reviewed by any physician thinking about prescribing prescription pain relievers.

3. Communication by the physician to the patient should include his or her preliminary conclusions based on the history and physical exam and the proposed pain management plan. The patient should be clear about the options available to treat the pain, both those that involve medications and those that do not. The potential risks and side effects of any medication should be described, along with advice about what to do when or if they arise. Any limitations on activities such as driving, physical exertion, or the use of alcohol should be noted in detail.

4. There should be a clearly articulated plan for follow-up within a reasonable period to enable the physician to assess the patient's progress with the recommended treatment, note any problems encountered, and alter the treatment plan if necessary.

There are special concerns and considerations with regard to chronic noncancer pain patients, who receive their treatment almost exclusively in the outpatient setting. Although primary care physicians who are reasonably knowledgeable about pain management should be capable of caring for patients with chronic pain problems, the fact remains that many of them are not conversant with the latest policy statements and clinical practice guidelines, and there is a widespread perception among physicians that such pain patients are often difficult to work with and very demanding. If, as a chronic pain patient, you or a loved one for whom you may be an advocate encounter this type of behavior in a physician, you should feel free to request a consultation by or a referral to a pain medicine specialist. Some chronic pain conditions or special factors about the patient may present treatment challenges that do require the advice and counsel of experts. The goal, of course, is to arrive at an effective treatment plan that can then be comfortably maintained by the primary care physician. However, a treatment plan that involves a long-term course of high-dose pain medication (e.g., an opioid analgesic such as OxyContin) may not be within the comfort zone of some primary care physicians. In such cases, the patient must be referred to another physician who is comfortable with this mode of treatment.

It has become increasingly common for physicians who provide long-term opioid therapy to insist that their patients sign an "opioid agreement" or "opioid contract." National clinical practice guidelines recommend such contracts to physicians caring for pain patients with a current or prior addiction problem. Nevertheless, out of an abundance (or excess) of caution, more and more physicians impose such contracts as a blanket precondition to initiating long-term opioid therapy for any patient, regardless of the addiction risk they might pose. Some of the provisions in typical contracts are straightforward statements about the goals of treatment, the anticipated benefits and potential risks associated with such medications, the expectation that there will be both a reduction in pain and an improvement in the level of function, the importance of taking the medication only as directed, and the need for regular follow-up visits. Other provisions that are common but may raise issues or concerns for some patients include the insistence that the patient fill all prescriptions at a single pharmacy, that the patient not obtain pain medication from any other physician during the course of treatment, and that the patient submit to regular but random urine drug screens to ensure that he or she is taking the prescription medications as directed and is not taking any other drugs that have not been prescribed. Patients who are required to sign such agreements should have a clear understanding of what is expected of them, what the physician is committing to, and what the consequences will be if any provision of the agreement is violated. Patients experiencing significant pain at the time they are asked to review and sign such an agreement should insist on adequate time to review it and ask questions, and if at all possible, they should enlist the support of a relative or close friend as an advocate.

Palliative Care: Pain and Symptom Management at the End of Life

It was once a common assumption that whatever fears physicians harbored about the risk of addiction to pain medication or the potential for adverse side effects from it became secondary and much less problematic in the case of patients confronting terminal illnesses who were not expected to live more than six months. Unfortunately, studies began to emerge indicating that many cancer patients were experiencing severe pain because the type and dosage of the medications they were prescribed by their oncologists (physicians specializing in the treatment of cancer) were woefully inadequate. These studies, by highly respected members of the medical community, were a wakeup call to cancer physicians and the patients who learned of the studies. Besides the cancer itself, many of the medications and procedures used to treat it may be a source of pain and distress to patients. In the past ten to twenty years, the medical community has gradually recognized that regardless of whether a patient continues to receive therapies targeted to the underlying condition (disease directed), he or she also should receive medications and other measures targeted at pain and other forms of distress (i.e., palliative care). This strategy, sometimes also referred to as *simultaneous care*, is a balanced approach to patient management recommended for virtually all treatment settings – everything from the intensive care unit of a hospital to a skilled nursing facility or even home health care.

When it comes to confronting the end stage of a terminal and irreversible condition, surveys reveal that people fear pain and suffering even more than death. Clearly, these patients are most in need of family or other loved ones to advocate for their interests, and those interests surely include the relief of pain and suffering. State-of-the-art palliative or hospice care can effectively alleviate a dying patient's distress in at least 95% of cases, although a difficult balance may have to be struck between a level of awareness that allows the patient to interact with others and a level of analgesia and sedation that ensures he or she is not suffering. How that balance should be achieved is a decision that should be made by the patient or, if the patient can no longer direct his or her care because of mental confusion or deterioration (as with Alzheimer's), the patient's spokesperson, based on his or her assessment of what the patient would want. Much of the distress experienced subjectively by the patient during the dying process is related in significant and unambiguous ways to the physiological burdens of his or her terminal illness and the deterioration of his or her body. However, there also are psychosocial, spiritual, and existential components to suffering that some commentators in the professional literature claim are not clinical in origin or nature and hence should not be addressed through clinical measures such as sedation when other efforts to relieve the distress have proven ineffective or inadequate. This dispute within the medical community becomes relevant to dying patients and their families only in the small percentage of cases (5%) in which the usual and customary palliative measures fail to make the patient comfortable.

High-quality end-of-life care is provided most consistently under the direction of specialists in hospice and palliative medicine. However, it also is true that this type of care often is a team approach, and members of the team may include nurses, psychologists, social workers, pastoral counselors, and others. The focus of care is the whole patient and his or her family, not just the underlying disease or its symptoms. In a small percentage of patients in the advanced stages of terminal illness, the usual means of addressing pain and suffering prove inadequate to ensure their comfort; therefore, extraordinary palliative measures must be considered. These measures sometimes are referred to as *palliative options of last resort*. Some are controversial, not only among health care professionals but also in the larger society. Nevertheless, patients, their families, and particularly those taking on the role and responsibility of a patient's formal surrogate or informal advocate need to be aware of what is or should be available in the most challenging cases.

It is debatable whether very high doses of pain medications, alone or in combination with other medications – such as those intended to reduce anxiety – should be considered among the options of last resort. As we noted previously, there remains a great deal of myth and misinformation among health care professionals (doctors, nurses, pharmacists) concerning the risks such medications pose for causing or hastening a patient's death – for example, by reducing his or her breathing rate. At least among thought leaders in palliative medicine, these risks are highly exaggerated, and obsessive concern about them is misplaced when a patient is within hours or days of an inevitable death from a terminal condition. The actual risk of impairing a patient's ability to breathe adequately is outweighed by the professional responsibility to minimize suffering. Discussions about the care of these patients often invoke the term *double effect*, a reference to an ethical principle maintaining that if the intent of the care provider is to relieve suffering, in the rare instance in which medications hasten a patient's death, the conduct is not wrongful because the death was a foreseeable but unintended consequence of the necessary palliative measures.

For some patients with uncontrollable and distressing symptoms, the only effective means of relieving their suffering is to administer sedating medications to induce a state of complete unconsciousness. This procedure sometimes is referred to by the unfortunate term *terminal sedation*. The term is unfortunate because it mistakenly suggests that the patient is sedated for the express purpose and with the direct result of causing his or her death. It is true that total sedation rarely, if ever, is provided to patients who are not in the advanced stages of a terminal condition. However, when the medications are properly administered and monitored, nothing about the sedative measures causes or even hastens a patient's death. A variation on total sedation, which usually is initiated only in cases of extreme and unmanageable distress, is known as *respite sedation*. As the term implies, total sedation is induced for a limited period to give the patient a break from experiencing the considerable burdens of advanced disease, in the hope that when the sedation subsequently is discontinued, the patient's suffering can be managed without sacrificing consciousness.

When total sedation is administered with no intention of discontinuing it, including after respite sedation has failed, a separate decision must be made about nutrition and hydration (food and water). Totally sedated patients cannot consume adequate nutrients and liquids to survive unless these are provided artificially, usually through a tube inserted through the nose into the stomach or by means of a tube surgically implanted directly into the stomach. Many patients for whom total sedation is considered can no longer make decisions for themselves; thus, determining whether to initiate or continue artificial nutrition and hydration is the responsibility of the patient's designated surrogate or spokesperson. Totally sedated patients cannot experience hunger or thirst, so the only reason to provide artificial nutrition and hydration would be to prolong the patient's biological life. It falls upon the surrogate to determine whether the patient would wish to have his or her body's functions continued in this way when he or she is near death and will never regain consciousness.

The law in two states (Oregon and Washington) allows physicians, at the formal request of a patient with a terminal condition, to prescribe medication (usually a barbiturate) the patient can take to end his or her life at a time of his or her own choosing. In Oregon, where this law has been in effect for more than ten years, a very small percentage of all patients who die each year elect to secure and use such a lethal prescription. The demographics of patients who choose this controversial approach are interesting because they stand in stark contrast to the dire predictions made by the opponents of the Oregon ballot initiative. The vast majority of Oregon patients who seek a lethal prescription are enrolled in hospice and presumably receiving quality palliative care. Opponents had argued that only patients without access to hospice and palliative care would (in desperation) pursue this option. Almost all these patients have health insurance, whereas opponents predicted it would be the poor and uninsured who would be left with no option but to seek assistance in hastening death as a release from untreated suffering. Finally, most of those who take a lethal prescription have education beyond high school, in contrast to the opponents' belief that the uneducated would pursue this option because they would not be as well equipped to navigate the complex and confusing networks of health insurance, provider networks, and regulations that characterize modern health care.

Another surprising insight from the Oregon experience is that undertreated pain and the inability to effectively manage other disease-related aspects of terminal illness are not the primary motivating factors in seeking a lethal prescription. Rather, the three most commonly cited reasons are more psychosocial or existential in nature – loss of autonomy (96%), loss of dignity (86%), and inability to engage in activities that make life enjoyable (86%) – which actually are the most controversial reasons for providing palliative sedation. Indeed, some prominent national professional organizations, such as the American Medical Association, recently adopted policies declaring that palliative sedation is never appropriate for so-called existential suffering, which has been characterized as "nonclinical" in nature. This policy position is controversial and in marked contrast to guidelines proposed by palliative care professionals. Particularly in this state of flux and uncertainty, patients whose end-of-life suffering and distress are vulnerable to being labeled "merely existential" need persistent and assertive advocates. Health care providers who loudly declaim the immorality of otherwise legal palliative options of last resort may well have a conflict of interest between their personal morality and the needs of their patients. In such situations, they have a moral and professional responsibility to recognize that conflict and disengage from decisions about treatment. Under no circumstances should they be allowed to bully or coerce patients or their spokespersons from pursuing their own sense of the patient's needs and best interests.

In most states, physicians who provide a terminally ill patient with a prescription they know or reasonably believe he or she intends to use to bring about his or her death are at risk of criminal prosecution and/or discipline by their state medical board. Some patients for whom the burdens of continued life significantly outweigh the benefits choose to stop eating and drinking as a means of hastening their approaching and inevitable death. In the medical literature, articles have begun to appear in which palliative care specialists consider this phenomenon. They report widespread confusion regarding what these patients experience. In patients whose terminal disease is in an advanced stage, the body's capacity to process nutrients and fluids is substantially reduced, so they do not experience hunger and thirst to a degree that even remotely resembles what a healthy person would experience going without food and water. Furthermore, the health care professional's ongoing duty of care requires that he or she at least offer palliative measures to these patients to manage any distress they might experience after declining nutrition and hydration.

Conclusion

In a Dickensian sense, this is an exasperating "best of times and worst of times" period in pain and symptom management and end-of-life care. It now is more likely than ever that, whether you are visiting your primary care physician's office or the local hospital's emergency department, a nurse will ask you not only if you are in pain but also to rate your pain level on a scale of 1 to 10 and will then note your responses in your medical chart. However, this apparent initial attentiveness may actually mask a serious ongoing systemic failure in American health care to take unrelieved pain seriously and to use readily available means to relieve it. Therefore, it is up to the individual patient and/or his or her spokesperson or family advocate to insist that the initial inquiry about pain is more than just a routine checking of boxes for the Joint Commission surveyors or a state licensing authority. Yes, there are many policy pronouncements about a patient's right to prompt and attentive pain care, but whether those pronouncements prove to be true for you as a patient will depend largely on whether you are the beneficiary of your own or someone else's persistent advocacy.

Another exquisite irony of our current health care situation is that the more determined and persistent you are in asserting your rights, especially if you are afflicted with a source and type of pain that calls for a trial of strong pain medication, the greater your risk of being labeled a difficult, malingering, or perhaps even drug-seeking patient. This catch-22 has been problematic particularly for chronic pain patients who, through hard-won lessons and insights as well as diligent self-education, may actually know more about what works for them (and what does not) than the physician from whom they are seeking competent and compassionate care.

These warnings are not intended to discourage you as a patient or family advocate, but rather to alert and empower you to overcome the persistent barriers to effective pain management. Most health care professionals have good intentions, but they are hindered by their lack of basic training in the assessment and management of pain and, too often, confused or intimidated by regulators who seem to be more intent on addressing the problems of drug abuse and diversion in society than ensuring that real patients with serious problems receive appropriate medical care. Such care is entirely consistent with the core values and professional responsibilities of physicians and nurses, and it is the moral and legal right of every patient.

EIGHTEEN

The Hardest Decisions

When Treatment Stops Working

– Timothy E. Quill and Mindy Shah

Living with a potentially life-limiting illness usually brings with it a series of difficult decisions. Beyond the impact of the initial diagnosis, new and tough choices arise when:

- Available treatments no longer are very effective
- The disease itself worsens despite proper treatment
- Complications cause a setback
- Your ability to get up and around declines
- You have trouble eating and drinking enough

Such events sometimes happen in rapid succession, and everyone (you, your family and friends, and medical providers) is so busy stamping out fires, nobody pauses to get the big picture. However, in general, choices about treatment need to be considered in terms of two things: prognosis and goals.

Let's look at prognosis. We've all heard stories about someone who was told he had six months to live, only to be mowing his lawn two years later, or the person who was never supposed to walk again striding across the stage to get her college diploma. Unfortunately, although these exceptions do occur, the more discouraging truth is that they are relatively rare, and most of the time, physicians overestimate rather than underestimate prognosis. The reasons for this overestimation are complex, but they are related, in part, to the fact that no doctor wants to deprive a patient or family of hope, and most patients (and their families) generally don't want to hear the reality of really bad medical news.

The problem with trying to maintain hope by holding back the truth is that it may undermine good decision making, in terms of both medical treatment decisions and the pursuit of personal goals. Someone who wrongly thinks he likely has years to live might continue to put off that trip to Europe to visit his sister. A patient with advanced cancer who thinks cardiac resuscitation would give her time to see her grandson's graduation might put herself, and her family, through unneeded suffering. On the other hand, if a young father's goal is to prolong his life to be with his family, he might jump at the chance for a therapy with tough side effects even if the best-case scenario would add only a few months to his life.

The purpose of this chapter is to talk directly about some of the hardest decisions sick people, and their families, face. Hopefully, it will provide a framework to guide you and your family through your own dialogue as well as through conversations with your physicians.

Advance Care Planning

Being diagnosed with a potentially life-limiting illness should trigger some serious advance care planning if you haven't done this already. *Advance directives* are documents to guide future treatment in the event you lose the ability to make decisions for yourself. They are activated only if you are too sick to make your own decisions, and their purpose is to keep you in the driver's seat if that happens to you. Most (but not all) people want their treatment to be much more comfort oriented and less disease directed if they lose decision-making ability, and advance directives give you the opportunity – whatever your philosophy – to make your wishes known. There are two kinds of advance directives:

A *health care proxy* is an individual you appoint to make medical decisions for you if you become unable to make your health care wishes known. Often, people choose their spouse or next of kin as health care proxy, but the proxy does not necessarily have to be a relative. In fact, sometimes close relatives have a hard time making tough decisions (like stopping treatments) because they don't want to lose someone they love. Whomever you ultimately appoint as your proxy, it's important to discuss with that person any limitations you might place on your care; it's their job as proxy to represent *your* wishes, not their own, so they need to understand your thoughts on medical treatments.

A *living will* is a document that describes your wishes and preferences regarding health care in the future if you lose the ability to make these known yourself. Many people use an attorney to create a living will, but this is not necessary in most cases. In a living will, you can communicate your preferences regarding treatments such as cardiopulmonary resuscitation (CPR), artificial nutrition and hydration (feeding tubes), dialysis, and ventilators. The living will is meant to serve as a guideline for your health care providers, family members, and health care proxy if they have to make future medical decisions on your behalf; in itself, it cannot serve as an official do-not-resuscitate (DNR) order (see later) and generally cannot overrule the decisions made by your designated health care proxy.

Experimental Treatments

You've tried all the normal treatments for your illness, and they have stopped working. What about experimental treatments and drug trials? After all, what do you have to lose?

Experimental treatments and drug trials can offer hope by providing the option of doing something when it seems all the other doctors have given up. After all, such studies are how new and effective treatments are discovered and developed. However, it is vital to understand what is being offered.

What Exactly Is the Treatment?

A once-a-day, well-tolerated pill with a low likelihood of harm, even if it has little chance of working, might be worth a try. An aggressive series of radiation or chemotherapy treatments with predictable serious side effects is a different matter. What is the likely effect of the particular treatment on the quality of your life?

What Does the Treatment Involve?

Frequent trips to the hospital to get blood draws or x-rays may be taxing and take up a lot of precious time and energy. If time is short, you might rather spend it at home or another more comfortable setting. Frequently, such trials are done at large academic medical centers in urban areas, which might mean travel expenses as well as time away from friends and family.

What Are the Possible Side Effects, and How Likely Are They to Happen?

An early trial may not have a lot of data on possible adverse effects and their likelihood, but clinicians usually have some idea about how toxic or well-tolerated a treatment will be from preliminary studies done before it became available for a clinical trial.

What Are the Possible Benefits, and How Likely Are They to Happen?

In most experimental clinical trials, the likelihood of benefit for an individual patient is small. For some, the "benefit" may involve contributing to science or helping others in the future. For others, the main hope is to find a treatment that might work even though the odds are small. It comes down to your personal goals; if you value quality of life over life extension, a small chance of gaining a few extra weeks of life might not be worth a treatment with a high likelihood of causing adverse symptoms such as fatigue, nausea, or vomiting. If you want to explore every possible way to extend life, even if there may be serious side effects, then experimental treatment may be worth considering.

Can I Drop Out of the Trial If I Have a Lot of Side Effects or If It Doesn't Seem to Be Helping Me for Any Reason?

The answer to this question is an unequivocal yes, so you may consider an experimental therapy a time-limited trial to see how you respond to it. If you feel worse at any time, you can choose to stop.

In general, if an experimental treatment doesn't involve a lot of time on your part, is easy to take, is convenient, and has a low probability of bad side effects, there probably isn't a real downside to giving it a try. If it doesn't work, you can stop it. If an experimental therapy is risky, has a lot of potential side effects, and requires a lot of time in the hospital or doctor's office, think carefully about it before beginning because it likely will require a lot of your precious time and energy.

Do-Not-Resuscitate and Do-Not-Intubate Orders

A DNR order means that medical personnel are not to attempt CPR if your heart stops beating in a way that can support life. Likewise, a do-not-intubate (DNI) order means they are not to put in a breathing tube (intubation) and put you on a breathing machine if you lose the ability to breathe on your own. CPR and intubation are done *by default* unless these DNR and DNI orders, respectively, are in place.

What Is Resuscitation?

When discussing DNR orders, the term *cardiopulmonary resuscitation* means using chest compressions, artificial ventilation (mouth-to-mouth, with a mask, or through a breathing tube), and possibly defibrillation (shocks delivered to the heart) to try to revive a patient whose heart has stopped pumping effectively. Chest compressions are done to try to temporarily support someone whose heart has stopped or is beating in a way that does not effectively provide blood to the body. While CPR is being done, medications often are provided to try to get the heart to work properly. Artificial ventilation is always given in this setting. Defibrillation may or may not be done during resuscitation, depending on the type of problem the heart is having. CPR tends to be a very invasive process, associated with broken ribs from the chest compressions, a sore chest from the electrical shocks, and a sore throat from the breathing tube. It should be attempted only if there is a reasonable chance it will revive the patient.

What Is Intubation?

Intubation means placing a breathing tube into the trachea (windpipe), then hooking the tube to a ventilator (breathing machine). This kind of treatment is always done during resuscitation and also may be done for serious lung problems (e.g., emphysema and pneumonia). The ventilator itself doesn't usually treat a problem; rather it supports breathing while medications or other therapies are used to fix the underlying lung problem. For people with a temporary breathing problem (e.g., pneumonia) and otherwise relatively healthy lungs, this process can sustain them temporarily until their lungs recover enough for them to breathe independently. For patients with severe chronic lung problems (e.g., severe emphysema or advanced lung cancer), their ability to breathe independently after being put on a breathing machine may be very unlikely, prompting some to refuse to go on the machine in the first place.

How Long Would I Be on a Ventilator?

Sometimes people can come off a ventilator in a few days if their underlying problem is quickly identified and treated, as is the case for some types of pneumonia. Other times – such as in cases of advanced emphysema or lung cancer, in which the underlying disease is progressive and not easily treated – there may be no end in sight. Also, regardless of the main lung problem, a coexisting illness such as heart failure, emphysema, or cancer can make it harder for a patient to get off the ventilator. Oftentimes, doctors already have a good idea which patients likely would have a struggle getting off a ventilator. Other cases are harder to predict.

One of the problems with going on a ventilator is figuring out what to do if you don't get better. Many (but not all) people would not want to be on a ventilator indefinitely, as life on a ventilator has significant limitations. With a breathing (endotracheal) tube in, you would not be able to talk or eat normally. You might need sedating medications to deal with the discomfort of being on the ventilator. If you need to be intubated for a prolonged period (usually two or more weeks), the endotracheal tube is switched to a tracheostomy A tracheostomy is a hole in the front of the neck that goes into the trachea, through which a small tube is placed that hooks up to the ventilator. With some training, many people with tracheostomies can talk while on a ventilator. However, eating is still impossible unless you can tolerate being off the ventilator for an extended period. Otherwise, nutrition is given through a tube going into the stomach (more on that later).

If I Weren't Getting Better, Would My Family and Doctors Just "Pull the Plug"?

If you want to give a ventilator a try but don't want to be on one indefinitely, one option is a time-limited trial. In this scenario, you (or your health care proxy) decide on a time for the treatment to be reevaluated (and maybe stopped) according to certain end points defined by you or your proxy as well as your physicians. Families and patients often choose this option when they feel they've tried everything yet don't want to indefinitely continue treatments that aren't working. The idea of stopping a ventilator may seem frightening to patients and their families, but when someone is removed from a ventilator and not expected to breathe well on his or her own, he or she is given medication to treat any breathlessness or other symptoms that might arise. In short, people don't feel as if they're suffocating (a very common fear).

Shouldn't Everyone Get Resuscitation and Intubation?

The general public has a lot of misconceptions about how well resuscitation works. For individuals with acute cardiac disease in whom resuscitation can be started quickly (within seconds or minutes) and whose underlying medical problems can be quickly treated, resuscitation may have a good outcome. For example, a man goes to the hospital with a heart attack, and his heart stops beating while he's in the emergency department. CPR is started immediately, and the patient gets medications that restore his heartbeat within a few minutes. He then receives further treatments to address his heart disease.

An entirely different situation arises in the setting of chronic or terminal illness. When a person's body is already weak because of multiple chronic illnesses, advanced pulmonary disease, cancer, and/or advanced age, it tends not to respond to CPR. In this case, the odds are extremely low that resuscitation will be successful (i.e., will restore effective heart function, allowing the patient to leave the hospital at some point); therefore, the burden of CPR is harder to justify for many people.

Would I Be a Vegetable?

No one can predict with absolute certainty what you would be like if you survived CPR. When resuscitation is done promptly, and if a pulse is regained within minutes, neurological deficits may be small or even absent. On the other extreme, if resuscitation efforts are prolonged (and especially if you have multiple medical problems to begin with), in the unlikely event you survive, you might end up with severe brain injury or even be brain dead. Also, the result may be somewhere between those two extremes, leaving you debilitated and perhaps requiring a lifetime of nursing home care.

Would I Be Giving Up If I Choose DNR or DNI?

Most people who are seriously ill still want to receive potentially effective treatments, but they don't want to undergo invasive procedures that have little or no chance of helping them. CPR and intubation fall into this category of very invasive measures that are not likely to help. Even if you choose DNR and/or DNI, all other potentially effective treatment options are still on the table for you to consider with your doctor. In that context, choosing is in no way giving up on effective treatment.

Transitioning to Hospice

Deciding to enroll in hospice often is a very challenging transition. Accepting hospice means coming to terms with a certain reality – the reality that treatment is not working and that one's time likely is limited. It usually means giving up hope on being cured and getting better. It means not going to the hospital for each thing that goes wrong. It may mean ending relationships with medical staff you've known for years. On the other hand, hospice provides many benefits that make most people glad they made the transition after it is done.

What Is Hospice, and Where Does It Occur?

Hospice is a comprehensive plan of care for terminally ill people focusing on maximizing comfort and improving quality of life, without further treatment of the underlying disease process. Although most people think of hospice as a place that cares for dying patients, hospice care may be given in the patient's home, in hospice houses, in nursing homes, or in the hospital. Actually, most hospice care takes place right in one's own home.

Isn't This Just for People Who Are on Their Deathbed?

This is a common misconception. To qualify for home or nursing home hospice, you need an average prognosis of six months or less (if the illness runs its usual course). This means some people may qualify for hospice when they're still up and about and enjoying life. If the average is six months, that means some patients may live as long as a year or two if the disease progresses slowly, whereas others may die in a matter of days to weeks, depending on their clinical situation. People who are less acutely ill may not need much help from hospice workers at first – perhaps just some medical equipment, a nursing visit once a week, or a number to call if they have questions. However, as their disease progresses, they'll already have established relationships with the hospice nurses and other personnel, and a plan will already be in place for dealing with the changes that accompany worsening disease.

Other sites of hospice care, such as hospitals and hospice houses, generally take people only with shorter prognoses, although rules may vary from region to region.

What Can Hospice Do for Me?

Hospice programs are designed to maximize quality of life for terminally ill patients. They employ specially trained physicians and hospice nurses to manage pain and other symptoms. If needed, home health aides help with basic personal care (e.g., bathing, feeding) and sometimes light housework. Social workers assess patient and family needs, coordinate services, and provide supportive counseling. Chaplains provide spiritual support. After death, bereavement coordinators help link survivors to grief support services, if needed. Most medication costs are covered by hospice, as are the costs of medical equipment (e.g., hospital beds and commodes). Finally, many patients and families are reassured by having a central contact person to call with problems or questions.

What Won't Hospice Do?

At home, hospice can provide as much as two to four hours of home health aide help; it does not provide twenty-four-hour care, so the bulk of care must come from family members and/or friends. In general, hospice programs won't cover hospitalization (unless needed for acute symptom management) or active treatment of the underlying disease. So, if you want more chemotherapy in hopes of remission or cure, hospice probably isn't for you. Also, if you want intravenous (IV) fluids or antibiotics, or if you want to return to the hospital for aggressive medical treatment if you get sicker, again, hospice probably isn't the right choice. Hospice attempts to help you live "as well as you can for as long as you can," with special emphasis on enhancing quality of life all the way through the final stages of your illness. Hospice policy regarding hospitalization and IV treatments varies from region to region; therefore, if the possibility of being hospitalized or receiving IV therapy is important to you, you should ask your local hospice agencies about their specific regulations.

Opioid Pain Medications

What Meds Are We Talking About?

Opioids include morphine, hydrocodone, oxycodone, hydromorphone, fentanyl, and methadone (otherwise known as narcotic pain medications). These medications are among the best available for controlling pain and shortness of breath.

Aren't They Too Strong?

These drugs are stronger than other pain medicines, such as aspirin, ibuprofen, and acetaminophen, but are indicated when these milder medications are ineffective. They can be started safely in people who haven't used them before if they are started at low doses and increased carefully as needed.

Will I Become Addicted?

This is a common concern and a reason some people hold off on using opioid pain medication. *True addiction* (the erratic use of these medications to get high rather than to treat symptoms) is very unlikely when opioids are used as directed. People with a history of past addiction are at higher risk for re-addiction but can still use opioid medications if needed for pain under the guidance of a pain management or palliative care specialist. *Tolerance*, when the body needs more of a certain medication to get the same effect, may develop with use of these pain medications but can be managed with dose or medication changes; it is not the same as addiction. *Physical dependence*, when the body shows withdrawal symptoms if the medicine is stopped suddenly, often develops with the use of opioid medications; it can be avoided if dose reductions are made gradually. Again, it is not the same as addiction.

Shouldn't I Save Them Until I Really Need Them?

There is no reason to delay using opioid pain medication if it can help you feel better. Some people may need their dosage increased over time to get good pain control, but there is no upper limit to the amount you can take (as there is with acetaminophen and ibuprofen). The only thing that sometimes limits the dosage is development of side effects. Furthermore, you can change from one opioid to another if the first one becomes ineffective.

What Side Effects Might I Experience?

Constipation tends to be the most bothersome side effect of opioids and, if not treated, it occurs almost all the time. Therefore, while on opioids, you'll probably need to take laxatives and stool softeners on a regular basis. Unfortunately, constipation usually lasts the whole time you're on pain medications. Other, less common side effects are nausea, sleepiness, itching, and difficulty emptying the bladder. Nausea tends to decrease over time. If you experience significant nausea, your doctor can put you on anti-nausea medicines for a few days until it lessens. Itching may be relieved by antihistamines. Sleepiness also may decrease after the first few days on the medication; if it persists, the dosage may need to be reduced.

Will They Hasten My Death?

Opioids can affect the body's drive to breathe, which is why big overdoses of pain medications can be fatal. However, *respiratory depression* hardly ever occurs without the patient getting very sleepy first. If you, your doctor, or your family notices severe drowsiness, the dosage should be reduced (or the medication stopped altogether). In an emergency, medications can be given to instantly reverse the pain medication. Serious overdoses are very unlikely when medications are prescribed by an experienced provider and the patient follows prescription instructions.

If symptoms of pain or shortness of breath become severe, sometimes high doses of opioids are required. Unfortunately, rapidly increasing doses may lead to increased sleepiness. Some people are willing to tolerate some discomfort to be more awake, whereas others want to be in as little pain as possible, even if that means they're pretty sleepy. What's more, many people change what they're willing to tolerate symptom-wise over time; someone might place a higher value on being alert when he or she still has important things to do (e.g., taking care of a will, seeing relatives) and then not mind being sleepy once these tasks are done. It's a very individual choice and one you should discuss with your doctor if the need arises.

At the very end of life, breathing patterns normally change; breaths may become shallow, irregular, or far apart. Some physicians and family members may be reluctant to use opioids in this situation for fear they may hasten death by further reducing the body's drive to breathe. Although there is a very slight chance using opioids may hasten death by a matter of hours, these medications generally shouldn't be withheld if they're needed to make the dying process more comfortable. Furthermore, if a patient has needed opioids up to this point to control symptoms, the medicines should not be discontinued because those symptoms likely would return, and additional symptoms from sudden withdrawal might make the situation worse.

Artificial Nutrition and Hydration

What If I Can't Eat Enough because of Lack of Appetite, Aspiration, Swallowing Issues, or Nausea?

What to do depends on your prognosis and your goals. If you have an illness from which you're likely to recover (or at least improve), it may make sense to accept artificial nutrition and hydration to get over the rough patches. For example, you may get artificial nutrition and hydration during chemotherapy treatments if you have severe nausea, after abdominal surgery until your gut heals, or during treatment that temporarily interferes with swallowing (e.g., head and neck cancer therapy). Such artificial means of sustenance include IV fluids, feeding tubes (inserted either through the nose into the stomach or directly into the stomach through a relatively minor surgical procedure), and total parenteral nutrition (TPN). Each method has drawbacks. IV fluids may increase swelling if you already have fluid overload. Feeding tubes may involve a surgical procedure, some initial pain at the site, and possible complications of the tube becoming dislodged or not functioning correctly. TPN involves the risk of fluid overload as well as potentially serious infections.

Aspiration (i.e., when food goes down into the lungs rather than the esophagus) is a complicated problem, as it often is recurrent. In these cases, a feeding tube sometimes is recommended as a safer way to provide nutrition. However, it is important to remember that aspiration can still occur with a feeding tube – the liquid food that goes through the tube can back up from the stomach, or normal mouth secretions may find their way into the lungs.

A big problem arises when eating and drinking become difficult near the end of life. Lack of appetite is a frequent symptom of cancer and may be hard to overcome. Pain and nausea also make it difficult to eat enough. Aspiration may occur as the body weakens, causing frequent pneumonias. Although managing symptoms certainly is important, starting TPN or a feeding tube frequently is counterproductive because of the added risks of these interventions and the low likelihood they'll provide any real benefit. In most situations, people in later stages of terminal illness don't get more energy or live longer with these treatments. Even simple IV fluids can increase swelling in the hands, feet, and abdomen and lead to fluid buildup in the lungs, all of which may cause discomfort and, in some situations, even hasten death.

Won't I Starve to Death?

Across nearly all cultures, the reflexive response to people who are ill is to feed them. Preparing and serving food is a powerful way to show love. It also is a way for people to express their care when words seem awkward or inappropriate. Certainly, small bites of favorite foods (if desired) can provide enjoyment for you and satisfaction for your family. The challenge for families becomes finding ways to show love and support that don't emphasize food, such as backrubs or massages, reading aloud, playing music, talking, praying, or simply sitting quietly together. Furthermore, lots of people worry about starving to death. From what people who have gone without food tell us, the experience of dehydration and fasting is not uncomfortable as long as the mouth is kept moist. Small sips of water or damp sponge sticks can prevent a dry mouth. It's important to remember that death eventually comes, not as the result of not eating or drinking but of the underlying illness.

If Dying Gets Too Hard

Most deaths at home or in a nursing home can be peaceful with attentive caregiving and careful symptom management. In a few cases, however, symptoms such as pain, breathlessness, nausea, and agitation become severe in the face of usual palliative therapy and need more aggressive treatment. If this happens to you, one option is to come to the hospital or inpatient palliative care or hospice unit for IV medications and intensive nursing care to make you more comfortable.

Tradeoffs between Pain and Sedation

Most of the time, pain and shortness of breath can be managed with medication that in no way hastens death. In fact, there are data showing that good pain and symptom management tends to extend life rather than shorten it. However, occasionally there are circumstances in which pain or shortness of breath accelerates as death approaches, and a patient may have to make tradeoffs between pain and sedation. Relatively early on, some patients may accept some extra pain to be more alert, but as death approaches, they may consider accepting more sedation to be freer from pain. There is wide acceptance that this tradeoff is permissible, as the intention of both clinician and patient is to relieve suffering and not to hasten death; in fact, the risk of hastening death is extremely small if it exists at all.

What If Even Hospitalization Doesn't Make Me Comfortable?

As mentioned previously, most deaths occur peacefully with minimal intervention. However, a few people must go to an inpatient setting for more intensive treatment of symptoms as death approaches. However, if suffering persists, another option is "palliative sedation to unconsciousness for treatment of otherwise refractory symptoms." Because a person can't eat or drink while unconscious, ultimately this type of sedation does end in death unless IV hydration is provided (which for most patients makes little sense because they are actively dying). Because there is debate about the ethical nature of sedation to unconsciousness, some physicians feel uncomfortable providing it. If this is an option you might be interested in, discuss your thoughts with your doctor. In most cases in which sedation to unconsciousness is being considered, it's worthwhile to get the involvement of a palliative medicine specialist or other physician expert in end-of-life care to ensure that all alternatives have been explored.

What about Physician-Assisted Suicide or Euthanasia?

There has been a long and continuing debate over physician-assisted suicide (in which the doctor provides a patient with a potentially lethal dose of medication for patients to take themselves) and euthanasia (in which the doctor administers a lethal dose of medication at the patient's request). Currently in the United States, physician-assisted suicide is legal only in Oregon and Washington state; euthanasia is illegal in all states. Although this chapter's purpose is not to make arguments for or against these practices, it's important to recognize that fears about dying badly and thoughts of suicide are common in terminal illness – about one in fifty terminally ill people in Oregon talks about assisted suicide with his or her doctor and one in six talks with family members about it. Only a tiny fraction of these people ever act on their thoughts (in Oregon, where physician-assisted suicide can be pursued openly subject to safeguards, it accounts for only 1 in 1,000 deaths). However, these conversations can help identify patients' (and families') biggest fears and serve as a stimulus to a better understanding of patient values and priorities. The take-home message: if you're thinking about ending your life, talk to your doctor.

Although there is a lot of public discussion over physician-assisted suicide, euthanasia, and other extreme measures, the reality is that most symptoms can be controlled by conventional medical practice. *Palliative care*, a medical subspecialty that focuses on symptom control in serious illness, is becoming increasingly available and can help patients in any stage of illness and alongside other treatments. For terminally ill patients who no longer desire or qualify for curative treatment, hospice usually is the most effective and comprehensive program for staying comfortable in a variety of settings. No matter what treatment approach you choose, dealing with the uncertainties and fluctuations of serious illness requires teamwork by you, your family, and your physician. Talk with your physician, and make sure he or she is committed to staying the course no matter what the future holds. If you, or your doctor, have misgivings about your ability to work together, ask to be referred to another provider.

NINETEEN

What You Need to Know about Disasters

– Griffin Trotter

In trying to impart essential knowledge to you about disasters, I run into several challenges. First, it seems somewhat presumptuous to assume the posture of an educator on this topic. There is perhaps no major human endeavor for which the knowledge gap between laypersons and experts is as small as it is for disasters. Both ordinary citizens and expert planners know, with almost indelible accuracy, the most basic, abstract features of disasters – they are compressed in time and typically also in space, they present acute dangers to individuals and communities, and they involve significant damage to social structures. The two groups also share similar and often mistaken impressions about human behavior in disasters and how disasters ought to be managed. Although it is true that expert planners typically have more tidbits of information about disasters, and a broader knowledge of existing disaster resources, they also tend to cling more tightly to erroneous beliefs (which, unfortunately, they possess in greater quantities). Although there is much detailed knowledge about disasters, especially in the realm of disaster sociology, neither disaster planners nor ordinary citizens typically are acquainted with much of it. In trying to formulate guidance for you, the general public, I am acutely aware that frequently you are the ones who shine brightly in disaster responses, whereas the so-called experts flounder in a labyrinth of rigid, maladaptive protocols.

Second, there is no distinct body of relevant information that will apply equally to all of you. What counts as essential knowledge varies considerably among citizens living in different locations. In my early medical training in St. Louis, Missouri, clinical mentors often said, "When you hear hoof beats in Missouri, think of horses not zebras." The general message here is universally valid: common things are common, uncommon things are uncommon. However, the rule about thinking of horses is very context-dependent. Someone in Kenya would be better advised to think of zebras. The same applies to disaster. When an alarm bell sounds in Topeka, one should be wary of tornadoes. When it sounds in Seattle, earthquakes and volcanic eruptions are more likely. In neither case, however, is it very wise to think of smallpox infections or atom bombs – which are probably even less likely than stampeding zebras escaped from the local zoo.

Third, the most important virtues in facing a disaster – thinking adaptively and embracing common sense – are not the sort of things you will acquire by reading a short essay. Although I can offer general tactical guidance, I cannot teach you these virtues. Fortunately, most of you already have them, and during times of crisis they usually intensify. Indeed, the greatest and most egregious of all disaster myths is that people typically panic. Panic is irrational behavior motivated by fear. Of course, disasters bring danger, and danger elicits fear. Fortunately, however, the fear we experience in disasters generally is more likely to heighten our strengths rather than our weaknesses. When we behave wrongly, it typically is because of ignorance rather than irrationality.

So, I refrain from the usual condescending advice to "remain calm" and instead provide you with information you may find useful in preparing for, and responding to, common disasters. If you want to put this advice into action, you will need to interpret it in light of your own personal circumstances.

What follows is divided into two sections. The first section explores the concept of risk – what it means, how it is assessed, and how you should think about it. The second section covers information you can use to construct a family disaster plan, including commentary on basic tactics and helpful gear. Seven priority areas are identified, with brief comments about how each one applies to different disasters and circumstances.

Risk

In our day-to-day lives, most of us are inconsistent in our management of risk. On the road, where most people experience their greatest immediate perils to life and limb, we drive at dangerous speeds, so close to vehicles in front of us that their fatal collision would surely cause our own death as well – all the while calmly chatting on our cell phone as if we were sitting at home by the fireplace. Influenced by the media, which regard violence as synonymous with newsworthiness, most of us are far more frightened by remote risks of terrorism or criminal attacks.

As I write this chapter, the Mumbai terrorist attacks, in which 165 innocents were killed, still takes up several pages of the *Wall Street Journal* after five days of extensive coverage. It is not the economic destruction or the death toll but rather today's headline – "Survivors Tell of Terror" – that consummates the terrorists' mission. In distinction, the cholera epidemic in Zimbabwe that so far has killed 425 people – also presumably innocent – has to this point received only a one-sentence blurb in the "World-Wide" news column.

The fact is, even during the month of September in 2001, more people died unnecessarily in the United States because of poor motor vehicle operation than because of terrorist attacks. Terrorists could pull off attacks of 9/11 magnitude every single month from now until eternity, and terrorism still would not exceed motor vehicle operation as a public health problem. Furthermore, if citizens were as unconcerned about being attacked as they are about dying in traffic accidents, terrorism would no longer terrorize and hence would probably cease.

Risk is the probability of some negative event, given certain existing conditions. Because these conditions and their cumulative interactions often are difficult to pin down, many risk estimates are educated guesses at best. As Lee Clarke[1] has argued, many descriptions of risk, including estimates of disaster risks, are best viewed as efforts to render fearful uncertainties into bits of scientific knowledge that are manageable by experts. We may find solace in such efforts, but they are not scientific in any rigorous sense.

The approach to smallpox is a case in point. The U.S. government has barred its citizens from obtaining smallpox vaccine, based on the reasoning that both the risk of a smallpox attack and the importance of freedom of choice are too small to justify the risks of immunization (which kills about one in a million who receive the vaccination) in the ordinary citizen. Interestingly, however, the government worries about smallpox epidemics enough to spend billions of dollars protecting against them. If a significant proportion of the population were immunized, smallpox risk would dwindle, and so presumably would the costs. In the deliberations of the Advisory Committee on Immunization Practices (ACIP), uncertainties about risk and feelings about reasonable risk tolerance are clothed in the rhetoric of scientific calculation. But, what qualifications do the scientists on the ACIP have to determine the proper equilibrium between the uncertain but tiny immunization risks and the peace-of-mind benefits that immunization brings to citizens who are deeply concerned about smallpox? None, of course. Expertise in such matters is a fiction.

There is, then, a lot of nonsense in the public sphere about risk – posturing by authorities, the presumption that value issues are scientific matters, and skewed assessments by a general public that often fears remote but exotic dangers more than the mundane dangers that regularly kill them in droves.

To set the stage for the guidance that follows, a few basic observations about disaster risk will be helpful. First, although the risk of dying in a natural disaster is uncertain, it is certainly less for most people than the risk of dying in other types of accidents, such as motor vehicle collisions, falls, house fires, and swimming accidents. Before you get fully energized on your family disaster plan, it is a good idea to check your fire alarms, fire extinguishers, and fire escape plans. Motor vehicle safety, swimming pool safety, and proper firearm storage also are probably higher priorities.

Second, the greatest disaster risks come from natural disasters that vary geographically. In my current abode, in farmland near St. Louis, the most substantial threats come from tornadoes, floods, and earthquakes (the last being far less common than tornadoes and floods, but potentially more devastating). In our neck of the woods, threats may be different. Generally speaking, the threat from terrorist attacks, publicized as it typically is, is much smaller than the threat from natural disasters. For residents of high-profile cities like New York, Jerusalem, and Washington, D.C., however, terrorism is a substantial threat.

Third, small-scale disasters are far more common than large-scale disasters and a more likely source of altered access to water, food, shelter, and transportation. On the other hand, large disasters tend to be the major killers. Although, on average, there are about 80,000 deaths worldwide each year from natural disasters, the fatality numbers multiply in years when a large swath of the world is struck by a major disaster. In 2004, for instance, 240,000 people died in natural disasters, primarily as the result of the tsunami in South Asia.

Underdeveloped countries typically suffer the greatest number of casualties. For instance, in 2007, twenty-three natural disasters were reported in the United States (the most of any country in the world) and seven in Mexico; yet, there were 1,858,058 reported disaster victims in Mexico compared with only 668,451 in the United States. In recent decades, the incidence of natural disasters has increased by about 7.5% annually, largely because of the increased frequency of hydrological (floods) and meteorological (storms) disasters.

The Family Disaster Plan

Optimum family preparations for disaster depend not only on the geographically most likely threats, mentioned earlier, but also on the setting in which you live and on the degree of support you can expect from your community in the event of a disaster. If you live in an urban area, you typically will have less access to natural food and water sources, but you may have better access to disaster relief services. Urban apartment dwellers may be at special risk of losing shelter if their buildings are damaged by earthquakes and tornadoes. In a rural area, the damage to residences may be extensive, but homes and apartments typically are spread out enough that sufficient shelter is likely to remain. Furthermore, if you own significant property, you may be able to construct adequate ad hoc shelters even after your home is virtually destroyed. Those living in trailer courts, on the other hand, are particularly vulnerable.

Disaster relief is a mixed bag. The outpouring of volunteers and donations during a significant disaster typically is immense – in fact, so much so that the logistics of managing large numbers of volunteers and supplies is one of the most challenging aspects of disaster management. Many lives have been saved through the dedication of disaster workers and the generosity of those who donate time and resources to the cause. Unfortunately, much current public disaster planning is based on a poor understanding of what is likely to transpire and how problems should be managed. This is especially true for time-compressed disasters, in which the need for effective intervention is immediate. In some cases – the public response to chemical nerve agent attacks being perhaps the outstanding example – the enactment of many existing community disaster plans is more likely to harm than help you. Chemical agent attacks pose a special problem, which I discuss later.

For those constructing family disaster plans, the best situation is to reside in a low-risk area, in a sturdy private dwelling with significant

surrounding property containing a water source and plentiful edible
flora and fauna. My own situation is not far from this, except that I
currently live in an area that experiences frequent tornadoes and is
near a major fault line. I grew up in rural Montana and Washington
State and have been an avid outdoorsman since youth, acquiring skills
that would be useful if I ever had to survive under adverse conditions
after a major disaster. Survival training in the military augmented that
experience. In general, my thoughts about surviving after a disaster are
shaped as much by this outdoor training as by my training in medicine
or disaster management. Hence, I suggest you consider reading a
survival manual, such as the currently available *U.S. Army Survival
Manual*,[2] which covers several different environments, or a manual
tailored to the particular terrain in which you live. Unfortunately,
there is insufficient space here to address survival techniques at any
length.

Regardless of your type of home or location, you should address
certain general categories of concern in planning for a disaster. These
are, in roughly descending order of priority:

1. Immediate physical safety
2. Shelter and temperature control
3. Water
4. Food
5. Medical treatment and routine health maintenance
6. Communication
7. Transportation

If you cover each of these seven bases, you are well situated to cope
with a disaster. Let us briefly consider each, with special attention to
the first.

Priority #1: Immediate Physical Safety

Protecting yourself from immediate hazards – that is, the physical
dangers posed by earthquakes, hurricanes, bombs, and so forth –
is your top priority, because it is a prerequisite for surviving long
enough to enact other priorities. Vast stockpiles of food, medicines,
and survival gear are of no use if you die in the first few minutes of a
disaster.

With natural disasters, there often are warning signs of an impending event. Public warnings are the rule before hurricanes and other
storms, although the precise location of the worst hazards will not be
known. Even tornadoes rarely strike without some advance notice of

danger. On the other hand, earthquakes and related events, such as tidal waves, are more difficult to predict. Plane crashes and industrial accidents are never correctly forecast, and human attacks are planned in secrecy. The more advance warning an event typically receives, the more amenable it should be to management by protocol. Evacuation, for instance, may be feasible before a hurricane but is unlikely to have much bearing before a tsunami or tornado and has no advance applications whatsoever to biological or chemical terrorism. Evacuation procedures are among the most important coping tools in certain disasters. Whether you should heed a call for evacuation is beyond the scope of this paper; however, assuming survival is your highest priority, in most cases you should evacuate in the manner advised by knowledgeable public authorities.

When evacuation is not feasible, or for some other reason has not occurred, you may be caught in the throes of a natural or human-made disaster. What to do will depend on the nature of the hazard. In an earthquake, for example, the Red Cross advises that if you are indoors, you should find a safe place where it is unlikely anything will fall. It recommends a "drop, cover, and hold on" tactic and advises that families practice it twice a year in safe places identified for each room of the family dwelling. (I confess I know of no families who actually do this – but even thinking about it, or practicing one or two times, could make a difference.) Pre-hazard preparations include bolting tall, heavy structures such as bookcases to studs and securing the water heater to wall studs with steel straps. If you are outdoors during an earthquake, you should drop to the ground in a clear spot away from buildings, trees, and power lines. If you are in a car, you should drive to a clear spot and stay until the shaking stops.

During a tornado, or when a tornado warning is issued, the Red Cross advises that if you are outdoors, in a car, or in a mobile home, you should try to get to the basement of the nearest sturdy building. If this is not possible, you should find a ditch or depression and lie flat. If you find yourself in a conventional home, you should identify a place that is central, likely to be shielded from flying debris, and in the lowest floor of the dwelling (preferably the basement). Practical guidance on preparations, tactics, and post-event recovery for each common type of natural disaster is provided, free of charge, by the Red Cross in easy-to-read pamphlets and on the Internet (www.redcross.org). After identifying likely natural hazards in your area of residence, a prudent next step would be to consult the Red Cross sources.

Guidance on immediate safety tactics during a human-made disaster, such as a bioterrorism, nuclear, or chemical attack, is perhaps more controversial than for natural disasters. Bioterrorism and natural epidemics typically begin as mysteries that unfold gradually, so immediate action to secure personal safety is not possible. Nuclear and chemical events are another story.

Large-scale chemical disasters likely come from toxic vapors, because liquid chemicals generally threaten only a small area. These may be caused by industrial accidents (as in Bhopal, India) or by terrorist attacks (as in Matsumoto and Tokyo, Japan). The most likely agents cause almost immediate symptoms, although mustards and vesicants (other than lewisite) are an exception in that symptoms are delayed for several hours. You will be alerted to such an event when you develop symptoms or, more likely, when you observe others in the vicinity exhibiting symptoms. With a nerve agent such as sarin, which was used in the Matsumoto and Tokyo terrorist attacks, some people may experience severe symptoms, even sudden death, in close proximity to others who remain relatively free of symptoms. Any attempt to render aid to collapsed victims in such an event is useless and will result only in your own death or serious injury. Nerve agent and other vapor attacks inevitably occur in crowded public spaces. In such an event, you should flee the area quickly – preferably to a place upwind of the apparent epicenter of the attack.

After successfully evacuating the site of a vapor attack in which you see victims quickly developing symptoms, if you remain symptom–free, you probably are safe. Vapors will be inhaled into the lungs and, barring a high-enough lung exposure to cause symptoms, there is no chance the concentration of toxin on clothes is enough to pose a serious threat in and of itself. Once arriving in a safe area, you should remove all clothing, including underwear, and if possible secure the clothing in a plastic bag, such as a garbage bag, which should in turn be secured in one or two more plastic bags. If modesty makes you hesitant about removing underwear, consider wearing one of the bags as an overgarment, removing everything underneath. Then go home and shower.

This advice differs radically from what you are apt to hear from public authorities. Unfortunately, in their planning for chemical attacks, some authorities have things badly, even lethally, wrong. The typical protocol for a vapor attack in an urban area is to 1) secure the boundaries of the "hot zone" (the area where toxic concentrations of the vapor exist), 2) remove victims from the hot zone, 3) decontaminate victims in a nearby "warm zone," using various contraptions to wash them, and 4) transport victims who need medical attention to a hospital, taking care that casualties are evenly distributed and no hospital gets overloaded. On the basis of such protocols, many hospitals assume they will have to decontaminate only small numbers of casualties and will not be severely overloaded with cases.

The probability that events will actually transpire in accordance with such protocols is near zero. First of all, there is almost no chance most affected victims will be "secured" at the attack site for decontamination. In virtually all terrorist attacks, 80% or more of victims self-evacuate before the attack zone is contained. It would not be possible to decontaminate most victims at the site, and it would not be possible to transport them in an orderly fashion via ambulance. This feat was not even achieved in a bombing in Israel in which the attack occurred next door to an emergency services station. Hence, second, we should expect hospitals to be overloaded with contaminated victims. Most hospitals are equipped to decontaminate only a few people (typically fewer than twelve) per hour, and some have no decontamination capabilities whatsoever. However, even in a relatively unsophisticated attack such as the sarin attack in Tokyo, in which only twelve people died – and only three of those ever made it to the hospital – thousands of victims and concerned bystanders streamed into the nearest hospital emergency department. The vast majority of these people would have been perfectly fine if they had followed the advice I outlined previously. However, and this is the third problem, by crowding together in the vicinity of a hospital, they greatly increased their exposure to the toxin. At Kyoto University, more than 70% of the doctors and many emergency medical service personnel were temporarily incapacitated by symptoms that developed because inadequately decontaminated individuals were kept in close proximity. It is undetermined how many citizens became ill simply because they reported to a hospital for treatment.

In summary, after exposure to a vapor attack, if you have no symptoms, you should quickly flee the attack site, going upwind if possible, quickly disrobe once you arrive in a safe area, and evacuate to a place where you can shower – as far away as possible from other victims. The very last place you should go is to a hospital or medical clinic. If you have minor symptoms, such as mild headache, runny nose, eye pain, or trouble with visual focusing, you will need to see a doctor but are probably not in need of immediate attention. If there is a secondary assessment center in your community – that is, a place other than a hospital or clinic where citizens are told in advance they can go for medical treatment and supplies in the event of a disaster – this is an excellent place to report to if you need attention. Unfortunately, most communities have not designated such sites.

The preceding guidance also may be the best advice for an attack with an aerosolized mustard agent – if it is the fastest way to get a very good shower with a steady water stream. However, with mustard agents, symptoms are not immediate and the need for thorough decontamination is much greater. Also, the threat from vapors given off by other victims is much less. Therefore, if public decontamination is available in such cases, it is the way to go.

One commonly dispensed piece of advice is that if you are at home during a chemical or biological attack, you should shut off the vents and seal windows, doors, and other sites of entry with plastic sheets and duct tape.[3] Although it would be great to have some duct tape around during a disaster, this advice won't be much help. With a biological attack, the agent will have diffused long before anyone becomes aware there has been a biological attack. This likely will be the case with chemical attacks as well. However, it is possible that someone indoors at home might observe people collapsing in the streets outside. In such an unlikely event, duct tape and plastic sheeting may be of use – although it is important, especially in a small living space, not to asphyxiate yourself by keeping these items in place too long.

Nuclear events and attacks also require evacuation, preferably upwind, and sometimes very thorough decontamination. Occasionally there also is minor danger from crowding in with others who need decontamination (if they are contaminated by radioactive particles), but typically other exposed victims pose no threat. The proper response to a radiological or nuclear event requires advanced knowledge of the pathological agent, the weather conditions, and the medical alternatives. You should seek decontamination, assessment, and treatment by trained clinicians whenever there is a possibility you have been exposed to radio-nuclear agents.

Priority #2: Shelter and Temperature Control

If you manage to survive the initial onslaught in a major disaster, you are apt to find yourself in a hostile environment. You may be away from home, with few prospects for adequate shelter. If you are home, you may be cut off for days or weeks from utilities such as electricity, gas, and water. If it is very cold, very wet, very windy, or very hot, your first priority will be to secure adequate shelter.

This task may not be as daunting as it seems. Using inexpensive equipment, I was able to live fairly comfortably for long periods in very harsh Arctic climates during my days as a mountaineer. A healthy person with ordinary outdoor supplies can live almost indefinitely practically anywhere. Provided one has access to an intact dwelling and plenty of warm covering, cold weather is not a serious threat to life and limb. To prepare for a prolonged period without heat, the most important things to do are 1) keep plenty of warm clothing, 2) have extra blankets and/or sleeping bags for everyone, 3) keep several alternative light sources – such as lanterns and flashlights with extra batteries – that can be used without electricity, and 4) keep adequate supplies of nonperishable, high-calorie foods (caloric intake needs to be increased with prolonged exposure to cold). With adequate shelter, fires are not necessary, but they can be a pleasant luxury.

Hot weather is more difficult to control (you can always add layers of insulation or clothing, but the process of taking them off terminates abruptly when you are naked). Heat waves are major killers, even in areas where air conditioning is a normal household appliance. When large populations face hot weather during a utility breakdown, the danger exceeds that of an ordinary heat wave. A generator in your home (with adequate fuel) can provide up to a few days of emergency power for an AC unit, but eventually you will have to adapt to the heat (frequent dips in a tub or pool, with air cooling, can help) or find a suitably air-conditioned environment outside the area of the power outage. For the elderly and those with health problems, the latter option should be arranged as soon as possible.

Priority #3: Water

An adult human needs a minimum of two quarts of water daily to maintain normal activities; this requirement increases with hot weather, strenuous exercise, and illness, and in children and nursing mothers. Healthy adults can survive many days without food, but such is not the case for water. Hence, maintaining water intake is a very high priority.

There are many mechanisms through which normal water supplies may be damaged or cut off in natural disasters and terrorist attacks. Fortunately, almost any environment provides ample opportunities to obtain water, and contaminated water generally can be made drinkable through purification by fairly simple methods.

One of the standard components of any home disaster plan is to store extra water – at least three days worth, assuming a gallon of water per day for everyone in your household (some advise a two-week supply, but that would be seventy gallons for a family of five). When water supplies are low, it is better to drink what you need rather than rationing, and then find more when it is needed. Several household reservoirs may be useful, including the hot water heater (make sure the incoming water is not contaminated and that the gas or electricity is shut off when the water heater is empty) and the reservoir tank of the toilet; typically, there are multiple outdoor sources as well.

If the water is contaminated with bacteria, public health authorities most likely will issue an order to boil the water before using it. If you have no contact with the authorities after a disaster, you should assume a boil order is in effect. At sea level, water should be boiled for at least one minute, and a minute should be added for every 1,000 feet above sea level. Water also may be purified with liquid household bleach. The Red Cross advises the following routine: "Add 16 drops of bleach per gallon of water, stir, and let stand for 30 minutes. If the water does not have a slight bleach odor, repeat the dosage and let stand another 15 minutes."[4] Although the Red Cross discourages the use of water purification products sold in camping stores, the light portable filters sold in these stores may be very useful for someone who is on the move, as they will effectively filter most bacterial pathogens that are likely to foul water supplies. However, they will not remove toxic chemicals and viruses. You also can easily construct improvised filters to clear dirty water, but you still must purify the water after filtration.

Priority #4: Food

Food probably will not be a problem for those with the foresight to store extra food in their home and vehicle. Because of their long shelf life, canned foods are ideal for extra food supplies, although there is little reason a family stuck at home could not dine on most of the usual foodstuffs. To prepare for dining without electricity, a manual can opener and a grill or camp stove with extra fuel are good items to have. Fatty food is best for piling on the calories, but it may increase your water requirements.

The conventional wisdom among hikers is that light, dehydrated food is best for someone on the move, because it doesn't weigh you down and can be rehydrated at the time of preparation with water obtained near the campsite. However, I have lived for days in the wilderness on precooked canned food alone; I feel the extra weight is offset by not having to carry cooking gear. Furthermore, a quick canned meal gives me more time for fishing (presumably not a major worry during a disaster, although access to a fishing hole may be an excellent way to round out a tasty disaster menu). For cooking outdoors, you will need waterproof matches or a grill lighter, so you should include these items in your disaster kit.

Priority #5: Medical Treatment and Routine Health Maintenance

If you have ongoing medical problems requiring prescriptions or other medical supplies, it is important to keep at least a two-week supply on hand at any time. Some disasters are accompanied by acute conditions, particularly traumatic injury or, in the case of a natural epidemic or successful biological attack, a dangerous infectious disease or toxic reaction.

In an epidemic or biological attack, if the agent is identified as something transmissible (contagious from human to human) and you have not been exposed, it is best to remain where you can minimize social contact (preferably at home). If you are ill or fear you have been exposed to a pathogen, it is desirable to find a source of medical treatment where crowds are unlikely. Mobile medical clinics are ideal but are not available in every locale. The next best alternative would be a small neighborhood assessment center. Unfortunately, few local disaster planners have identified such centers or notified the general public of their location. Given the typical lack of appropriate advance planning, if you are seeking treatment, you will have to stay in communication with authorities – always be wary about going somewhere that might be crowded. In such cases, hospitals and major medical clinics are, again, about the worst places to go. Home antibiotic supplies are a consideration, especially where there is no state-sponsored physician monopoly on dispensing them. Unfortunately, stocking the right antibiotic is not that easy to do, and stocking a broad array is expensive (especially if one wants to avoid exceeding the expiration date). With nontransmissible biological agents, such as the anthrax and tularemia microbes and the ricin and botulinum toxins, whether or not you are exposed is a matter of chance. When you need treatment, there is no special danger in going to get it.

If the condition requiring urgent treatment is not a contagious illness, there is little risk in reporting to a hospital or clinic. Better yet, you could contact public health authorities for advice on the best place to get immediate medical attention.

Priority #6: Communication

Experts commonly advise that families arrange a meeting place in the event they are separated during a disaster and unable to return to their home. Our family has not done this, for a few reasons. First, our schedules and local movements are complex, so in our case it is difficult to predict where we would be. A fixed meeting point could be a hindrance if it were far removed from our actual locations. Second, although it is tempting to select an alternate meeting place close to home, if we are unable to get home, it seems unlikely that we would be able to get to such an alternate meeting place. Third, if it were possible to get to a meeting place close to home, then it would be possible to get close to home – and we likely would meet up during our disappointed efforts to return home. Finally, it is far more important to avoid immediate hazards than it is to reunite quickly. People are likely to expose themselves to hazards (e.g., by traveling downwind of a radio-nuclear event) while they are heading to a fixed-point rendezvous.

For these reasons, I have advised family members to focus on their own personal safety during the immediate aftermath of a disaster, and later (only when their own safety is secured) to either return home (if that is feasible) or seek information about a likely meeting point by coordinating family communications through out-of-town relatives. Families with vulnerable dependents who might get separated during a disaster (e.g., young children at day care or school) need to make arrangements with the people who will be looking after them.

This plan depends on access to telecommunications, which may be difficult to obtain in disasters. Phone lines may be down and cell phone communications may be difficult or impossible. Evidently, text messages have a higher likelihood of getting through than phone calls. With this in mind, I have advised my kids to use their Uncle Carmen as the point of contact if they are unable to reach their mother or me during a disaster. Uncle Carmen is their only adult relative under thirty-five years of age, which qualifies him to send and receive text messages. For the rest of us, thoughts of successfully navigating a text message can be more fantastical than phobias about trampling zebras. I trust, however, that – with help – we will find a way.

Priority #7: Transportation

Even when evacuation is not possible, transportation can be important. It is frequently advised that you keep a full gas tank – and obviously that would be nice in a disaster. However, in the immediate aftermath of a disaster, foot travel may be the only or the best means of getting from place to place. Disaster relief personnel generally target transportation sources early in their efforts. If the normal means of transportation are not available, public officials likely will offer alternatives – and when mass transportation is needed to get people out of a dangerous area, the provision of such will undoubtedly be a major priority for rescuers. If you can establish lines of communication with disaster workers, you should eventually be able to arrange needed transportation.

Conclusion

Nations, states, cities, and hospitals have disaster plans – and so should we all. Although perishing in a disaster is not apt to be among the greatest perils you face, nor among your most pressing concerns, you are almost certainly vulnerable to some natural and human-made disasters. With a little study and advance preparation, you can greatly increase your odds – and those of your loved ones and dependent family members – of surviving a major disaster.

REFERENCES

[1] Clarke L: *Mission Improbable: Using Fantasy Documents to Tame Disaster* (Chicago: University of Chicago Press, 1999).
[2] U.S. Department of Defense: *U.S. Army Survival Manual* (New York: Dorset Press, 1994).
[3] Frist B: *When Every Moment Counts* (Lanham, MD: Rowman & Little-field, 2002), p. 27. This book is, in general, a very good source of advice for ordinary citizens on the threat of bioterrorism.
[4] American Red Cross: *Food and Water in an Emergency* (ARC-5055). Federal Emergency Management Agency, FEMA-L210 (1994).

TWENTY

Making the Internet Work for You

Researching Your Health Questions

– Bette Anton

Consumer health information is in great demand, and the widespread availability of such information has both positive and negative aspects.

Many types of information may be found on the Internet, ranging from condition-specific organizational websites, associations, and self-help groups, to organizational and commercial Web portals ("webliographies") and freely available, up-to-date medical literature. The amount of health-related information on the Web is overwhelming, and if you wonder whether or not it is reliable, you're not alone. This chapter focuses on a few excellent health websites and on techniques for evaluating other health information sites you may find in your explorations.

Although the Internet is a significant resource for finding health information, it is very important to evaluate the information you read and/or use. Therefore, part of this chapter is devoted to skills for evaluating health-related websites. This chapter is not meant to be comprehensive. Indeed, with the overabundance of health websites aimed at consumers, it would be impossible to cover them all. However, it does point you toward good sites for answering many consumer health questions and should give you confidence in your ability to judge health information you encounter while searching for health information for yourself or others. Knowing where to look for information, and how to evaluate and interpret it, may allow you to take more control of your health.

The Pew Internet and American Life Project (Pew) provides a very interesting background on the use of the Internet for finding health information. In 2006, Pew reported that 80% of Internet users had searched for health information.[1] This means that approximately eight million American adults look online for health information each day.

Pew reports the following categories as the most popular among people looking for health information online: a specific disease or medical condition; a medical treatment or procedure; diet, nutrition, vitamins, or nutritional supplements; exercise or fitness; prescription or over-the-counter drugs; health insurance; alternative treatments or medicines; a particular doctor or hospital; mental health issues; and environmental health hazards.

Other relevant findings of the same Pew survey are that almost half of what are referred to as "health seekers" search for health information for someone other than themselves, and that more than half report that the information they found had an impact on their own or someone else's care. Another important finding that has bearing on the need for evaluation is that most people, approximately 75%, do not consistently check the source and date of the information they find.

With these findings as a background, the goals of this chapter are to help you become comfortable conducting an online health information search, learn to explore and become familiar with several reliable health websites, and understand and apply evaluation techniques to unfamiliar health websites.

Getting Started

Following are several broad categories, with specific suggestions and questions to keep in mind when searching for important health information.

Know what you're looking for. Determine who the information is for – is it for yourself or a family member, friend, or child? – and what kind of material or level is required and appropriate. Use a dictionary, anatomy book, and health encyclopedia first. Check spellings and clarify the diagnosis or terminology. Are you looking for support as well as factual information? What, if any, information have you already been given by your health care provider? If you don't have enough information, call your health care provider for more.

Think about the kind of information you want or need. Do you need information about a disease, a drug, or alternative treatments? Is it about the causes (etiology) or outcome (prognosis) of a condition or disease? Do you want information on the treatment for or on the care of a patient with a condition or disease? Would you like information on a support or advocacy group for the condition or disease? Do you require background information, or something in greater depth? Consider which organizations or associations might provide information.

Become familiar with the general health information–finding tools you believe are reliable. When you find sites that look relevant, use the evaluation criteria discussed later in this chapter to help you decide whether the information is credible, timely, and useful. If you don't find good information the first time, try again, perhaps by using a different search strategy or viewing a new website. Finally, remember that even the best "evidence" may not pertain to a particular individual.

Use some basic strategies that can help filter your search. This is of utmost importance when using a general search tool such as Google or Yahoo. Always read, and try to use, the advanced searching features. Read about how you can combine terms, or avoid others, to make your search more relevant to your needs. Also, try using the specialized health sections of commercial search tools if they are available. For example, try Yahoo Health (http://health.yahoo. com).

Better yet, and especially if you are a frequent searcher for health information, have your own list of high-quality resources. Become familiar with tools that are produced by known, reliable institutions. Several of these are described in the following sections.

MedlinePlus

MedlinePlus, a website of the U.S. National Library of Medicine (NLM), is a high-quality resource for consumer health information, with great breadth and depth, and one of the best such resources available for finding answers to some common and not-so-common questions. It is an excellent place to begin your search for health-related information. Besides being a comprehensive, one-stop site, MedlinePlus has several other advantages that make it a useful resource for health information. In addition to its sponsorship by the NLM – the world's largest medical library – it also is a service of the U.S.

National Institutes of Health (NIH), and much of the information it provides comes directly from the NIH. The information on MedlinePlus is both authoritative and up to date; in fact, the site is updated daily. Importantly, there is absolutely no advertising on MedlinePlus. Its only purpose is to provide authoritative information – as opposed to many commercial sites, regardless of their quality, for which advertising is an integral part. MedlinePlus's Quality Guidelines are clearly stated at http://www.nlm.nih.gov/medlineplus/criteria.html. In addition to health topics, it has extensive information on drugs and supplements and includes a dictionary as well as an illustrated encyclopedia. Much of this information also is provided in Spanish, and some of it is available in more than 40 languages other than English.

In addition to printed information, MedlinePlus contains dozens of easy-to-understand tutorials on diseases or conditions (e.g., diabetes – meal planning), tests and diagnostic procedures (e.g., colonoscopy, newborn screening), surgery and treatment procedures (e.g., LASIK, hip replacement), and health and wellness (e.g., back exercises, managing stress). There also are videos of actual surgeries, if you are inclined to watch one.

The latest health news is reported almost daily; news sources include press releases from major medical organizations and reports from conferences. You can receive daily news updates by signing up for delivery via e-mail or RSS feeds.

A good way to begin using MedlinePlus is to take the online tour: http://www.nlm.nih.gov/medlineplus/tour/tour.html.

There will be times, however, when MedlinePlus won't fully answer your questions, or you may feel a second opinion is necessary. There are literally thousands of health sites available, and it will be useful to become familiar with the very best of them. Following is a brief review and exploration of additional reliable government and nonprofit health websites and the types of questions that can be answered using them. All are important sources of information for commonly asked questions. Some are the result of collaborations between the NLM and other government entities. You may use these sites as a supplement or alternative to MedlinePlus, although several are linked to or can be accessed through MedlinePlus. In particular, they can answer many of the questions the Pew identified as those most commonly asked by health seekers. The sites mentioned in the following sections are high-quality health care information resources that can address many health-related questions.

National Library of Medicine Collaborations and Other U.S. Government Health Sites

NIHSeniorHealth

http://nihseniorhealth.gov

One resource that links right from the MedlinePlus welcome page is NIHSeniorHealth.

The goal of NIHSeniorHealth, a joint project of the NLM and the National Institute on Aging, is to provide health-related aging information to the public. NIHSeniorHealth is good for many of the same reasons that make MedlinePlus good. It contains reliable and reviewed information, it is updated frequently, and, importantly, it was developed using research on the cognitive changes in older adults, making it especially suitable for this population.

In general, seniors are at greater risk for health problems. This site deals specifically with the ones that are most common in older adults. It makes no assumptions about the user and provides answers in understandable language, with links to further information if the user requires it. Its features include short videos, quizzes, and FAQs about specific conditions; the language is simple, pages are short, and searching is simple.

NIHSeniorHealth may be used, and may be the best place to begin, to look up information on diseases most commonly found in seniors. It can answer queries such as "I want the latest information on . . . [Alzheimer's, arthritis, cancer, macular degeneration, etc]." It is especially useful for those who may have vision or hearing problems – it uses large text as well as sound and enables users to change the contrast. All these features make NIHSeniorHealth an appropriate resource for older people.

The following three resources are linked from the "Other Resources/Databases" section of MedlinePlus.

DIRLINE

http://dirline.nlm.nih.gov

DIRLINE, the Directory of Health Organizations, is produced by the NLM. This site allows users to search by a disease or condition, or by an organizational name or acronym, to find support and research organizations; some of this information is provided in Spanish. It's a good place to search for both known and unknown health organizations. DIRLINE also has a feature called "Health Hot-lines," an online database of hundreds of organizations that have 800 numbers.

Use DIRLINE to answer questions such as:

- I think I've been exposed to asbestos. Are there groups I can contact for further information?
- Does the American Thyroid Association have a toll-free number?

Genetics Home Reference

http://ghr.nlm.nih.gov

Genetics Home Reference contains consumer information about genetic conditions and the genes or chromosomes responsible for those conditions. Board-certified medical geneticists are among those who choose the information to be included in this resource. The site includes a handbook titled *Help Me Understand Genetics*, which contains easy-to-understand explanations of how genes work and how mutations cause disorders. Also of note are the "Resources" section and extensive information on genetic testing.

Use Genetics Home Reference to answer questions such as:

- My sister has breast cancer. What are the chances that my daughter or I will have it too?
- What genetic testing is usually done in pregnant women?
- Where can I find more information on Parkinson's disease?

healthfinder.gov

http://www.healthfinder.gov

Developed by the U.S. Department of Health and Human Services and other federal agencies, healthfinder.gov is a very comprehensive website geared toward consumers. Its information, in both English and Spanish, is provided through links to other federal agencies and state government sites, nonprofit and voluntary organizations, educational institutions and libraries, and a limited number of commercial resources. The "myhealthfinder" feature allows anyone from eighteen-year-olds to seniors to receive personalized health recommendations. Another useful healthfinder.gov feature is "Health Calculators," interactive tools for men's and women's health issues, nutritional intake, and more.

Use Healthfinder.gov to answer questions such as:

• Where can I find free or low-cost health care?
• Am I at risk for diabetes?
• Is my mother eligible for Medicaid?

Following are two important NIH databases.

Household Products Database

http://householdproducts.nlm.nih.gov

Household Products Database contains information about thousands of brand-name household products and their potential health effects. It provides information on specific chemical ingredients and their quantities in common household products, manufacturers' names and contact information, acute and chronic effects of chemical ingredients, and links to other toxicology information.

Use Household Products Database to answer questions such as:

• Is my toilet cleaner harmful to my dog?
• Could my rash be caused by my aftershave?
• Is the glitter my kids use for their art projects dangerous?

Tox Town

http://toxtown.nlm.nih.gov

Tox Town is an interactive guide to commonly encountered toxic chemicals, as well as to public health and environmental topics. Users can search both by location and by chemical. The results are presented in nontechnical language, in both Spanish and English, and include links to further information on the chemical's possible impact on human health.

Use Tox Town to find answers to questions such as:

• How can asbestos exposure harm my health?
• My brother's house was painted two years ago. Should he worry about lead exposure?
• What are the health hazards of working in an auto shop?

National Center for Complementary and Alternative Medicine

http://nccam.nih.gov

We frequently have questions related to alternative therapies and herbal medicines. The National Center for Complementary and

Alternative Medicine (NCCAM) defines complementary and alternative medicine (CAM) as a group of "diverse medical and health care systems, practices, and products that are not presently considered to be part of conventional medicine." Usually, there are fewer studies on the efficacies of the treatments and safety of CAM, but in the United States, approximately four in ten adults and one in nine children – that is, those age seventeen and under – are using some form of CAM. These therapies include acupuncture, aromatherapy, chiropractic, herbals, homeopathy, hydrotherapy, Feldenkrais therapy, massage, naturopathy, and many more. Some may be so common we don't even think of them as alternative any more. Integrative medicine combines mainstream medical and CAM therapies for which there is some high-quality scientific evidence of safety and effectiveness. The NCCAM is one of the NIH's twenty-seven institutes and centers. Its mission is to support rigorous scientific research on complementary and alternative healing practices, to train researchers in CAM, and to disseminate information to the public and professionals on which CAM therapies work, which don't, and why they don't.

The NCCAM is a good resource to find answers to questions such as:

• My daughter is taking St. John's wort for depression. Does it really work?
• Will echinacea keep me from getting a cold?
• Is garlic a good treatment for diabetes?

Cancer Information

Another common topic for consumer health searches is cancer. There are three excellent organizations to keep in mind when searching for this information: the National Cancer Institute (NCI; http://www.cancer.gov), the American Cancer Society (http://www.cancer.org), and the University of Pennsylvania's Oncolink (http://www.oncolink.com). I will focus on the first one, the NCI.

The NCI is part of the NIH. Its comprehensive cancer website includes information on many different types of cancers, coping strategies, alternative therapies, statistics, clinical trials, support and resources, and more. On this site, users can find information on cancers, from the most common to the rare, and by body section or system. It provides quick links to support groups and useful dictionaries for terminology one might encounter when receiving a cancer diagnosis. It also gives users several options for contacting an NCI professional for answers to specific questions.

Use the NCI website to find answers to questions such as:

- My mother was diagnosed with stage IIA cervical cancer. How can I find out more about it?
- Will I have chemotherapy or radiation treatment for my non-Hodgkin's lymphoma?
- How common is prostate cancer?

Drug Information

Although there are several reliable drug websites, one of which is discussed later, keep in mind that most drug websites are commercial in nature, simply advertising for pharmaceutical companies or particular drugs. Over the past several years, direct-to-consumer advertising of drugs has become quite common. Unfortunately, advertising, particularly for drugs, can be misleading in several respects. Many ads provide no information about the name and symptoms of the condition or disease for which the drug is being promoted. Few ads include information on the success rate of a drug, the necessary duration of use, possible alternatives, or less expensive treatments. Direct marketing takes place whether or not scientific consensus has been reached on a drug's effectiveness. Sometimes, misconceptions about both the disease and the possible risks of the drug are promoted along with the drug itself. The United States and New Zealand are the only countries in the developed world in which there is no governmental control or review of drug advertising.

One reliable drug site, DrugDigest (http://www.drugdigest.org), has many useful sections:

The "Drug Library" includes extensive information about the most commonly prescribed drugs as well as vitamins, herbs, and supplements. It also allows users to view pill images and find information about the proper use of some types of medication, such as eye drops and inhalers. Some of these instructions have accompanying videos.

The "Check Interactions" section allows users to learn about drug–drug interactions as well as interactions of drugs with food and alcohol.

Users can compare drugs and drug side effects in the "Compare Drugs" section.

A browsable list of conditions or diseases with explanations, treatment, causes, risk factors, and more is found in the "Conditions & Treatments" section. This section provides extensive information about current treatments and possibilities for future ones.

The "Interactive Tools" page includes a medication checklist with questions users can ask themselves about each of their prescriptions.

It also enables users to make a customized medication or emergency contact card and to assess their risk for several diseases or conditions.

Use DrugDigest to answer questions such as:

- Are there interactions between St. John's wort and Zoloft?
- What treatments are in development for glaucoma?
- What are the differences in side effects between Lexapro and Prozac?
- Is arnica gel effective for healing bruises?

Lab Information

We frequently want to know which laboratory tests might be ordered for a particular condition, what to expect during the test, and what the test results mean, or we want information about routine screenings. A common question we ask is whether or not a certain test result is "normal." For many tests, there is no single number that is considered normal, but rather a range of values. The age and sex of a person also may make a difference. Lab Tests Online (http://www.labtestsonline. org) is an excellent place to find answers to queries such as these. Its purpose is to help patients and caregivers understand clinical lab tests, both those that are part of routine care for a particular disease or those that may be used in diagnosis and treatment. It was created by the clinical laboratory community and contains several excellent features. It is formatted with at-a-glance results in tabbed sections for general information about a lab test, including what is being tested and how the sample is collected; further information about the test, including what the test results mean; and answers to common questions regarding the test and the condition. The site also allows users to ask further questions if they do not find what they are looking for. Users can search by test, conditions or diseases, and normal screenings by age groups and during pregnancy.

Use Lab Tests Online to answer questions such as:

- My doctor says my cholesterol is 210. What does that mean?
- My newborn grandson was given a hearing test in the hospital. Is that normal, or do they suspect he might have hearing problems?
- What will my glucose test for diabetes be like?

Finding Hospitals and Doctors

Over the past several years, we have seen a trend toward health "report cards" that evaluate the quality of hospitals, physicians, health plans, and other health providers. The U.S. Agency for Healthcare Research and Quality (AHRQ) has designed the Health Care Report Card Compendium (http://www.talkingquality.gov/compendium), which is a good starting point for those seeking such information, although it is not comprehensive. When judging the quality of these report cards, one should ask several questions, such as, Who created the report card? What questions were asked? Who gave the answers? How many people were surveyed? Is the information reported of interest and applicable to me? Is terminology defined? How old is the information?

Evaluating Health Websites

Consumers have access to more medical information than ever before. The Web and its sophisticated search tools have resulted in a greater number of patients accessing Internet health information. At the same time, many groups and individuals are creating health-related websites. Several research studies were performed recently evaluating the ease of searching, information gained, and the quality of health information on the Web. Almost all these studies show that the quality of health information on the Web varies tremendously: there are valuable nuggets of information amid a vast amount of junk.

Here's what we know about consumer searching behavior. Consumers use search engines rather than health or medical portals or libraries. When assessing the credibility of a website, consumers claim to look primarily at the source, whether it has a professional design or official touch, the language, and the ease of use. However, under observation, none investigated "about us" sections, disclaimers, or disclosure statements.[2]

The best way to find health information on the Web is to go to the sites we know have reliable, accurate, current, and unbiased information. The websites mentioned earlier are such sites. However, there are times when we will use Google or another commercial search tool. When we do this, we must have a way to ensure that the information we find is the best possible; therefore, we must develop good evaluation skills.

Five Criteria for Evaluation

Content on the Web is unregulated; therefore, *anyone* can publish *anything*. As mentioned earlier, there is sound health information and there is dangerous information, and we must be able to tell the difference. There are five basic criteria for evaluating health websites: accuracy, authority, bias, currency, and coverage. The next section explains each criterion and how to use it. By using these five criteria together, we have sound guidelines for evaluation. Even before using the five criteria, there are preliminary steps you can take to evaluate health web pages.

Read the Web address (URL) carefully. Ask yourself if the site is someone's personal page (look for ~ or %; a personal name). Although personal pages are not necessarily bad, you will need to investigate the author very carefully; on personal pages, there is no publisher or domain owner to vouch for the information presented.

Generally speaking, information that has the backing of an organization or institution has better quality control than material from an individual. The domain (*.gov* for a government website, *.edu* for an educational institution, *.org* for a professional organization, *.com* for a commercial website, etc.) should be appropriate for the content. Determine whether the information source is the most reliable for the needed information. Who is the "publisher"? The publisher generally is the agency or person operating the server from which the document is issued and usually is identified in the first part of the URL. For example, in the URL http://www.nih.gov/PHTindex.htm, a web page on hormone replacement therapy (HRT), the publisher is the U.S. National Institutes of Health. Ask yourself whether you have heard of this entity, whether it corresponds to the name of the site, and whether it *should* correspond. For example, on the NIH website, is HRT a topic you would expect the NIH to report on?

Once you've opened the site, scan the perimeter of the page and think about these questions: Why did the person create the page? What's in it for him or her? Is he or she trying to sell something? In other words, what is the purpose of the site?

Using the Five Criteria

Accuracy

For the most part, Web standards to ensure accuracy do not exist, although there have been several attempts to institute them, especially for health information. Many, if not most, web pages are neither reviewed nor verified by editors or peers. Ask yourself the following questions to determine whether the content is accurate: Are the sources of information clearly given? If the information is drawn from the writer's own experience, was it based on observation or on carefully designed research? If the content is factual, are the facts accurate? You may need to check other sources for comparison.

Authority

Often it is difficult to determine the authorship of a web page. An unsigned piece of information does not have the authority of a signed one. If a name is listed, the author's qualifications frequently are absent. The more information an author provides about himself or herself, the better. Remember that anyone can put something on the Web very quickly and cheaply. Be skeptical about names of organizations that sound prestigious and reputable but could be operated out of someone's basement. Always try to find an "about us" link to determine a site's authority and agenda.

Look for the same information you would for an author of a book or journal article. Ask yourself these questions: Who is the author, institution, or agency that claims accountability and is responsible for the content? Health sites may have advisory boards or consultants. Knowing who these people are might give you more information about the quality of the website. An e-mail address is not enough, although you can try to e-mail the person for further information. If the page is unsigned, was it found in a usually authoritative place, for example, on the NIH website? What can you tell about the author and his or her credentials? Is the author a physician, student, machinist? Does the information appear to be accurate? Why or why not?

Bias

A web page can merely be a platform for someone trying to make a point. Signs of this include exclamation points, huge fonts, and sensational photographs and stories. It is important to check to see whether the author's goals are clearly stated. Ask the following questions to determine whether the content is biased: Does the author bring any biases in posting the information? For example, an evaluation of a drug is questionable if it is posted on the website of a competing pharmaceutical manufacturer. Is the author's purpose to persuade you or sell you something? Is the person presenting the information independently, or does he or she have a reason to be presenting information in a particular way? Above all, ask yourself who paid for or sponsored the web page; this information should be fully disclosed.

Currency

Given how rapidly medical developments occur, health information more than five years old may be outdated, incomplete, and/or inaccurate. Therefore, for most health websites, up-to-date information is desirable, although there may be times when currency is not an issue. Dates frequently are not included on web pages. When a date is provided, sometimes it is not clear whether it is the date the page was created, the date it was revised, or the date it was placed on the Web. Some web pages are dynamic and will post the date the site was accessed. The date of the information, and any revisions, should be clearly posted. Ask these questions regarding the information: Is it current and timely? Is it dated, or can you tell from the content when it was written? Is it likely to change? Is it recent enough to be useful? Is it time sensitive? For example, statistical information *must* be dated to be meaningful.

Coverage

Many health websites are not comprehensive. The material provided may be accurate, but important information may be left out. At times, you may need to vary your approach to searching to find relevant information. One way to determine whether the coverage is adequate is to look at other sites on the same topic. These questions may help you determine whether the coverage is sufficient: How does the information compare with other sources on the same topic? Is a better source available? Does the site have a disclaimer that describes the purpose, scope, currency, authority, and any limitations of the information?

Links to websites that can help you determine whether information may be a hoax or even worse – fraud – are provided on the Canadian website http://chis.wikidot.com/hoaxes.

Evidence Matters

During the past two decades, practice in health care has moved toward an evidence-based model. This involves making health care decisions using current evidence, the efficacy of which has been demonstrated, taking an individual's needs and particular circumstances into consideration. It is meant to integrate a clinician's knowledge and skills with the "best" evidence from current research.

Although approximately 40,000 articles are added each month to PubMed, the NLM's international database of scientific health-related literature, very few can be considered clinical evidence. There is a hierarchy of evidence, ranging from reports of research, through opinions and editorials, to case reports, clinical trials, and finally summaries of clinical trials. Because most of the articles are related to basic research, and the fewest are reports of clinical studies, the body of evidence sometimes is referred to as a pyramid. At the top of the pyramid are randomized clinical trials, and above that, those publications that discuss combined results of many trials, systematic reviews, and meta-analyses. These are the types of publications considered to contain the best evidence.

When you are trying to determine whether information is reliable, keep the evidence pyramid in mind. *Randomized controlled double-blind studies* (also called RCTs) are the gold standard for medical research. What does this term mean?

- *Randomized* – participants are randomly assigned to intervention groups so that the groups can be compared
- *Controlled* – there is a comparison group, one that does not receive the treatment or intervention
- *Double-blind* – neither the study participants nor the researchers know who is receiving the treatment or intervention

Systematic reviews are summaries that use objective, reproducible methods to identify evidence-based studies and analyze them. Meta-analyses combine the data from several different studies. In both cases, you can usually get a better overview of a particular topic than is available from any single study. Why is it important to know about the evidence pyramid? It is important to know what kinds of study or research were used in drawing conclusions about the possible quality of the research. It is very important, however, to remember that even the best evidence may not pertain to a particular individual. As with all health information, it is up to the health care provider to determine whether the information is relevant to an individual patient.

The Cochrane Collaboration (http://www.cochrane.org) is an international group that disseminates evidence-based health care information. Two of its major contributions are the systematic reviews and meta-analyses it produces on health care interventions. Most Cochrane reviews are based on randomized controlled trials and use other evidence when appropriate. Although the full content of the reviews and meta-analyses are available only for a fee, the abstracts and plain-language consumer summaries of the reviews are browsable or may be searched using keywords at http://www.cochrane.org/reviews/index.htm. These summaries provide important evidence-based health information.

Another evidence-based website containing consumer health information is Informed Health Online (http://www.informed healthonline.org). Much of the information on this website looks carefully at evidence from systematic reviews of the Cochrane Collaboration. This website not only provides and promotes evidence-based health information, but also clearly explains its value. It has an A-to-Z list of health topics, which is frequently updated, and sections that may be browsed according to anatomic system or topic category, such as prevention or cancer.

Further Points to Remember about Evaluation

Beware of phrases such as *miraculous cures, exclusive product, secret formula,* and *ancient ingredients.* Also remember that certain phrases that are used commonly may suggest something they are not. For example, *contributes to, is linked to,* and *is associated with* do not mean *causes. Doubles the risk* is meaningful only in the context of what the risk was in the first place. If the original risk was one in a million, doubling the risk is only two in a million; if the original risk was one in one hundred and it doubles, that is a larger risk. *Significant* is not the same as *statistically significant.* A finding is statistically significant when the association between two factors has been found to be greater than might occur at random, determined by mathematical formulas. The media, however, often use the word to mean *important.* An important assertion later may be found to be flawed or incorrect. With regard to information about drugs, particularly from drug companies, keep the following in mind: *may* does not mean *will.* Scientific studies gather evidence in a systematic way, but one study taken alone seldom proves anything. Personal testimonials, even those from "medical experts," are not evidence. Finally, breakthroughs happen only rarely. The discovery of penicillin and the development of the polio vaccine were true breakthroughs, but not everything referred to in this manner truly are.

We are moving into the era of "Health 2.0." This involves using the Web in an interactive way in which information or content sharing, collaboration, and social networking are converging to make finding personalized health information ever easier. Social networking sites, blogs, wikis, interactive websites, and news feeds, to name just a few possibilities, have become common; new applications are being created, such as personalized health-tracking websites and online calculators. In the near future, we may be maintaining and controlling our own health records. Although these are welcome enhancements that allow consumers of health information to participate more fully in their own health care, they come with challenges as well as potential. Knowing how to search for, evaluate, and apply health information can be very empowering, as can be the proficient use of new tools. However, the final interpretation of health information found on the

Internet should always be made in discussion with one's own health care provider.

REFERENCES

[1] Pew Internet & American Life Project: http://www.pewinternet.org/~/ media//Files/Reports/2006/PIP_Online_Health_2006.pdf.pdf.

[2] Eysenbach G, Kohler C: How do consumers search for and appraise health information on the World Wide Web? Qualitative study using focus groups, usability tests, and in-depth interviews. *BMJ* 2002, 324(7337): 573–577.

Patient Individual Profile

– J. Westly McGaughey, Ruchika Mishra, and Alexis Lopez

Dear Patient:

This book began with a letter to you, and it is fitting that it ends with one as well. It is evident throughout the chapters that there are two realities of contemporary health care: 1) Your health providers want to take care of you and your health needs in the best way possible, and 2) there is less and less time available for them to spend with each patient. To address these conflicting realities, we offer the Patient Individual Profile form as a way for your health care providers – principally, your doctors and nurses – to learn more about you – your background, values, and preferences. Having this information will help them go beyond treating just your body – it will let them look at you as a person.

This form is a way to talk about things that matter to you most. The questions are intended to give you an opportunity to share the sort of information with your health providers that does not commonly arise in the course of treatment but does have a bearing on who you are. The questions are intended to provide a personal portrait that goes beyond you as a patient, but you should use them as you wish. Feel free to leave any questions unanswered or substitute others you believe are important, and take advantage of the note at the end to tell your providers anything else you want them to know.

As part of your medical records, all the information in the Patient Individual Profile will be treated confidentially. Give a copy of the form to your doctor and keep one for yourself. Give a copy of the form to anyone who will treat you and anyone who will speak on your behalf. To keep the form current, change your responses to any questions whenever you need to; however, notify your health care providers, or anyone else you give it to, of any changes. Be sure to take the form with you if you change your primary care physician or visit a hospital.

The Patient Individual Profile exists simply to assist your health care providers in helping you when you need them. Whether you prefer to use the written form, as provided here, or the information it covers as the basis for conversations with your health care providers, the profile adds an important dimension to your health care.

Patient Individual Profile

Full Name : _____   **Date:** _____

What you wish to be called (if different from above): _____

Contact address: _____

Home Phone: _____   Cellular Phone: _____

E-mail Address: _____

YOUR PERSONAL AND FAMILY BACKGROUND

About You

Your date of birth: _____

Where were you born? _____

_____

Where did you grow up? _____

_____

What is the highest level of education you have completed?

☐ Primary School/Less than High School

☐ Secondary School/High School

☐ Some College/Junior College/Associate's Degree

☐ College Graduate/Bachelor's Degree

☐ Graduate School/Advanced Degree (MA, PhD, etc.)

How would you identify your race? _____

How would you identify your ethnicity? _____

Are you:

☐ Married/Domestic Partnered   ☐ Separated

☐ Unmarried, Living with Partner   ☐ Widowed

☐ Divorced   ☐ Never Married

What do you do for a living? _____

_____

Are you:

☐ Employed Full Time   ☐ Employed Part Time

☐ Unemployed   ☐ Retired

☐ Student   ☐ Self-Employed

Your Father   ☐ No Information

Place of birth: _____

Occupation: _____

Religion: _____

What is the highest level of education your father completed?

☐ Primary School/Less than High School

☐ Secondary School/High School

☐ Some College/Junior College/Associate's Degree

☐ College Graduate/Bachelor's Degree

☐ Graduate School/Advanced Degree (MA, PhD, etc.)

Your Mother   ☐ No Information

Place of birth: _____

Occupation: _____

Religion: _____

What is the highest level of education your mother completed?

☐ Primary School/Less than High School

☐ Secondary School/High School

☐ Some College/Junior College/Associate's Degree

☐ College Graduate/Bachelor's Degree

☐ Graduate School/Advanced Degree (MA, PhD, etc.)

Do you have brothers and/or sisters? ☐ Yes ☐ No   If so, how many? _____ Brothers _____ Sisters

What are their ages?

_____

Do you have children? ☐ Yes ☐ No   If yes, how many? _____ Males _____ Females

What are their ages?

_____

Do you have grandchildren? ☐ Yes ☐ No   If yes, how many? _____ Males _____ Females

What are their ages?

_____

YOUR LIFE

Do you live alone?   ☐ Yes ☐ No

If no, who lives with you?

_____

What language(s) do you speak at home? _____

If you speak a language other than English, would you want an independent translator?

☐ At the Hospital   ☐ At Your Doctor   ☐ In All Cases

Or do you have someone you would prefer to translate for you?   ☐ Yes ☐ No

If yes, whom? _____

How may we contact them? _____

What do you like to do in your leisure time?

_____

_____

Does your family have a place in your life? If yes, please tell us of their involvement.

_____

_____

_____

_____

Do your friends have a place in your life? If yes, please tell us of their involvement.

_____

_____

_____

_____

What dietary preferences do you have, if any?

_____

_____

_____

YOUR RELIGIOUS PREFERENCES AND BELIEFS

What is your religious or spiritual background?

☐ Buddhist

☐ Christian

☐ Hindu

☐ Islamic

☐ Jewish:

    ☐ Conservative

    ☐ Orthodox

    ☐ Reform

☐ Native American

☐ Orthodox Christian

☐ Other Eastern

☐ Protestant:

    ☐ Denomination: _____

    ☐ Inter-Nondenominational

☐ Roman Catholic

☐ Agnostic

☐ Atheist

☐ Spiritual but not formally religious

☐ Other _____

_____

How often do you attend religious services?

☐ Not Applicable

☐ Less than Once a Year

☐ Once a Year to Several Times a Year

☐ Once a Month to Several Times a Month

☐ Once a Week or More

Would you want a chaplain (religious or spiritual representative) to visit you if you are admitted to the hospital?

☐ Yes   ☐ No

Would you like us to notify your own religious or spiritual contact if you are in the hospital? ☐ Yes   ☐ No

If yes, who? _____

How may we contact them? _____

_____

Is there anything else about your religious or spiritual background that you would like your health care providers to know?

_____

_____

_____

_____

_____

YOUR HEALTH DECISIONS

If you are not able to speak for yourself, who do you want to speak for you? _____

How can they be contacted? _____

Do you have an advance directive? An advance directive is a document that you complete to make sure your health care wishes are known and considered if for any reason you are unable to speak for yourself.   ☐ Yes   ☐ No

If yes, who has a copy? _____

If yes, what kind is it?

☐ Advance Directive   ☐ Living Will
☐ Durable Power of Attorney ☐ Other _____

If no, would you like to make one or have assistance in making one? ☐ Yes ☐ No

Have you ever been cared for in a different health care system? ☐ Yes ☐ No
If yes, where? _____

YOUR CONTACTS

Did someone assist you in completing this form? ☐ Yes ☐ No

If yes, what is their relationship to you? _____ Their name: _____

Would you like this person to be a contact for you? ☐ Yes ☐ No

If yes, under what conditions, if any?

_____

_____

If yes, please provide their telephone number(s): _____

Is there anyone in your family you regularly speak with/consult regarding your health issues and/or decisions?

☐ Yes ☐ No   If yes, whom? _____

Would you want us to contact this person? ☐ Yes ☐ No

If yes, under what circumstances? _____

If yes, please provide their name and contact details: _____

Are there any friends in particular that you regularly speak with or consult regarding your health issues and/or decisions?

☐ Yes ☐ No   If yes, whom? _____

Would you want us to contact this person? ☐ Yes ☐ No

If yes, under what circumstances? _____

If yes, please provide their name and contact details: _____

Is there anything about your health decisions, values and preferences you would like to tell us that we have not asked?

_____

_____

_____

Is there anything regarding your health that you would like to share with us that we have not asked?

_____

_____

_____

_____   _____
Signature   Date

Index